CHILD HEALTH PSYCHOLOGY

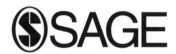

CHILD HEALTH PSYCHOLOGY

A BIOPSYCHOSOCIAL PERSPECTIVE

JULIE M. TURNER-COBB

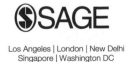

Los Angeles | London | New Delhi
Singapore | Washington DC

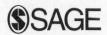

Los Angeles | London | New Delhi
Singapore | Washington DC

SAGE Publications Ltd
1 Oliver's Yard
55 City Road
London EC1Y 1SP

SAGE Publications Inc.
2455 Teller Road
Thousand Oaks, California 91320

SAGE Publications India Pvt Ltd
B 1/I 1 Mohan Cooperative Industrial Area
Mathura Road
New Delhi 110 044

SAGE Publications Asia-Pacific Pte Ltd
3 Church Street
#10-04 Samsung Hub
Singapore 049483

Editor: Michael Carmichael
Editorial assistant: Keri Dickens
Production editor: Imogen Roome
Copyeditor: Sue Ashton
Indexer: Cathryn Pritchard
Marketing manager: Alison Borg
Cover design: Wendy Scott
Typeset by: C&M Digitals (P) Ltd, Chennai, India
Printed and bound in Great Britain by Ashford
Colour Press Ltd

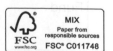

Library of Congress Control Number: 2012955657

British Library Cataloguing in Publication data

A catalogue record for this book is available from
the British Library

ISBN 978-1-84920-590-0
ISBN 978-1-84920-591-7 (pbk)

In memory of my wonderful mother,
in love and appreciation of her generosity, kindness and sense of humour

CONTENTS

LIST OF FIGURES

LIST OF TABLES

ABOUT THE AUTHOR

Julie Turner-Cobb is a health psychologist with an active research interest in psychoendo-crinology and an established publication record in the area of child health psychology. She is a Chartered psychologist and an associate fellow of the British Psychological Society, a registered Practitioner psychologist with the Health and Care Professions Council and an associate editor for the *British Journal of Health Psychology*. Currently a senior lecturer in the Department of Psychology at the University of Bath, she is Director of Studies for the MSc in Health Psychology. She has published extensively in the areas of acute and chronic illness in children and in adults, with a particular focus on the family context and the role of social support and coping. She has been investigating the effects of psychosocial stress on hypothalamic-pituitary-adrenal (HPA) axis functioning for over 20 years, and has been involved in advancing the theory and measurement of cortisol testing in children. A major theme which carries through much of her work is the application of the common cold as a paradigm for the influence of psychosocial factors on acute illness in otherwise healthy children. She has made frequent contributions on radio, talking about her research, and has been a consultant for television documentaries requiring cortisol expertise. She lives in Bath and is a mother of two daughters.

ACKNOWLEDGEMENTS

This book has been waiting to escape for many years and is a culmination of a variety of research interests and a range of teaching experiences. Writing a textbook of this type is both an enormous endeavour and a thrilling journey of discovery. There are numerous brilliant people who have inspired and influenced the development of my ideas and research over the past 20 years or so, too many to mention, but thanks in particular are due to David Spiegel, to my research colleague David Jessop, and to the Westminster Stress Research Group.

I do not care to admit how long it has taken to complete this text, but suffice it to say I am indebted to my colleagues at the University of Bath for their patience and confidence in its eventual completion. I am very grateful to the University and the Department of Psychology for affording me a period of sabbatical study to move ahead with my writing. I would particularly like to thank my health psychology colleagues Ed Keogh, Paula Smith and Karen Rodham for their wise words and advice on topics that I found myself branching into but which were not my original area of specialty. Thank you for letting me tread on your turf, so to speak: I enjoyed our discussions and look forward to engaging in some of the potential collaborative research that emerged.

Special mention goes to Tim Gamble for his insightful and somehow always timely suggestions for fascinating nuggets of news and relevant websites. Thanks also to my clinical collaborator, Mike Osborn: talking with you has the effect of unleashing new ideas and ways of looking at health interventions. Much appreciated and by no means least is the assistance of my hard-working team of postgraduate students, including Fiona Begen, Tara Cheetham, Steve Dean, Lifang Neo and Carmen Skilton, for literature searches, compiling tables, proof reading and all-round, positive enthusiasm.

PART I

AN INTRODUCTION TO CHILD HEALTH AND WELL-BEING

INTRODUCTION: WHAT IS CHILD HEALTH PSYCHOLOGY?

1

Covered in this chapter

- Definition of child health psychology
- The psychosocial context of child health
- The developmental context of child health
- The mind–body link: from medieval to modern-day views
- The mind–body connection in modern times
- Health-related behaviour and social cognition models
- The changing face of health threats
- A worldview on child health
- Communicating health

Interest in the promotion and enhancement of health in children reflects a central human drive to protect and nurture, often in the hope of improving life chances and well-being for future generations. In this chapter, I begin by defining what is meant by *child health psychology*, and look at where it fits within the framework of psychology, health and medicine. I then start to consider what, how and why psychological factors might be important in relation to physical health in children and the impact of psychological factors across the different stages of development from infancy to adolescence. The role of psychological influences on physical health in children is introduced from an historical perspective in order to set in context our modern-day approach. Biomedical advances are discussed in the context of past, present and future physical health threats and challenges to child and adolescent health. Whilst this book focuses on health in the Western world, we will also consider threats to health in developing countries and contrasts between health threats across the globe.

DEFINITION OF CHILD HEALTH PSYCHOLOGY

In its broadest sense, the discipline of health psychology as defined by the British Psychological Society's (BPS) Division of Health Psychology (DHP) relates psychosocial factors to physical health and illness in order to (i) promote and maintain health; (ii) prevent and manage illness; (iii) identify psychological factors which contribute to physical illness; (iv) improve the health care system; and (v) help formulate health policy (see www.health-psychology.org.uk). The term 'psychosocial' refers to any combination of psychological and social factors and their interplay. Psychological factors include the way a person thinks (cognitions), their coping responses, attitude and their temperament or personality (sometimes termed individual differences). Social factors include the social resources available to an individual, which are embedded within their culture and position within society and within their more immediate social network.

Child health psychology, then, is the specific application of health psychology research and practice to physical health in children, as well as the implications and applications of psychosocial influences during childhood development on subsequent health in adulthood. In this book, I use the term 'childhood' to cover the full age range of child and adolescent years from zero through to 18 years old, with specific age groups highlighted as different issues are covered. In some chapters, the boundaries of this age range are extended at either end of the spectrum in order to consider prenatal health issues during pregnancy or the transition from adolescence to adulthood and what this means for access to health services, as well as the implications of childhood experience on adult health in middle and older age. As the focus throughout this book is on biopsychosocial interactions, important questions relate to how the physiological response systems of the body might be shaped, both positively and negatively, by early life experience, and how these influences map onto health during childhood and through to adulthood. This begs the question of what the potential might be for interventions to repair or 'normalize' the response systems in cases where early psychosocial experiences have created a physiological imbalance. These are not easy questions to answer, and research in this area has a long way to go, but we can go part way in answering some of these questions based on research findings to date (as well as debunking some more spurious ideas that have developed along the way).

In many respects, these are exciting times for health psychologists interested in child health. An important change in perspective, or paradigm shift, is beginning to emerge across the many related scientific disciplines of health and illness, which reflects a greater understanding of the impact of early life adversity on physical health right across the whole gamut of different life stages. This gives recognition to the idea that early life experience from conception through to childhood can have a large influence on health outcomes throughout the lifespan or course of life. I will return to this life-course idea throughout the book but, to introduce it here, it is based on an increasing amount of evidence which has found a whole range of adult health conditions to be associated with childhood experiences. The influence of psychosocial factors on children is central to health psychology and related disciplines because of the lifespan implications. The full

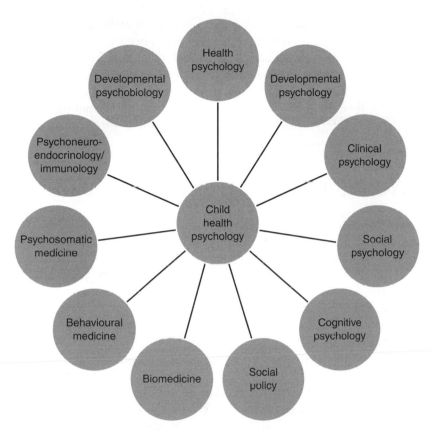

FIGURE 1.1   Disciplinary links to child health psychology

circle of implications is important, considering not just childhood itself but the longer-term perspective into adulthood and across the lifespan, as well as prenatal influences on child health.

There are also several overlapping disciplines specific to childhood that directly acknowledge psychosocial influences on physical health, including developmental psychology and the field of developmental psychobiology, as well as other broader fields, such as clinical psychology and biomedicine, from which the topic of child health psychology draws. Figure 1.1 gives an idea of these disciplinary links and influences which I will be drawing on throughout this book. It is by no means intended to be exhaustive but may be useful to consider whilst reading the following chapters. Think of it as a conceptual drawing board rather than a definitive conceptual model: you may want to add further areas or links between the disciplines given.

In connection with this, in recent years there has been a sea change in the use of positive terminology relating to 'wellness' rather than the more historical terminology of 'illness' and 'ill health'. This, of course, fits with major advances in medical technology and pharmaceutical development. This shift has, on the whole, been presented as an optimistic paradigm change. Yet, at the risk of appearing cynical, this could, in part, be due to a reluctance to face the negative side of ill health realistically. The positive or optimistic approach of health psychology is, first and foremost, to recognize the negative impact and turmoil brought about by ill health and to use this knowledge and understanding to build prevention programmes and interventions where possible, but also to provide care and support in the face of chronic or terminal illness.

THE PSYCHOSOCIAL CONTEXT OF CHILD HEALTH

There are two main concepts that I want to introduce in relation to the psychosocial context of child health: these are the concepts of social support and socioeconomic status. The concept of *social support* encompasses both psychological and social aspects: for example, the size of a person's social network, or having a family member or friend who can offer emotional support (someone to talk to or share emotions with), financial support (providing money for a school trip) or practical support (ensuring a safe lift home from a late-night party). These latter two types of support may be practical in origin, but whether or not help is available or perceived to be available is also likely to be bound up with emotional meaning and significance, as it is for emotional support itself. As will become obvious, harnessing the power of social support is an important tool in interventions to improve physical health outcome. The concept of social support is discussed in detail in Chapter 2; the methodological aspects of social support assessment are covered in Chapter 3; and various forms of support are mentioned throughout the remaining chapters.

The second of these concepts, *socioeconomic status*, is the term used for an individual's position in society and is measured in a number of different ways, including household income, a person's marital status (or for children that of their parents), access to/level of education, family size, or whether or not a household owns a car. In particular, socioeconomic status is relevant in situations where childhood experience has its roots in social and economic disadvantage or poverty. Childhood socioeconomic status has been implicated in an impressive array of examples of causes of death (mortality) during adulthood and the occurrence of a variety of adult health conditions from depression to cardiovascular disease (Braveman and Barclay, 2009).

The strength of this association between low socioeconomic status and poor physical health has been demonstrated across a range of racial groups and ethnicities. Using family income as the measure of socioeconomic status, Braveman and Barclay (2009) illustrate the consistent nature of socioeconomic status in its impact on health in a sample of children aged 17 years and under in the United States. For each of their three categories of race/ethnicity, a clear pattern was found which indicated that the lower the family income, the poorer the physical health of the children. Within this income–health pattern, they also demonstrate variability in health outcome between the race/ethnicity categories, with

Hispanic children showing a larger proportion 'in less than very good health', followed by black/Hispanic children, and white/non-Hispanic children showing a larger proportion in good health.

It has long been accepted that investment in early education is a key area for reducing social deprivation and breaking the cycle of poverty, and extensive education research exists in this area. This has emerged from an increasing awareness and acceptance of the effects of early life stress on physical health outcomes, coupled with the understanding that socioeconomic disadvantage (i.e., lower income, poorer education) can influence health via the numerous potential stressors that it may create. Individuals living in a poorer environment are more likely to experience stressful events relating to various disruptions in their personal, family, community, or school life, including personal maltreatment, parental conflict, and violence in their neighbourhood (Shonkoff et al., 2009). There is increasingly compelling evidence for a process of 'biological embedding' in which the experience of early adversity primes the physiological systems, setting the scene for vulnerability to negative health outcome following subsequent life stress (Shonkoff et al., 2009). This is a theme I will return to later as we consider the theories and mechanisms by which this might operate (Chapter 2), how this can be applied to the experience of intra-uterine stress during pregnancy (Chapter 4), and the effects on childhood health and illness later in life (Chapter 5). Of course, just as low socioeconomic status *per se* does not cause ill health, disease and illness are not solely the domain of those with low socioeconomic status. Indeed, the effects of stress and anxiety on underlying physiological mechanisms associated with ill health are often a curse of the middle classes in the developed world. Disease and illness are seen throughout the socioeconomic classes, but having low socioeconomic status during childhood carries with it an increased chance of ill health, particularly for certain types of conditions as described above. Gaining an understanding of how and why these health differences exist, and the interactions between these social factors and psychological factors, is of much interest to health psychology and related disciplines.

The implication of this life-course perspective is that early intervention is essential if health disparities later in life are to be minimized. The factor that has enabled this to receive attention and move the field forward is the potential economic impact for healthcare provision. The current thought is that providing health investment in adult care is expensive and limited, whilst investment in improving the physical and social environment of children will pay dividends through a reduction in their health-care needs throughout their life. This perspective goes beyond the idea that investment in childhood poverty will merely improve health-related behaviours such as diet and exercise, important though they are, to the notion that reducing stress in early life will physiologically alter the developing child and consequently improve their health outcome over time as well as that of future generations. This may all sound rather far-fetched, and it is unrealistic to think that inequality, stress and adversity can be eliminated, but aside from the very real practical improvements in health outcome, the theory and supporting evidence for alterations in this way provide a sound theoretical basis for understanding the powerful mechanisms behind mind–body links and their central importance in the application to child health.

THE DEVELOPMENTAL CONTEXT OF CHILD HEALTH

It is vital to consider the developmental context in which health and illness are set. There are many excellent developmental psychology textbooks which document the biological, cognitive, language and social development during childhood (e.g., see Parke and Gauvain, 2009). Of particular importance with respect to child health psychology are the ways in which these developmental changes impact upon understanding and expression of the concept of health and illness and the degree to which children may be more biologically vulnerable or resistant to disease. In Chapter 2, we consider the developmental progression of children's cognitive understanding of health and illness, particularly through the earlier part of childhood. In conjunction with this, we also examine the biological development of the immune system and the endocrine system, which help explain patterns of resilience and vulnerability in childhood as a critical period in the setting of the stress response systems, the outcome of which can influence adolescent responses and development.

Within the developmental context of child health, the concept of attachment is particularly relevant. Attachment is very much a cornerstone theory in the field of developmental psychology, central to understanding social relationships across the lifespan. Whilst the focus in this book is on health psychology rather than developmental psychology, one of the compelling aspects of health psychology, as suggested above, is its interaction across several different strands of psychology and beyond. The theory of attachment also underlies the key concepts of social support and supportive relationships. Attachment theory was originally associated with mental health outcomes and psychopathology, but it is intimately bound up with an individual's ability to give and receive social support and, as such, is a recurrent theme which underlies many of the physical health issues discussed throughout this book.

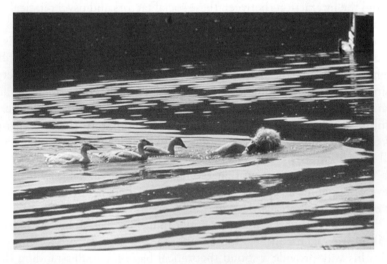

FIGURE 1.2 Konrad Lorenz swimming with imprinted goslings

Source: www.flickr.com/photos/pluriverse/3403875417/sizes/m/in/photostream/.

Attachment theory was first put forward by John Bowlby, a psychiatrist with a background in psychoanalysis, almost half a century ago in 1969. He built on the incredible work of ethologist Konrad Lorenz (1937) who was the first to show the process of 'imprinting' in action. Using goslings, Lorenz discovered that, during the critical period shortly after hatching, if he was the first figure they saw and bonded with at this time, the young goslings would imprint or attach to him as their object of affection and this bond would remain with them throughout their life. Figure 1.2 shows imprinted goslings following Lorenz, their 'mother-goose', out swimming.

Imprinting experiments with newly hatched ducklings are still used as a powerful teaching tool on some undergraduate courses in psychology. The process of imprinting has also been popularized in film and fiction: for example, the story 'Fly Away Home' in which goslings imprint on a young girl who is able to fly the geese to safety as they follow her microlight plane. The term 'imprinting' is also still attracting attention as a concept in recent popular teen vampire fiction, albeit an altered use of the term not to be confused with original Lorenzian theory. Bowlby's theories on attachment, particularly mother–child bonding, attracted an international following in psychology and, with the contribution of other theorists and practitioners in this area, led to work which is still influential across many branches of psychology as we know them today.

So what is attachment? Attachment is described as a 'strong affectional tie that binds a person to an intimate companion' and is a 'behavioral system through which humans regulate their emotional distress when under threat' (Sigelman and Rider, 2009: 406–7). Being close to the attachment figure creates security, and being away from the attachment figure can create separation anxiety. It stems from the initial bonds formed with parents or close attachment figures at just a few months of age, and in different forms early attachment plays out in all subsequent attachment relationships experienced throughout life, particularly in close relationships with significant people, including romantic relationships. Sigelman and Rider (2009) describe the longevity of attachment from a lifespan perspective: there are 'basic similarities among the infant attached to a caregiver, the child attached to a best friend, and the adolescent or adult attached to a mate or lover' (2009: 407), although we develop different ways of expressing this attachment and of coping with separation from the attachment figure and regulating the emotions this produces. The theory of attachment comes up again when we consider developmental aspects below, and as applied to separation anxiety as a source of stress in Chapters 2 and 5, as well as in Part II when we consider issues of death and dying.

THE MIND–BODY LINK: FROM MEDIEVAL TO MODERN-DAY VIEWS

Every age of man has in some way expressed an awareness of the influence of the human psyche in illness and disease or rather, in health, as modern thinking would have it.

Historically, the relationship between mind and body has had a somewhat chequered career in Western medicine. In the ancient world, belief in the healing powers of non-medicinal or spiritual forms abounded, often in the shape of myths or legends (Box 1.1).

BOX 1.1

The legend of King Bladud

In the world heritage city of Bath, home to many things ancient, including the ancient Roman spa visited for its healing waters, the legend of King Bladud persists to this day. As long ago as 863 BC, Bladud, prince and heir to the throne, had returned home after studying Latin in Athens. Yet there was no rest from his years of study as health was on his mind. He had contracted leprosy during his travels abroad and was keen to make sure his condition did not cause his inheritance to be overlooked by his father, the king. In order to hide, he disappeared from the comfort of the palace, disguised himself as a swineherd, and sought refuge in the countryside near Bath. The pigs he tended also contracted leprosy but, much to Prince Bladud's surprise, they were cured after rolling in the hot, muddy waters around Bath's springs. Bladud followed suit, rolling in the hot, muddy water, and he too experienced the miracle cure. He went on to become king and was so delighted at the curative powers of the area that he founded the city of Bath, dedicating the healing waters to the Celtic goddess Sul (the city becoming known as Aquae Sulis to the Romans).

   It may be just a legend but it demonstrates enduring interest in the power of non-medicinal healing. Incidentally, the legend is still very much alive in the city of Bath (see www.kingbladudspigs.org/).

Together with the Greek philosophers Plato and Aristotle, most writings document the birth of medicine as stemming from the thinking and scholarship of the ancient Greeks (Nutton in Porter, 2001), particularly the work attributed to Hippocrates and his disciples, written approximately 300–500 BC. Notorious in this work is the humoral theory which proposed four humours, that of bile, phlegm, blood and black bile, synonymous with the four mental states or temperaments: choleric, phlegmatic, sanguine and melancholic. The influential work of Galen, an ancient Roman of Greek origin, built on these ideas in the second century AD, advancing knowledge with his practice of animal dissection; he can be thought of as an early pioneer of stress-related illness (Nutton in Porter, 2001). This mind–body view persisted, the mind being associated with mental illness rather than physical illness, and observations of mind–body links being explained as witchcraft, magic or even demon possession well into the seventeenth century (Box 1.2).

BOX 1.2

Medieval ducking stool

This instrument of social control and public humiliation was used to punish those believed to be witches (as well as nagging wives). There persists a fascination with such forms of extreme social ostracism, with medieval relics and reconstructions still attracting captivated crowds today. The ducking stool (Figure 1.3) can be seen as an icon of the mind–body connection since it represents a misunderstanding of the link between psychological processes and physical events. Those thought to be witches, usually women, were accused for a range of reasons and these included the belief that they had inflicted disease or caused stillbirth, or simply because they had a skin condition or birthmark (for more on what constituted witchcraft in medieval times, see www.witchcraftandwitches.com). In other words, they were thought to exhibit a link between the human psyche and physical ills. In this way, the ducking stool symbolizes a fear of the mind–body link and an intrinsic fear of social evaluation and rejection if suggestion was made as to such a link.

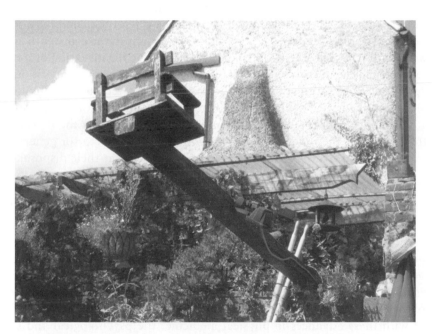

FIGURE 1.3   Medieval ducking stool over the River Stour in Canterbury, UK

It was René Descartes, renowned French philosopher (he of 'I think therefore I am' fame) and early physiological psychologist, who refined mind–body dualism, subsequently referred to as Cartesian dualism (Descartes, 1984). Amongst other things, Descartes identified the connection between mind (or soul) and body as physically occurring in the pineal gland of the brain via retinal nerves from the eye (Leahey, 2004). It is also vital to consider the role played by organized religion in the development of medicine and health, a role which has shown a typically conflictual 'approach–avoidance' relationship through the ages (the psychological notion of moving forward with something whilst at the same time being held back by fear). In many respects, religion was often seen as holding back medical advances (i.e., 'avoidance') due to the fear of science and the unknown, retaining a strict distinction between body and soul and being in favour of persecuting evil in the form of witches and magic. Yet in other respects, religion promoted the idea of divine healing and welcomed it (i.e., 'approach'), embraced the tolerance of physical suffering as a coping technique, and was central to the provision of psychosocial concepts such as social support. One does not have to search very far to see this debate continuing today (for example, see Dawkins, 2006; McGrath and Collicut McGrath, 2007) and I am not about to resolve it here. Yet it is important to bear in mind the role of religious beliefs, at both a personal and a cultural level, when considering the historical context of health psychology, particularly relating to children and the role of the family as a social unit.

Treatment of physical illness progressed exponentially in the eighteenth and nineteenth centuries with scientific and medical advances, including the invention of tools such as the stethoscope and the microscope, an increase in knowledge about bacteria and antiseptics, the development of vaccinations (e.g., against smallpox, tetanus and diphtheria) and the advancement of surgical ability made possible by the application of anaesthetics such as ether and chloroform (Porter, 2001). An important change in the delivery of primary health care during the nineteenth century was the family doctor or general practitioner, although they had relatively few effective medical tools at their disposal, bloodletting being one of the most commonly used (Shorter in Porter, 2001). From the 1850s onwards, the provision of hospital care for children grew rapidly, with Great Ormond Street Hospital for Children leading the way in the UK (1952) and the New York Hospital for Women and Children in the US (1954), resulting in dedicated children's services provided in most major cities in the developed world today. Similarly, advances in obstetrics and gynaecology in the nineteenth century saw a decline in the previously high death rates of mothers and newborns, with the advent of anaesthetics, antibiotics, delivery methods and hospital provision. (For a fascinating illustrated account of medical history, documenting a timeline of medical advances, see Porter et al., 2009.)

Yet with these advances in physical medicine, the psychological and social person-centred approach was largely overlooked, perhaps even feared (again, we are reminded of the duckings tool), in the struggle to move forward in scientific recognition. The twentieth century saw the development of psychosocial schools of thought, namely psychoanalysis, psychosomatic medicine, behavioural medicine, psychoneuroimmunology and health psychology. The human need for consideration of psychosocial aspects in health created a shift from the biomedical model to a biopsychosocial model of health and illness. Physicist Sir Isaac Newton's third law of motion that 'for every action there is an equal and opposite reaction' is a useful analogy: in this case, the extent of the shift is made possible due to

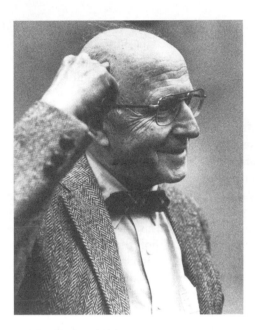

FIGURE 1.4   George Libman Engel lecturing in 1987

Source: Edward G. Miner Library, University of Rochester Medical Center, New York.

the reduction in resistance enabled by the cultural readiness for more person-centred medicine. This shift towards the inclusion of psychosocial factors was significantly advanced by George Engel's work, and is beautifully articulated in his influential paper over three decades ago (Engel, 1977; see Figure 1.4). His seminal paper argued for a need to move from the reductionist dualism of the then pervading medical model of disease (mind and body being separate entities never to interact with one another) to a more holistic, integrated approach. This new approach put forward was the biopsychosocial model, which incorporated psychological and social factors, along with physical factors, in consideration of health, illness and treatment. It is well worth taking a look at Engel's original paper which skilfully explains the two positions, setting them in historical context. Interestingly, Engel, in particular, notes the role of Western religion in the evolution and maintenance of the biomedical model (1977: 131), due to the Church's belief in the separation between the body and the soul.

THE MIND–BODY CONNECTION IN MODERN TIMES

The biopsychosocial model is now a major contributor in modern-day health care and pervades thinking about health and well-being at a cultural and society level, although the battle with reductionist dualism is far from over. It is interesting that in advocating and advancing such new ways of thinking about health and illness, examples of child health are often used. For example, Engel used the case of a traumatized infant female patient, called Monica, whom he and his colleague Franz Reichsman studied in depth over the course of 25 years (Reichsman et al., 1957; Engel et al., 1979; Dowling, 2005). This represents an early documented example of the longitudinal effect of childhood trauma, an idea we will come back to in subsequent chapters.

This is the point at which, in a lecture, I would probably be interrupted and bombarded with questions from those who have a background or interest in psychoanalysis. You may also have noticed that I have already referred to the field of psychoanalysis when introducing the work of Bowlby above. In considering the historical context, it would be remiss of me not to mention that Engel's work took much of its influence from psychoanalytical thinking and, indeed, the work of Sigmund Freud also used examples of mental neuroses in children resulting in a range of physical health symptoms (Brown, 1972). Psychoanalysis was, after all, influential in psychology in the mid-twentieth century. For the purposes of this book, however, I point to this merely to the extent of showing an early and important milestone of the biopsychosocial concept in the study of child health.

However, since the discipline of psychology is traditionally associated with mental health and psychological well-being, it is often difficult to shift or extend this view to include an understanding or appreciation of the impact of psychological factors on physical health outcomes. I seem to spend a lot of time doing exactly this, explaining how psychosocial factors can affect physical health to people who are simultaneously surprised that there is a science which looks into this, yet are intuitively in agreement from personal experience. In fact, once the subject is mentioned, people are often only too keen to recount numerous examples where they have seen mind–body influences in action. There is, of course, significant overlap or co-morbidity between physical health and mental health. Whilst mental health issues and psychopathology are referred to in this book, the focus is on physical health as an outcome and intervening physiological dysregulation.

In Chapter 2, I look in more depth at definitions of health and illness, as well as definitions of stress and coping and the processes and mechanisms through which psychosocial factors influence physical health. Before we go there, it is important to understand the essence of the mind–body relationship. The best way to explain the mind–body link is with a quote from leading therapist and academic, David Spiegel, who sums up one of his editorials linking psychosocial factors and cancer progression in adults by saying that 'it is not simply mind over matter, but it is clear that mind matters' (Spiegel, 1999: 1329). In other words, disciplines which incorporate psychosocial factors in physical health are not purporting some kind of magical 'think positive' influence of mind over physical matter. Instead, they are providing strong scientific evidence for the importance of the mind in physical health through recognized physiological routes.

I come back to the mind–body issue several times throughout the book, so it is worth taking a few moments to think about what is meant by this in scientific terms before continuing, in order to grasp the concept thoroughly. Related concepts, such as immune conditioning and areas of research such as psychoneuroimmunology, are also described later in the book (see Chapter 3). The reason I am making such a song and dance about grasping the scientific meaning of mind–body relationships is because the influence of psychological factors has frequently been misunderstood and consequently misinterpreted or unrealistically portrayed, particularly in the media and in popular self-help texts. For example, positive thinking (see Box 1.3) has often been over-interpreted as the 'cure all' for a host of conditions, including cancer, sometimes to the extent of having the damaging effect of blaming patients for their own illness. For an in-depth critique of the 'think positive' campaign, see Barbara Ehrenreich's (2009) book devoted to the broader theme at a cultural level.

In this book, we will be adhering closely to the scientific reality that psychological state is important in physical health, not through some magical means, but as evidenced through careful consideration of the processes, mechanisms, models and theories underlying mind–body connections. These processes and mechanisms are central to child health, and child health is key to understanding the theories and models linking psychosocial factors and health outcome across the lifespan.

BOX 1.3

Positive thinking cures all?

Think about the news articles, advertisements (see Figure 1.5), TV programmes and children's stories related to health that you have recently read, heard or seen. Consider the following questions:

What message do they convey?
What does the product promise to deliver?
Can positive thinking be a barrier to improved health outcome?
How might these messages shape the health attitudes, health-related behaviours and understanding of the link between stress and illness in children?
Think about not just the direct effect on children but the indirect effects via parental influence.

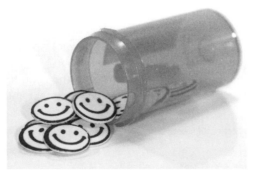

FIGURE 1.5   Happy pills
Source: Shutterstock_1572633.

BOX 1.4

Ring a Ring o' Roses

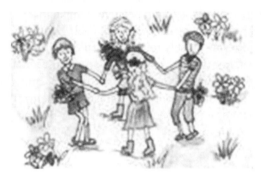

FIGURE 1.6   Children's nursery rhyme 'Ring a Ring o' Roses'
Artist: E. Cobb.

Ring-a-ring o'roses,

A pocket full of posies,

A-tishoo! A-tishoo!

We all fall down

The Great Plague of London (1665) was caused by bubonic plague or the Black Death. The children's nursery rhyme 'Ring a Ring o' Roses' (English version; 'Ring around the Rosies' in the US version) symbolizes the fear and misunderstanding of the time surrounding contagious disease. The words 'ring o' roses' reflect the rosy red skin rash characteristic of bubonic plague, and in the English version 'A tishoo' represents the symptoms of violent sneezing. The 'pocket full of posies' is a reference to the sweet-smelling herbs carried in order to ward off the plague, as people believed that bad smells were the cause of contagion (Alchin, 2009). Do the posies perhaps hint at an early form of homeopathy as we know it today, or do flowers simply symbolize the provision of comfort and hope in an otherwise seemingly helpless situation?

Children would typically hold hands in a circle to recite the song (Figure 1.6), possibly unintentionally symbolizing both the ease of contagion through contact and the importance of social support through friendship.

So what are we left with after considering this meandering pathway of medical and psychosocial evolution in the study of child health? Modern Western society uses the terms 'stress', 'coping' and 'social support' in everyday common parlance. These are considered in depth in Chapter 2, but here we ask the question of why they are so key to physical health – in fact, why are we even considering them? The answer in many respects is simple: because psychosocial factors have a scientifically measurable impact on physical health outcome. Ask any health-care professional, any member of the public – indeed, ask a child – and they will most likely be able to recall anecdotal evidence from their own experience of psychosocial factors affecting physical health.

It is intriguing to look at examples of how misunderstandings relating to health and illness have been tied up with trying to make sense of the influence that psychological factors might have on health. Aside from the medieval examples given above, examples have pervaded children's literature down through the centuries, seen in popular nursery rhymes, stories, legends and sayings, an example of which is the nursery rhyme 'Ring a Ring o' Roses' (see Box 1.4). Nursery rhymes and legends often reflect accounts of common misunderstandings, yet they also sometimes reflect understanding and knowledge about the relationship between psychological factors and disease prior to scientific evidence being available to explain the connection. As such, they may be bound up with magic and mystery, yet often contain essential truths which one generation felt important to pass on to the children of the next.

As you will see throughout the rest of this book, although we may hold these beliefs about the link between psychosocial factors and physical health outcomes, and while science has provided evidence to support them and Western medicine has gone a long way to incorporate these factors into health care, there is still a long way to go. The scope to develop these links further and to capitalize on them in order to improve health and prevent illness is enormous. In some respects, consideration of psychosocial concepts in physical health and illness could be viewed as an affluent modern addition for Western societies to adopt, or for the more affluent in those societies to improve their comfort and quality of life. It could be argued that the developing world has more life-and-death dilemmas to face and cannot afford to include such luxuries. This, of course, is true to a degree, but it could also be argued that we cannot afford to ignore psychosocial factors given their potentially powerful and cost-effective outcomes. Seminal work by House and colleagues (1988) demonstrates the power of one of these concepts – that of social support. In respect of mortality, lack of social integration was found to be comparable with risk factors such as smoking and serum cholesterol levels (House et al., 1988). Of all the research that has been published in the past quarter of a century, this is perhaps one of the most compelling and straightforward comparative examples of the influence of psychosocial factors on physical health outcome.

HEALTH-RELATED BEHAVIOUR AND SOCIAL COGNITION MODELS

Whilst the main focus of this book is on the physiological changes that occur under different psychosocial conditions and how early psychosocial experiences play out across the lifespan, it is important not to overlook some of the more practical influences of psychosocial factors on health outcome. In the past 25 years, psychologists have put much collective effort into improving health outcome by attempting to influence lifestyle factors, such as diet, exercise and sexual behaviour, in order to prevent or reduce the prevalence of ill health. Health intervention projects and promotion campaigns, often targeted at children or their parents, use a variety of techniques to alter behaviour. These techniques stem from a number of key theories in this area, which highlight beliefs and attitudes about, and intentions towards, performing health-related behaviours. Termed 'social cognitive models' or 'models of social cognition', the theories they generate help to explain some of the conscious and unconscious cognitive processes operating to influence behaviour: in other words, to explain why people do or do not take action towards averting illness or towards improving behaviour relating to their health.

Dominant theories in this area are that of the *health belief model* (HBM; Becker, 1974; Rosenstock, 1974; Becker and Maiman, 1975) and the *theory of planned behaviour* (TPB; Ajzen, 1985, 1991), along with its earlier, less famous relation, the *theory of reasoned action* (TRA; Fishbein, 1967, 1980, 2008; Morrison et al., 2002). For a detailed account of such models, you will be spoilt for choice over which health psychology text to consult (highly recommend for coverage of this topic is Morrison and Bennett, 2012). To summarize the concepts involved, the HBM attempts to predict behaviour based on the interaction of demographic factors, such as age and gender, with the socially constructed, learnt beliefs an individual holds. The beliefs held are driven by that person's perception of how threatening a certain behaviour is and the relevance it has for them, as well as their perception of the benefits of, and barriers to, performing the behaviour. The TPB incorporates social dimensions of health behaviour to include mediating levels concerned with a person's 'attitude' towards the behaviour, what their family and friends will think (termed 'subjective norm'), and how much control they feel they have over the behaviour (termed 'perceived behavioural control'). These, in turn, influence the intention an individual has to change their behaviour (termed 'behavioural intention') and, ultimately, the behaviour. So, for example, if aiming to engage in behaviours such as trying to lose weight, engage in more exercise or to practise safe sex by using a condom, an individual's success in meeting this behavioural goal or outcome will be determined by their own attitude to that behaviour, what others would think of them performing that behaviour, and how much control they believe they have in performing that behaviour. Admittedly, this is not rocket science, but towards the end of the 1990s and into the new millennium, these theories became exceedingly popular and, in particular, took the UK health psychology field by storm. The TPB became a key theory and was applied across numerous health-outcome studies, covering all manner of applications from breast/testicular self-examination (Steadman and Quine, 2004) to the safe storage of firearms in houses with children (Johnson et al., 2008).

The reason for the success of these seemingly 'common-sense' theories was due in part to the fact that they offered an intuitive explanation for why some people were more likely to perform health behaviours than others. Coupled with the later addition of the concept of *implementation intentions* (Gollwitzer and Oettingen, 1998) to explain the gap between intention and behaviour, this has been one of the most successful intervention-based models in health psychology. The intention–behaviour gap, as its name implies, addressed the issue that, despite good intentions, people often fail to perform the intended behaviour and need additional prompts to encourage them to do this. Implementation intentions involve individuals committing to when they will perform a behaviour and to locate a trigger to remind them to do it (e.g., taking a vitamin pill every morning with breakfast). Similarly, stage-based models which have enabled interventions to be individually tailored and targeted, based on the person's readiness for change, have also been incredibly successful in health psychology. The stage-based models known as the *transtheoretical model* (TTM; DiClemente and Prochaska, 1982) and the *health action process approach* model (HAPA; for applications, see Sutton, 2008) have shown significant cost-effective potential for intervention studies seeking to change behaviour. Since their inception, a plethora of publications has applied these theories across a range of health behaviours.

Yet of the thousands of papers published which are based on social cognition and stage-based models, a vast majority cater to adult populations, with only approximately 10 per cent being concerned with health behaviours in children or adolescents. Areas where they have been applied in child and adolescent populations include the full gamut of health and related behaviours, such as immunization uptake (e.g., against influenza and the more recently available human papillomavirus [HPV] vaccine);

BOX 1.5

Jamie Oliver's healthy eating campaign

In September 2006, a media storm hit pupils at a School in South Yorkshire following changes to the lunch menu as part of celebrity TV chef Jamie Oliver's campaign to improve nutrition in schools. A mother was captured on camera taking orders for junk food from the school gates. Seen as a 'backlash' against the introduction of healthier school lunches, this example demonstrates just how difficult it is to change behaviour and the many influences on that behaviour. From the mothers' perspective, reports suggested that there were concerns over whether the children were receiving a sufficient quantity of food and enough time to eat it within the new schedule imposed by the school.

TABLE 1.1 Examples of studies applying social cognition models to child health

Health behaviour	Population	Study	Model
Immunization			
Influenza vaccination	Adolescents in a rural area (n = 337; mean age 14 years)	Painter et al. (2010)	HBM
HPV vaccination	Physicians (n = 207) of adolescent girls aged 9–15 years	Askelson et al. (2010)	TPB
	Parents (n = 567) of adolescent girls aged 10–18 years	Brewer et al. (2010) See also Reiter et al. (2009)	HBM
Rotavirus (gastroenteritis) vaccination	Expectant parents/parents (n = 807) of newborns up to 6 weeks old	Dubé et al. (2012)	TPB
Diet and nutrition			
Childhood obesity	Mothers (n = 201) of children aged 2–5 years	Andrews et al. (2010)	TPB
Healthy eating	Adolescents aged 10–13 years (n = 261)	Hewitt and Stephens (2007)	TPB
Quality of diet	Mothers (n = 300) of toddlers aged 24–36 months	Swanson et al. (2011)	TPB
Physical exercise			
Physical activity	Low SES children aged 6–10 years (n = 77)	Armitage and Sprigg (2010)	TPB/implementation intentions
Active lifestyle (physical activity and 'screen time' behaviour (i.e., watching TV, DVDs, playing computer games)	Mothers (n = 162) of children aged 4–5 years	Hamilton et al. (2013)	TPB
Smoking			
Parental factors/smoking	Adolescents aged 10–14 years (n = 1070)	Harakeh et al. (2004)	TPB
Maternal communication/parental smoking	Children aged 8–12 years (n = 1478)	Hiemstra et al. (2012)	TPB
Medication			
Adherence to antiretroviral therapy	Parents of HIV-positive children aged 0.9–11.5 years	Steele et al. (2001)	HBM
Sun protection			
Encouraging sun safety	Adolescent girls and boys (n = 80) aged 13–16 years	White et al. (2010)	TPB
Sun protective practices towards children	Preschool staff (n = 245)	James et al. (2002)	TPB
Safety practices			
Safe storage of firearms	Married women with children (n = 185)	Johnson et al. (2008)	TPB
Use of car booster seats	Parents (n = 151) of children aged 4–8 years	Bracchitta (2006)	TPB

Note: HBM, health belief model; SES, socioeconomic status; TPB, theory of planned behaviour.

adherence to medication such as antiretroviral therapy; sleep and bedtime routines; parental use of booster seats in cars; encouraging physical activity and exercise; improving dietary behaviour and reducing obesity; smoking behaviour; and sexual health – in particular, condom use. Table 1.1 gives some specific examples of research in which the HBM and the TPB have been applied in child and adolescent populations across a range of health behaviours and age groups. These are just examples and many more can be found in the literature. As can be seen from the list of examples in Table 1.1, the applications in child and adolescent health have enormous potential, not least because the influences on attitude and habit formation may be greatest during the developing years. During this time, parental and peer pressure can exert considerable effect, creating an optimum environment for maximizing intervention, laying down foundations for lifelong attitudes towards, and habits associated with, health behaviours. An example from the media of the barriers faced in changing health behaviours in children and their parents is given in Box 1.5.

When considering the likelihood of changing a behaviour, it is important to bear in mind that not all health-related behaviours are equal in their resistance to change. Whilst the use of sunscreen by parents and children may be relatively simple to predict or to change based on these models, some behaviours, as can be seen in Box 1.5 above, are more difficult to change than others. More emotionally laden behaviours, such as condom use in adolescents, create different barriers and challenges. The gap between intention and behaviour is often the greatest for behaviours associated with actions that have a strong element of emotional and physical pleasure (e.g., sexual behaviour and condom use in adolescents).

Not only are the applications of these models relevant in their own right but, importantly, the social cognitions driving health behaviours are important in terms of biopsychosocial interactions. Health behaviours contribute to and interact with underlying psychosocial and physiological processes involved in health and illness. In other words, behavioural factors, such as medication adherence, may mediate between psychological factors, such as stress, and disease activity or progression in chronic illness (Gore-Felton and Koopman, 2008).

Without getting into a full-blown nature–nurture debate about the relative influence of genes versus environment on child health, some of these examples demonstrate the power of parental input on health outcomes in children. With the exception of cases of negative parental influences via deliberate neglect and harm, parental influences on health-related behaviours in children more frequently stem from good intentions, as seen above in the example of parents insisting on junk food for school lunches (see Box 1.5). A further example which very quickly spiralled into a major international news story, due to the understandable concern and anxiety of parents, is that of the combined vaccination for measles, mumps and rubella (MMR) described in Box 1.6. This vaccine is offered to children at 13 months, with a booster vaccination at 3 years and 4 months of age or shortly afterwards.

BOX 1.6

MMR health controversy

This story was cited by the media as 'one of the biggest health controversies in recent years' (BBC news, January 2010) following the publication of an article (Wakefield et al., 1998) in the much-respected medical journal *The Lancet*. The article claimed to have found evidence for a causal link between the MMR vaccine, autism and bowel disease, but the claims were not substantiated. There were numerous issues with this study, not least that it was based on a very small sample size of only 12 children referred to specialist clinics. The paper generated enormous media interest and great anxiety and concern in parents, which led to many parents choosing not to vaccinate their children. Despite a false scientific premise and inadequate evidence, as a consequence there has since been a significant rise in cases particularly of measles and mumps since the late 1990s. Figures continue to increase, with cases of measles in the UK being reported as having doubled between 2011 and 2012 (Health Protection Agency reported by BBC news, 24 August 2012). Not only do these viruses produce an unpleasant acute illness in children, they can also lead to serious complications, even death, and can cause birth defects if unvaccinated women who have not had previous exposure to the viruses become exposed to them during pregnancy. For an excellent and detailed account of this case and the pitfalls of the reported research, see Ben Goldacre's book *Bad Science* (2008). *The Lancet* has since retracted the article, and instead cites many articles which provide evidence against any link between the MMR vaccine and autism and bowel disease. Also, Wakefield has since been removed from the medical register by the General Medical Council (GMC). Attitudes and behaviours are less easy to change, however, and parental anxieties remain in the aftermath of such controversies; hence the continued rise of these conditions due to inadequate vaccination uptake.

The MMR controversy demonstrates how parental eagerness to promote health in their children, combined with fear of taking the wrong course of action, can in fact have negative consequences for health outcome. In other words, the result of actions generated by fear or lack of understanding of the risk associated with doing or not doing a certain behaviour (i.e., to vaccinate or not to vaccinate) often creates the greatest risks to health. The notion of risk perception features heavily in recent debates and in popular writing about child health and safety. In an attempt to protect children, many would argue that society has become so risk averse that children are overprotected or effectively 'bubble-wrapped' during childhood and adolescence to a degree that is detrimental to their development (for discussion of this topic, see Gill, 2007; Tovey, 2007; these types of ideas are cleverly articulated from a popular perspective in the novel *May Contain Nuts* by O'Farrell, 2005). Of particular note here is also the drive to purchase dietary products with the addition of omega-3 fish oils. Whilst the association between omega-3 and cognitive functioning is well substantiated, the introduction of products such as omega-3 milk and omega-3 supplements appeals to parents who believe that they are giving their children an advantage never before available. Of course, omega-3 fish oils have been around as long as fish have been available for consumption. Yet with the advent of new omega-3 products and peer pressure on parents to compete (i.e., 'subjective norm'), consumerism is able to cash in on parental concerns and fears about their children's health and related academic performance. For psychologists, this gives a perfect opportunity to observe parental behaviour in relation to child health, including that of parental overprotection.

THE CHANGING FACE OF HEALTH THREATS

It is important to keep in mind that health threats are constantly changing over time. Medications and vaccines are developed, viruses mutate and the rate of the spread of infection fluctuates according to many variables, from compliance with simple hygiene recommendations to global warming (a debate I am not going to enter, but it is a variable worth mentioning). As we will see in Chapter 2, when considering biological development, the status of the T-helper balance of the immune system during childhood contributes to vulnerability or resistance to certain types of disease. Due to the typical immune profile of early childhood, a greater incidence of conditions such as asthma and other atopic allergic reactions is seen. Similarly, younger children are less able to regulate their temperature and are more likely to develop fever and hence be less able to defend against viral invasion. Yet children are more resistant to certain types of diseases spread by parasitic invasion. In Chapter 2, there is a full account of the T-helper balance mentioned above.

Prior to the development of vaccinations and antibiotics in the twentieth century, the leading cause of disease was from infection, including smallpox, measles, tuberculosis, syphilis, diphtheria, meningitis, and malaria. Frequently appearing in plague proportions as epidemics (a plague across a specific region or country) or, indeed, pandemics (an epidemic that has spread across the globe), such diseases would often later become viewed as 'childhood illnesses': the reason being that adults who survived the disease were immune to developing the infection if subsequently exposed, but previously unexposed children were not immune so were more vulnerable to contracting these illnesses (Kiple in Porter, 2001). With the advent of vaccinations, there is now the potential to prevent contagion of these diseases, and that of other viral infections. A recent development in viral resistance is the development of a vaccine against the cervical cancer-causing human papillomavirus (HPV) now offered to teenage girls in most developed countries.

In Western countries where vaccines are routinely offered, uptake is not 100 per cent, even without health controversies such as that surrounding the MMR vaccine, which reflects the psychosocial context of parental decisions to vaccinate children. The advent of the HPV vaccine carried with it additional psychosocial issues relating to parental views on, and knowledge of, sexual activity in adolescence, sparking an array of controversies. The dilemma reflects parental concern to protect whilst at the same time addressing concerns over condoning and encouraging sexual activity amongst adolescents. Coupled with the drive for adolescent freedom to choose, and strong beliefs about whether or not adolescents should be or are sexually active, the introduction of the HPV vaccine has met with some strong opposition, particularly in the United States. Yet, by contrast, in developing countries, much-needed provision of vaccines is hampered by lack of financial aid rather than psychosocial and cultural choice. Thus, worldwide, a range of factors shapes the current landscape of disease prevalence in children.

The threat of pandemics from avian influenza (H5N1), commonly known as 'bird flu', and influenza A virus (H1N1), commonly known as 'swine flu', has dominated public awareness of infectious disease. They demonstrate the rapid spread of viruses, enhanced by viral mutation and exacerbated by modern global travel and lifestyle. Swine flu emerged as a pandemic in Mexico in the spring of 2009. In August 2010, the World Health Organization (WHO) announced that the virus was officially in a post-pandemic period. However, the threat from swine flu is certainly not over and it continues particularly as a seasonal health threat, especially for children under 15 years of age, a group which has shown particular vulnerability to the virus. The vaccine for swine flu is now included in the UK seasonal flu vaccine provided by the NHS, available to 'high-risk' categories of patients (such as the elderly, those with chronic conditions or those who have compromised immunity) or, where available, to those who choose to pay privately. Given the particular susceptibility of children to swine flu and the rise in cases seen from increased contagion at the start of the school term during winter months, a heated debate currently exists over whether the swine flu vaccine should be provided to all children, particularly those in younger age groups, as part of the standard vaccination programme. Whilst swine flu has not seen anywhere near a return to the numbers of deaths seen from plague in centuries gone by, such pandemics are a stark reminder of our continued vulnerability to viral infection despite modern medical advances. Exposure to viral infection and the psychosocial factors that influence susceptibility are a central theme of this book and are explored in depth in Chapters 3 and 5. It is worth being mindful of the landscape of infectious illness worldwide in order to appreciate how and to what extent interventions to increase resistance may be possible.

Human immunodeficiency virus (HIV) and the syndrome that results from this virus, acquired immune deficiency syndrome (AIDS), remains a significant health threat worldwide. The WHO estimated a staggering 3.4 million children under 15 years of age living with HIV worldwide in 2010 (WHO/UNAIDS, 2011). New infections of HIV in children aged under 15 years in 2010 are estimated at 390,000, with AIDS-related deaths in children estimated at 250,000 (WHO/UNAIDS, 2011). HIV/AIDS is a good example of a modern condition once viewed as a life-threatening pandemic in the 1980s, now defined in the Western world largely as a chronic condition which can be managed by antiretroviral medication. However, in developing countries where preventive measures are more limited, the HIV infection rate and death from AIDS-related illness are declining more slowly, and so it remains a life-threatening virus in these less affluent parts of the world. The WHO has made significant advances in providing antiretroviral treatment for children in developing countries in recent years (see www.who.int) in line with their HIV prevention and treatment policy. It is a target of the WHO to enable every child throughout the world to be born free of HIV by 2015. The race against time to develop an HIV vaccine continues, with research groups around the world making advances in this area.

A WORLDVIEW ON CHILD HEALTH

The World Health Organization states that 'over 40% of the global burden of disease attributed to environmental factors falls on children below five years of age, who account for only about 10% of the world's population' (www.who.int/en). Furthermore, the WHO points out that 'environmental risk factors often act in concert, and their effects are exacerbated by adverse social and economic conditions, particularly conflict, poverty and malnutrition' (www.who.int/en). Some of the major causes of childhood disease and death in developing countries include malaria, HIV/AIDS, pneumonia and meningitis. For example, the leading cause of death in children under 5 years old in developing countries is malaria. This treatable virus continues as an epidemic in Sub-Saharan African and Asian countries due to socioeconomic conditions, with malaria affecting predominantly poor women and children, perpetuating the vicious cycle of poverty under which they live. The WHO has set eight Millennium Development Goals (MDGs), with the aim of achieving these by 2015. At least four of these goals are directly related to improving the health of children worldwide. These are to (i) *eradicate poverty and hunger* (MDG 1); (ii) *reduce child mortality* (MDG 4); (iii) *improve maternal health* (MDG 5); and (iv) *combat HIV/ AIDS, malaria, and other diseases* (MDG 6).

In 2010, the WHO reported approximately 400,000 mother-to-child transmissions (MTCTs) of HIV. The successful achievement of MDGs 4 and 5 is supported by the WHO Partnership for Maternal, Newborn and Child Health (PMNCH). Initiatives generated by these goals include interventions to reduce and eventually to eliminate mother-to-child transmission of HIV (either pre-, peri- or postnatally) through the use of antiretroviral therapy (ART). Changes in the landscape of world health are demonstrated by the introduction of pneumococcal vaccine in several developing countries; for example, in early 2011, in Kenya. This vaccine protects against pneumonia which the WHO estimates is responsible for 1.6 million childhood deaths per annum worldwide, as well as protection against meningitis and sepsis.

Other environmental risks to children include those from unclean drinking water, poor sanitation, food and chemicals. Although we touch less on these types of health risk in this book, health psychology has a part to play in improving child health through changing attitude and behaviour at an individual and societal level. This links to child health psychology in improving provision of, and access to, health care, as well as uptake of the health care provided for children and adolescents. One chemical pollutant affecting children is that of second-hand smoke. The statistics on second-hand smoke exposure for children are staggering, the WHO reporting that 40 per cent of children worldwide are exposed to second-hand smoke at home, and 31 per cent of deaths from second-hand smoke are in children. Furthermore, exposure to second-hand smoking at home perpetuates the cycle of smoking behaviour as youth exposed are 1.5–2 times more

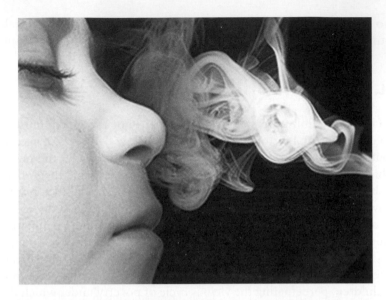

FIGURE 1.7   Advert from the World Health Organization's 'Tobacco Free Initiative' warning against second-hand smoke

Source: European Union, 'Protect children: don't make them breathe your smoke' (www.who.int/tobacco/healthwarningsdatabase/secondhandsmoke_children/en/). © European Union.

likely to start smoking themselves (see WHO, '10 Facts on second-hand smoke'; www.who.int/features/factfiles/tobacco/en/; Figure 1.7). Countries worldwide have made significant effort in tackling this issue through increased awareness, attitude change and legislation over the past decade.

COMMUNICATING HEALTH

In Chapter 2, we address children's understanding of health and illness, approximate ages at which different cognitions develop, and the context of these developments. Appreciation of a child's level of cognition and their context-relevant experience is vital for effective communication. In later chapters, we directly examine the effect of acute and chronic illness during childhood and the associated medical experience, including hospitalization. There have been huge advances in child-friendly hospital environments over the past half-century, which acknowledge the necessity to minimize stress or trauma relating to medical procedures. Stress responses generated from more routine health procedures, such as the heel-prick test in newborns or responses to minor surgical procedures such as circumcision, are well documented. Effective communication does not just entail age-appropriate verbal communication, but extends to the entire experience relating to health and health care. Communication takes on special importance when children are chronically ill, or when they are seeking to understand serious illness or death in a parent. Yet, central to this book is also the importance of appropriate communication about health and illness in healthy children, and the transmission of beliefs about illness across generations and cultures. Accurate understanding about the link between psychosocial and physical health influences from an early age places the child at an advantage in reducing health risk and maximizing physical health throughout the course of life.

CHAPTER SUMMARY

In this chapter, we have introduced some of the underlying psychosocial issues in child health. The psychology of child health has been defined and the various disciplines that contribute towards the interdisciplinary approach taken have been outlined. I have attempted to debunk the myth of positive thinking as a magical 'cure all' and instead introduced the scientific foundation behind the mind–body link. I have also explored some of the origins of psychosocial influences in health as they relate to children and adolescents, and pointed towards some of the developmental considerations inherent in understanding child health. The biopsychosocial model has been introduced as the key perspective that will inform the topics discussed throughout the book. In Chapter 2, we will look in more detail at health, illness and well-being, with a focus on the concept of stress and how this fits in with the concepts already outlined here.

KEY CONCEPTS AND ISSUES

- The biopsychosocial model
- Social support
- Socioeconomic status
- Imprinting and attachment theory
- The mind–body relationship
- Health behaviours
- Social cognition models
- Intergenerational transmission
- A life-course perspective

FURTHER READING

To read the original work on the biopsychosocial model by Engel is inspirational:

Engel, G.L. (1977) The need for a new medical model: a challenge for biomedicine. *Science*, 196(4286): 129–36.

For in-depth background on medical history, containing some very poignant illustrations:

Porter, R. (ed.) (2001) *Cambridge Illustrated History of Medicine*. Cambridge: Cambridge University Press.

More detail about the historical context of psychology:

Leahey, T.H. (2004) *A History of Psychology: Main Currents in Psychological Thought*, 6th edn. Upper Saddle River, NJ: Pearson Prentice Hall.

For a sound text on developmental psychology:

Parke, R.D. and Gauvain, M. (2009) *Child Psychology: A Contemporary Viewpoint*, 7th edn. New York: McGraw-Hill.

The original attachment work and related volumes on loss and separation (amusingly yet cleverly marketed by some booksellers as 'the attachment and loss trilogy'):

Bowlby, J. (1969) *Attachment and Loss*, vol. 1: *Attachment*. Harmondsworth: Penguin.

Bowlby, J. (1973) *Attachment and Loss*, vol. 2: *Separation, Anxiety and Anger*. Harmondsworth: Penguin.

Bowlby, J. (1980) *Attachment and Loss*, vol. 3: *Loss*. London: The Hogarth Press and the Institute of Psychoanalysis.

Current editions (1997/1998) published by Pimlico, London.

For a summary of Bowlby's work set in the context of research in ethology:

Van der Horst, F.C.P., van der Veer, R. and Ijzendoorn, M.H. (2007) John Bowlby and ethology: an annotated interview with Robert Hinde. *Attachment and Human Development*, 9(4): 321–35.

USEFUL WEBSITES

The British Psychological Society Division of Health Psychology: www.health-psychology.org.uk

The World Health Organization (WHO): www.who.int/en

For PowerPoint slides with clear illustration of global HIV/AIDS estimates, see UNAIDS World AIDS Day Report 2011: www.who.int/hiv/data/en

Health Protection Agency (HPA): www.hpa.org.uk

HPA's e-bug website for an interactive educational tool explaining the spread, prevention and treatment of infection: www.e-bug.eu

National Health Service (NHS) information on swine flu: www.nhs.uk/conditions/pandemic-flu/Pages/Introduction.aspx

DEFINING HEALTH, ILLNESS AND WELL-BEING

2

Covered in this chapter

- Definitions of health and illness
- Stress and coping: chronic versus acute stress
- The relevance of cognitive and social development in health and illness
- How can psychosocial factors influence physical health?
- Biological responses to stress
- How can the immune system be influenced by HPA axia regulation?
- Psychobiological theories of stress and coping
- Resiliency factors and individual differences

Having set the scene of child health psychology in Chapter 1, this chapter provides the more in-depth definitions and theories central to subsequent chapters. It begins with some basic definitions of health and well-being, before expanding into psychobiological theories of stress and illness. Whilst much of this information comes from the adult literature, it is not assumed that theories and models of stress in adults can translate directly to children. Instead, particular attention is given to whether or not and how these theories relate to children and to health outcomes in childhood. I consider the similarities and differences between adult and child stress responses and, in doing so, look at how stress plays out in health across the generations.

DEFINITIONS OF HEALTH AND ILLNESS

Most people would accept that 'health' is more than the absence of physical symptoms of illness and implies a positive balance between psychological well-being and physical health. According to the World Health Organization (WHO), health is defined as 'a state of complete physical, mental and social well-being and not merely the absence of disease or infirmity' (WHO, 1948). According to the Good Childhood Inquiry, a 2-year investigation into children's experiences of childhood in the UK, commissioned by the Children's Society, in order to 'flourish', children require the following (Layard and Dunn, 2009):

- Loving families
- Friends
- A positive lifestyle
- Solid values which give meaning to life
- Good schools
- Good mental health
- Enough money to live without shame

Whilst the Good Childhood Inquiry focused on the mental and social well-being of children, rather than on physical health, it is of interest here as the implication is that the psychosocial factors required for positive well-being are the same factors that translate into positive physical health outcomes. These seven characteristics that enable children to flourish map directly onto the types of variables examined in academic studies linking psychosocial factors with neuroendocrine and immune outcomes in health. These are the same familiar constructs that repeatedly stand out as the champions (and culprits) associated with health and illness: namely, social support, health-related behaviours, coping ability, including meaning-based coping, and socioeconomic status or environment.

There has been some debate in the literature over whether health and illness are two ends of the spectrum or overlapping concepts. Most health psychology literature now interprets these concepts as occupying separate but overlapping domains. Research suggests that in younger children (4–5 years old) their own understanding and definitions of illness are focused around the presence of illness symptomatology. By preadolescence (approximately 11–12 years old) this moves towards a more positive focus on health-related behaviours (Myant and Williams, 2005) and becomes progressively so throughout adolescence (Millstein and Irwin, 1987). Figure 2.1 shows a direct comparison between definitions of health and illness in a group of 83 UK children, aged 4–12 years, assessed across a number of illnesses (e.g., the common cold, chickenpox, asthma, toothache, a bruise, and broken bones). The children were given a series of six vignettes or stories about children with different illnesses, then asked a number of questions which tapped their understanding of illness, including how they would describe being ill (i.e., definition of illness) and what causes it. As you can see from the breakdown of children's definitions, the profile of health is quite different from that of illness: these concepts are not understood simply as opposite definitions of one another. With older children, the 'don't know'

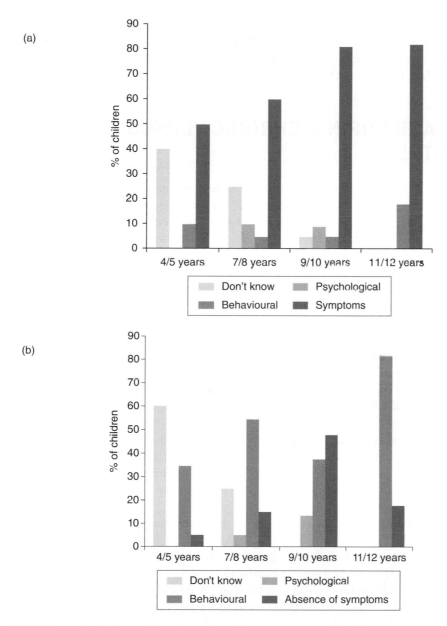

FIGURE 2.1   Definitions of illness and health in a group of 83 UK children aged 4–12 years

Source: Myant and Williams (2005: 810–11, fig. 1).

answers decreased and the definition of illness in terms of 'symptoms' increased, whereas psychological and behavioural definitions were much less likely to be used across all the age groups. By contrast, in defining health, behavioural factors were most popular with age groups of 7–8 and 9–10-year-old children, whilst the youngest age group was the most likely to respond with 'don't know' and the 9–10-year-old children most commonly defined health as the absence of symptoms (Myant and Williams, 2005). So children are able to make subtle distinctions between the concepts of health and illness, and the contrasts between the two differ with age.

STRESS AND COPING: CHRONIC VERSUS ACUTE STRESS

Everyone seems to know what stress is, since we have all experienced it in various forms. Yet the sources of stress and the responses to it differ widely across individuals (one person's stress is another person's relaxation, so to speak). To begin to understand the links between stress and health in children, we need a clear definition of stress as a starting point. The work of Lazarus and colleagues in the late 1970s onwards provides exactly this. Although not without criticism, their definitions of stress and coping became hallmarks of the stress and coping literature and are as applicable today as they were when they first emerged over a quarter of a century ago. In this work, termed the *transactional theory*, or transactional model of stress and coping (Lazarus and Folkman, 1984), the experience of stress is defined as 'the condition that results when person-environment transactions lead the individual to perceive a discrepancy – *whether real or not* – between the demands of a situation and the resources of the person's biological, psychological, or social systems' (Sarafino, 1998: 70, emphasis added). Similarly, Cohen and Herbert (1996: 119) later summarized stress as being 'when demands imposed by events exceed individuals' ability to cope'.

Lazarus and colleagues described a process of cognitive appraisal whereby individuals initially assess the meaning of a potential stressor (primary appraisal) to decide if the event or situation is stressful to them and, if so, in what way (i.e., what is the harm or loss that has resulted and what is the future threat or opportunity for challenge?). The process of secondary appraisal occurs simultaneously with primary appraisal and involves an evaluation of the individual's ability to cope with the stressor and the resources available to do so. This model is depicted in Figure 2.2 as shown by the boxes and arrows. An important but often understated development of this model evolved from work by Folkman (1997) in a study exploring the coping experiences of male caregivers for their partners with HIV/AIDS. In this modified version of the model, the importance of 'meaning' and 'benefit-finding' are exemplified as positive outcomes of an otherwise very upsetting chronic stress experience. Rather than an unfavourable or unresolved outcome necessarily leading to distress, this modification allows for meaning-based coping to lead to the outcome of positive emotion which further sustains the coping process through a reappraisal of the event or of the coping resources available to deal with it. The tinted boxes and arrows of Figure 2.2 show the model attenuated to include meaning-based coping. Here, we are considering how children cope with a range of stressors from everyday stress to more severe stress. To take this one step further and link it in with the

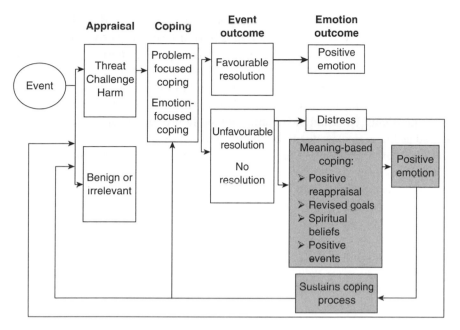

FIGURE 2.2   Revised positive states and coping with stress model

Source: Adapted from Folkman (1997).

caregiving role mentioned above, whilst the theme of parenting as a form of caregiving is mentioned throughout the book, in Part II we look specifically at the experience of children as carers, their coping resources and the impact on their health and well-being. The revised part of the model particularly comes into play when we consider stress and coping in children in these situations.

These definitions of stress and coping can be equally applied to children, although stressor types and coping ability are reflected in developmental stage. This begs the question of what the difference is between the terms 'stress' and 'stressor'. There are different ways to view this, but the clearest working definition is to understand 'stressors' as agents with potential stress-inducing abilities, and 'stress' as the result of the potential stressor successfully having created the psychophysiological experience of stress in the individual. This is a classic stimulus-response in some respects but, importantly, what constitutes the active ingredient of the stressor, or catalyst capable of creating the stress experience, is not the same for all individuals. It is the interpretation of the potential stressor by the individual that determines whether or not the stressor can realize its potential and cause stress to be experienced. In other words, it is the meaning of the event, not the event itself, which defines whether or not it is stressful. The psychosocial factors that determine this meaning are precisely what are being considered in this book.

There are, of course, differences in the magnitude of stress experienced. Later on in this chapter, I consider the difference between acute and chronic stress, but before doing that, it is worth taking time to navigate the various stress taxonomies that shape the study of psychosocial stress. One way to categorize different stressors is to distinguish between major life events (e.g., death, divorce, moving house, getting married), minor life events (e.g., changing jobs, taking a holiday) and daily hassles (e.g., losing something, being late, arguing with a friend). Put into the context of childhood stress, such life events include those relating specifically to the child, as well as to those responsible for their care, such as parents or guardians. For example, death, moving house, or starting a new school may all be classified as life events, as would be the birth of a sibling, parental divorce or separation and change in parental income. Questionnaires which assess everyday stress or 'hassles' in children include items which refer to stressors such as being teased in the playground, falling out with a friend, being told off by a teacher, or having an argument with a parent. Table 2.1 (see Box 2.1) gives examples of these different types of stressors. Although couched in child-relevant terms, the sources of stress are perhaps not that different from the everyday work, home or relationship stressors experienced in adulthood. Life-event rating scales became popular in the 1970s and assess number and severity of events, or ascribe a pre-assigned stress weighting to life events that have occurred over a given time period; for example, the Holmes–Rahe life-events inventory (Holmes and Rahe, 1967).

BOX 2.1

Examples of stress in children

TABLE 2.1   Examples of stress in children: major and minor life events and daily hassles

Major life event	Minor life event	Daily hassle
Death of a brother or sister	Increase or decrease in parent's income	Having a bad dream
Birth of a brother or sister	Change in parent's job so he/she has less time at home	Being teased at school
Being suspended from school	Joining a social organization	Best friend not wanting to be your best friend any more
Moving to a new school	Death of a pet	Losing something
Death of a close friend	Failing something at school	Having to give a talk in front of the class
Being admitted to hospital because of illness or injury	Being awarded a special prize for personal achievement	Parents arguing
Parent in hospital	Going away on holiday	Teacher angry because of your behaviour

Source: Based on items included in the Life Events Scale (Coddington, 1972) and the Children's Hassles Scale (Kanner et al., 1987).

> **Points to consider**
>
> How similar are childhood stresses to those in adulthood?
> What is the distinction between major life events, minor life events and hassles?
> Why are positive events sometimes experienced as stressful?

There was a trend in the 1980s, which were very much pioneering times for positive psychology, to examine 'uplifts' as well as 'hassles', acknowledging that the same source (e.g., the experience of parenting) could bring with it both hassles and uplifts (Kanner et al., 1981, 1987). This work suggested that it was the balance between the rewards of the uplifting aspects (e.g., the joy of parenting) versus the costs of experiencing the stress associated with that source or event (e.g., the demands of parenting) that may be important. Yet hassles and uplifts, much like positive and negative affect (mood or feelings), appear to be separate constructs. Rather than the positive aspects balancing out the negative ones, or vice versa, both positive and negative aspects (uplifts and hassles) can be experienced at the same time. Both positive and negative responses are important to consider in understanding a child's response to an everyday 'hassle' or life event. Current stress research tends to focus on negative aspects of stress rather than uplifts or positive life events, although positive psychology and meaning/benefit-finding, as mentioned above, are increasing in popularity.

A major factor in dealing with stress is the perceived and actual control that an individual has over the stressor. Perceived stress is a further measure of stress, which refers not to any specific event but instead to the general feeling of being under stress. To use a metaphor, since these abound in the stress literature, it is the degree to which an individual feels that the weight of the world is upon their shoulders, or the degree to which they feel burdened by events and demands. Since the stress experience is very closely bound up with notions of control, this is particularly relevant for children. In childhood, a double-edged sword exists, whereby children have less responsibility than they will have in adulthood, which may be seen as stress reducing, yet they also have significantly less control over life events (e.g., parents moving house, the decision to change school, parental conflict and separation). This lack of control, in the form of necessary parental and school authority, may cause a degree of stress in itself, particularly for children aged 5 years and upwards for whom emotional, behavioural and social elements start to take on greater meaning (Gunnar, 1992). Issues of control particularly come to the fore in the teenage years, contributing to a dynamic stress experience between adolescents and their parents.

Assessment of perceived stress in children is more complicated than in adults because of the difficulty in verbalizing the concept of stress, particularly in younger age groups. This is addressed in Chapter 3 when considering psychobiological assessment methods in health. It is worth noting here, though, that in a study of children's knowledge and understanding of stress in 4–11-year-olds, most (78 per cent) had heard of the word 'stress' and some could define the concept, although the sophistication of this

TABLE 2.2 Percentage and number of children able to define stress in each age group and elements/coping strategies mentioned at least once

	Age group			
	4–5 (n=11)	6–7 (n=13)	8–9 (n=13)	10–11 (n=13)
Definition of stress				
Appropriate definition provided	45% (5)	62% (8)	100% (13)	100% (13)
Definition included				
Behavioural elements	9.1% (1)	23.1% (3)	0	30.8% (4)
Cognitive elements	0	15.4% (2)	38.5% (5)	7.7% (1)
Emotional elements	27.3% (3)	53.8% (7)	61.5% (8)	100% (13)
Physical/biological elements	9.1% (1)	7.7% (1)	38.5% (5)	46.2% (6)
Other elements	9.1% (1)	7.7% (1)	15.4% (2)	15.4% (2)
Experience of stress				
Children with indirect experience	64% (7)	85% (11)	92% (12)	100% (13)
Children with direct experience	46% (5)	69% (9)	77% (10)	92% (12)
	4–5 (n=11)	6–7 (n=13)	8–9 (n=123)	10–11 (n=13)
Coping strategies				
Active coping	33.3% (3)	37.5% (3)	33.3% (4)	45.2% (6)
Distraction	33.3% (3)	12.5% (1)	8.3% (1)	38.5% (5)
Social support	11.1% (1)	37.5% (3)	33.3% (4)	15.4% (2)
Emotional expression	11.1% (1)	0	41.7% (5)	53.8% (7)
Problem focused	11.1% (1)	37.5% (3)	25% (3)	23.1% (3)
Emotion focused	0	0	41.7% (5)	23.1% (3)
Others (e.g., take tablets, relax)	11.1% (1)	12.5% (1)	58.3% (7)	7.7% (1)

Source: Valentine et al. (2010).

explanation increased with age (Valentine et al., 2010). By the age of 8 years and upwards, all of the sample of 50 children could define stress appropriately. Descriptions of stress became more complex with age, particularly for emotional content, and even in the youngest age group of 4–5 years almost half were aware of having experienced stress directly (Valentine et al., 2010). The use of coping strategies also varied with age, with emotional expression being used more in older children and active coping or distraction being favoured by the youngest children in the group (Valentine et al., 2010; see Table 2.2).

There is a further related concept in addition to negative stress and positive uplifts. This is the idea of 'positive stress' which originates from the work of Hans Selye (1974) in which he distinguished between 'eustress' and 'distress'. *Eustress* is essentially good stress, which is associated with positive or motivational states and controllable types or levels of stress. *Distress*, on the other hand, is the uncontrollable type or level of stress which causes discomfort and is usually what is being referred to when the term 'stress' is used. Eustress is often linked with improved performance, whether in public speaking, exams or running a marathon, demonstrating that some stress really can be good for you, indeed even desirable to perform well. It is when stress is perceived as uncontrollable and intolerable that the damaging, often immuno-suppressive effects endure and have a negative influence on health outcome. It is usually this uncontrollable or negative stress that is being referred to when the term 'stress' is used, but it is worth remembering that other, more positive aspects of stress exist and that not all stress is necessarily negative. Keeping this in mind is helpful in developing ways to deal with stress and to turn the distress experienced into a more useful direction, perhaps harnessing the power of eustress.

BOX 2.2

Examination stress

Examples of stress experienced in relation to examinations in school-aged children frequently hit the headlines. An example of this was a news article in June 2004 which reported the story of a 15-year-old girl who committed suicide because of anxiety about her exams. The teenager had taken an overdose of anti-malarial medication. Such extreme reactions are relatively rare but highlight the anticipatory stress experienced by adolescents with increasing competition in secondary school exams. In this instance, a clearly behavioural outcome (suicide) was observed, but in many cases the effects may be more subtle and go unnoticed. For example, the psychological pressure of exams may also present a challenge to physical health through endocrine and immune effects, and the influence of these stress experiences may have long-lasting implications. Such stress experiences are unlikely to decline with the pressure on adolescents to perform and compete, particularly within the climate of increasing fees for higher education. This presents a challenge to develop intervention strategies that target school-aged children, enabling them to develop appropriate health-enhancing psychological and physiological coping skills.

Source: http://news.bbc.co.uk

Points to consider

When does acute exam stress become a chronic stressor?
What interventions might be most beneficial and with which age groups?
How can the psychological and physiological effects of exam stress be observed?
What sort of interventions might be valuable in reducing the stress experienced around exams?

Examination stress in children and adolescents (see Box 2.2) has been particularly highlighted with the onset of regular national testing programmes in children from the age of 7 years upwards in the UK. Yet academic examinations have been documented as causing stress responses, altering immune functioning which may be an indicator of increased vulnerability to disease (Glaser et al., 1993; Deinzer et al., 2000). It is important to consider, therefore, not just how to avoid stress but how to cope with stressful events. In children, learning to cope with stressful events can create resilience in adulthood, both psychological and physiological (at an endocrine and immune level). Interventions to cope with stress and reduce exam anxiety have proved successful at both these levels (Kiecolt-Glaser et al., 2001).

Similarly, the stress taxonomy used by the National Scientific Council on the Developing Child (US) divides stressful events (i.e., the stress experience) into three types: (i) beneficial or positive stress; (ii) tolerable stress; and (iii) harmful or toxic stress (National Scientific Council on the Developing Child, 2005). Positive stress is associated with normal and natural development, and examples of stressors that might trigger this type of response are given as the experience of starting with a new child-minder or the response to an immunization injection. The experience of starting school, a subject covered in depth in Chapter 5 of this book, would also come under this category. Tolerable stress covers the major and minor life events described above which children can cope with over time and with sufficient support. Toxic stress is the most severe category of stress experience, in which children are exposed to physical or emotional maltreatment, abuse or neglect, or severe poverty. The effects of these toxic-level stressors are considered in more depth in Chapters 4 and 5.

So what makes stress stressful? As described above, there is a distinction between a potential stressor and the experience of stress itself. Anything could potentially be a stressor, but it is the experience and appraisal of an event that defines it as stressful or not. A further important distinction is between acute or short-term stress and

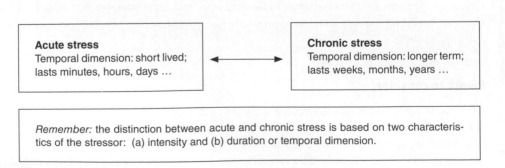

FIGURE 2.3   The distinction between acute and chronic stress

chronic or longer-term stress. This distinction is predominantly one of duration as well as intensity of the stressor, and is most easily viewed as a continuum as illustrated in Figure 2.3.

Acute stress is short lived, usually lasting minutes, hours or days. Sources of acute stressors in the natural environment, or hassles as described above, could include those events relating to life domains of school, work, home, friends, family, and social relationships. Due to common underlying elements associated with stress appraisal, including the threat of social evaluation (i.e., fear about judgements being made by others) and time pressure, their effects can also be simulated in an experimental laboratory setting. There are established protocols for inducing psychosocial stress in the laboratory, which include the acute stress associated with public speaking and arithmetic. One of the most well established, particularly in conjunction with reliable physiological assessment of stress hormone response, is the Trier Social Stress Test (TSST; Kirschbaum et al., 1993). The TSST involves performance in front of a panel of judges made up of the experimenter, who puts the participant under pressure to perform well, and two other individuals, who each take on different roles aimed at increasing stress associated with social evaluation (termed socioevaluative threat or SET; Dickerson et al., 2009).

Understandably, such experiments are designed for adults, and limited use has been made on children, although the TSST has been adapted for children (CTSST), using age-appropriate maths challenges and story-telling as the public-speaking task (Buske-Kirschbaum et al., 2003). We come back to methodology and, importantly, to the ethics of experimental design with children in Chapter 3, but here the significant point is that acute stress responses can be reliably induced in the laboratory setting, demonstrating key underlying characteristics of stressors which may be seen in everyday life. More extreme acute stressors include those that are sometimes termed 'cataclysmic events' (Morrison and Bennett, 2012), resulting from sudden events on a catastrophic scale as seen in natural disasters such as earthquakes and in terrorist attacks. These are acute as they cause a sudden, immediate stress reaction, although the effect(s) may also be long lasting and subsequently also become classified under chronic stress responses.

Chronic stress lasts weeks, months or years and is typified by the classic life-event stresses described above. Other chronic stressors include caregiving, the longer-term effects of natural disasters, terrorism and illness itself. These types of common major life stressors may on initial reading appear to belong more to the world of adults rather than children or adolescents. On closer inspection, however, this is not necessarily the case as chronic stressors such as bereavement, parental divorce or caregiving may be stressors which are faced in early life. When experienced by children, these events take on a greater dimension, often perhaps because it feels innately unjust and out of kilter with our view of life's trajectory; equally, it may be because there is a sense that chronic stress or severe life events in early life may have greater consequences in the long term as a result of the psychological and physical disruption caused. There are also specific life events and severe stress experiences of particular relevance to childhood, such as abuse and maltreatment, and we will consider these specific experiences in Chapter 5.

BOX 2.3

Highlighting research: modern-day stresses

Source: A. Schreier and G.W. Evans (2003) Adrenal cortical response of young children to modern and ancient stressors. *Current Anthropology*, 44(2): 306–9.

Study rationale and hypothesis: It takes time and physiological energy to adapt and learn to cope with stressors. Based on an evolutionary perspective, people should be better able to cope with stressors which have been around for many years than more recent or modern stressors.

Definition of terms: 'Ancient' stressors = chronic demands that have been with the human species since the beginning of time. 'Modern' stressors = new demands that have emerged in the past 10–12 thousand years (post-Neolithic age, i.e., since the dawn of agriculture).

Methods: Participants were 262 children with a mean age of 9.2 years, predominantly white, 46 per cent female, and their mothers. Interview with mother and child, plus life-event checklist answered for the child by the mother. Stressor severity was deduced and classification of stressors as 'ancient' or 'modern' was conducted. Overnight collection of urinary cortisol (8 p.m.–8 a.m.) as a measure of hypothalamic-pituitary-adrenal axis activity. Control variable = parental income.

Results: Mean frequency of stressors per child was 6.20 comprising 3.12 'modern' and 3.06 'ancient'. Controlling for income as a measure of socioeconomic status, modern stressors but not ancient stressors were significantly related to cortisol levels; i.e., greater exposure to modern stressors were associated with higher cortisol levels (see Table 2.3; Figure 2.4).

Conclusion: More modern stressors impose greater demands due to insufficient adaptation. As lifestyles continue to evolve, with ever faster technologies requiring greater adaptation, the stress response system will need to enable adaptation in order to cope with the new demands.

TABLE 2.3   Frequencies of the most common childhood stressors

Stressor	Sample frequency
Modern	
Close family member hospitalized for serious illness	142
Close family member away from home a lot	137
Parent has lost his/her job or has been unemployed	128
Ancient	
Child upset by family arguments	148
Close family members have had serious arguments with each other	112
Child has had to deal with people whose behaviour was frightening	98

Source: Schreier and Evans (2003).

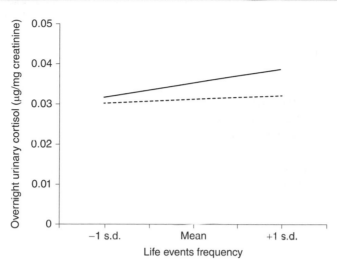

FIGURE 2.4 Regression plots of cortisol for childhood exposure to modern stressors (solid line) and ancient stressors (dotted line)

Source: Schreier and Evans (2003).

Points to consider

Can stressors be usefully divided into categories of ancient and modern?

How could this study be expanded: what other measures could be used to improve the comparison between older and more modern stressors?

Are modern stressors really that much more taxing or do we tend to view stressors of a previous age through rose-tinted spectacles?

Of course, life events and hassles rarely occur in isolation; in fact, life stress is best described by the well-known adage 'It never rains but it pours' since one life event often entails another, as in the case of death or divorce necessitating a house move, the house move bringing with it financial implications and disruption of social relationships.

THE RELEVANCE OF COGNITIVE AND SOCIAL DEVELOPMENT IN HEALTH AND ILLNESS

The overlapping but separate concepts of health and illness have already been described above. But how and when do children develop these concepts and what influences the beliefs they hold and the understanding they have of health and illness? Research into children's cognitive and social development with respect to illness has been most strongly influenced by the work of Bibace and Walsh in the 1980s. Their seminal work, published in 1980, specifically examined the development of illness concepts in children and was based on the cognitive staging theorists, Piaget and Inhelder (1947) and Werner (1948). Bibace and Walsh (1980) developed Piagetian concepts of cognition to embrace children's understanding of illness, based on children in the United States. These six stages and their application are detailed in Table 2.4 and are consistent with Piaget's pre-logical reasoning (ages 2–6 years), concrete-logical reasoning (ages 7–10 years) and formal-logical reasoning (age 11 upwards). Interestingly, Bibace and Walsh (1980) also point to an additional category of 'incomprehension' in some of the youngest (4-year-old) participants, which precedes the initial pre-logical, 'magical' level of thinking.

In the examples given in Table 2.4, the common cold is used to illustrate the developmental levels, but Bibace and Walsh (1980) also used several other illness examples to test their staging model, including 'heart attack', 'measles' and 'cancer'. The theory demonstrates a child's understanding of both cause and effect in relation to illness. Despite some very valid criticisms

TABLE 2.4   Developmental levels of the perception of illness

Magical level – explanations based on association

1 *Phenomenism.* The child describes the illness in terms of any phenomenon s/he has experienced as associated with the illness, without clear differentiation of cause and effect. 'A cold is from ... it's when your nose runs.'
2 *Contagion.* The child describes the illness in terms of body experiences or symptoms. S/he associates a specific external cause with the illness, but cannot explain how the cause leads to the effect. 'A cold is a runny nose and it's like from going outside in winter.' (How?) 'It's from being out in the winter time.'

Concrete level – explanations based on sequence

3 *Contamination.* The child describes illness in terms of experienced symptoms and explains its cause as originating in external acts or situations. The child explains how a sequence of causal events leads to the illness by contacting or involving the body as a whole. 'A cold is from when you're swimming in cold water or out in the snow. It stays in your body ... it goes up onto your chest.'
4 *Internalization.* The child describes the illness and explains how a sequence of mechanical actions leads to changes in specific internal body parts. 'A cold is when your nose gets stuffed up and you can't breathe. It's from the germs getting into your nose and lungs and clogging them up so you can't breathe. You sneeze to get the germs out.'

Abstract level – explanations based on interaction

5 *Physiological.* The older child or adult describes an entire internal disease process involving the interaction of multiple causes and effects on multiple body parts. 'A cold is a change within the body resulting in symptoms like coughing, sneezing, running nose, headaches and stuffed-up sinuses. You catch the germs that are all around us. Coughing and running nose are the side effects of the body's fighting them off; it makes mucus to carry away the dead germs.'
6 *Psychophysiological.* The older child or adult explains how multiple causes and effects interact by describing transformations at the cellular level. 'A cold is the collection of symptoms that define the immune system's response to an invading virus. The white blood cells ... And this happens when the person is experiencing a lot of stress.'

Source: Bibace, Schmidt and Walsh (1994)

of Piagetian staging theory *per se*, particularly surrounding the rigidity of the stages, the illness applications of Bibace and Walsh have remained relatively unscathed and this model has maintained a central place in thinking about children's understanding of illness. Other studies which followed found further evidence to support these stages in other illnesses (e.g., Eiser and Patterson, 1983; Eiser et al., 1983). Walsh and Bibace (1991), along with other researchers (e.g., Peltzer and Promtussananon, 2003, using a black South African sample), have similarly applied the categories to a child's understanding of the causal mechanisms in AIDS.

Developing this model further in relation to illness, attention has been drawn to the importance of experience and learning, as well as to differences between illness types. Importantly, subsequent work highlights that children may be more capable in their understanding of illness than these early applications allowed. Studies with clear-cut results in this area are few and far between. A study in the late 1990s emphasized the multidimensional nature of children's concepts of health, moving beyond staging to include the context of daily-life experience, variables associated with socialization experiences including age, socioeconomic status and sex differences in a sample of Canadian children (Normandeau et al., 1998). They report conceptions of health, in their group of 1,674 children aged 5–12 years, as being 'complex' and being composed of three constructs, which they termed (i) functionality (e.g., doing sports, activities and the absence of disease); (ii) mental health (well-being and relationships with others; e.g., looking healthy, feeling good); and (iii) lifestyle health behaviours (e.g., healthy diet, sleeping habits and body hygiene). Sex differences were not observed in the conceptualization of health, but several effects were found for socioeconomic differences with typically younger, middle-class, urban children having the greatest understanding of a healthy diet. Of course, it is important to note that conceptions of illness are just that, and as such may not translate into health-related behaviours in practice, but understanding how children think about health and illness is a critical starting point for informing and implementing health promotional activities and interventions.

The study by Myant and Williams (2005) mentioned above examined the understanding of specific illnesses in a group of 83 children aged 4–12 years, with a focus on illness definitions, prevention, time course and recovery, in addition to the more classic illness causality associated with infection or injury. Whilst the authors found age effects of understanding as you would expect, with more complex explanations emerging as age increased, they also report illness-specific differences in level of understanding across all ages (e.g., a greater understanding of causality for toothache than for asthma or the common cold). Interestingly, despite the common cold being a contagious illness that the children would almost certainly have had personal experience of, in this study children of all ages held misconceptions about its causality compared to knowledge of causality for other common childhood infections such as chickenpox. Yet they showed a high level of reasoning about definition, prevention and recovery regarding the common cold. There may be various sophisticated explanations for this concerning the nature of the symptoms of a cold and the fact that colds are often associated with the winter months (although prevalent all year round).

The learning environment at home and school may contribute to such misconceptions of causality through messages that are transferred or communicated from parents, teachers and the general cultural environment (e.g., children may be inaccurately told that 'being cold' can 'give' you a cold). These beliefs take on very strong influences in children's understanding of illness and become cognitively engrained. There is a wonderfully endearing children's book (which even common-cold researchers have been known to read to their offspring) entitled *Buster Catches a Cold* (1983, original author Hisako Madokoro). It tells of a cheeky puppy who ignores the warning of his mother not to go out in the rain because he may catch a cold. Sure enough, Buster goes out in the rain looking for a cold and comes back home sneezing or, to put it scientifically, exhibiting symptoms of the common cold. The universality of this is shown by the fact that the story is taken from a Japanese book translated into English for the US market. The common cold is a fascinating example which we will come back to many times in this book as it is one of my particular areas of interest (see Chapter 3 for more explanation as to why I have this peculiar fascination). To sum up, experience and the learning environment are important contributors to children's understanding of illness, and there is evidence that generalizability of conceptual stages, whilst a useful guide, cannot be assumed, and may vary according to experience, socioeconomic status, culture and illness type.

Whilst I have referred to cognitive and social development under the same umbrella, these are, of course, distinct areas of research in their own right. As can be seen from the examples given, cognitive conceptions of illness occur in a social context and, as such, it is essential for healthy physical and emotional development that cognition and socialization occur in tandem. Social well-being is internationally recognized as integral to health as evidenced in documents from organizations including the United Nations, the World Health Organization, and the European Union (Kohler and Rigby, 2003). Social development in the first few years of life is dependent upon parent/carer–infant interaction, with increasing input from school influences and peers as child development continues, until adolescence when a cacophony of competing social domains vie for attention. Social experience is a theme we will come back to in Chapter 5 when considering the effect of child maltreatment on physical health outcome, and in its many related forms of social relationships, support, connectedness, integration and isolation throughout the book.

HOW CAN PSYCHOSOCIAL FACTORS INFLUENCE PHYSICAL HEALTH?

In Chapter 1, I asserted that the influence of psychosocial state on physical health is more than mind over matter, and that a scientific rationale and evidence exist for this relationship. Stress influences physical health via biological mechanisms, developed and deployed for the purpose of escaping life-threatening situations in our evolutionary past. In humans, these mechanisms have now been co-opted to deal with non-physical, psychological stressors. The same physiological response results, although psychological threats do not necessarily require this same physical response. The result of this is the production of end immune altering hormones which often have very little functional utility in dealing with

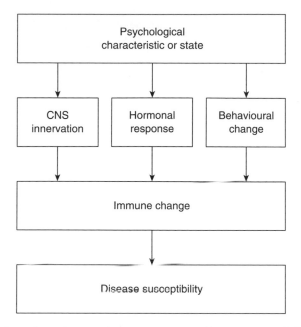

FIGURE 2.5   An outline of psychoneuroimmune routes to disease susceptibility

Source: Cohen and Herbert (1996).

the types of stressors that characterize the modern world. Figure 2.5 shows an early model by Cohen and Herbert (1996) which summarizes this process. In this biopsychosocial model, psychological characteristics or state influence disease susceptibility via three possible routes: (i) central nervous system (CNS) activation; (ii) endocrine or hormonal alteration; or (iii) changes in health behaviours. One or more of these routes then impacts on the immune system to influence the likelihood of becoming ill by altering susceptibility to disease. Cohen and Herbert (1996) point out that the arrows are in one direction only in this model, for the sake of simplicity, but that other connections are plausible.

Moving from this general model to a later, more detailed, biopsychosocial model, Lutgendorf and Costanzo (2003) developed the model proposed in Figure 2.6 which shows how the science of psychoneuroimmunology fits with the field of health psychology. Health outcomes in this model are categorized into (i) vulnerability or resistance; (ii) disease onset and symptoms; (iii) progression/exacerbation/recovery and quality of life; and (iv) survival and quality of life. Routes to these outcomes are via psychosocial processes, biological factors, and health behaviours or lifestyle choices, which influence neuroendocrine and immune mechanisms. Notice that an indirect route to neuroendocrine and immune alteration is via life stress, given as a separate box and including socio-economic status and early life experience. Interventions are also incorporated into this model as an influencing factor on health/illness outcome. Lutgendorf and Costanzo (2003) also make use of not just unidirectional, but also bi- and pluridirectional arrows to indicate connections between constructs.

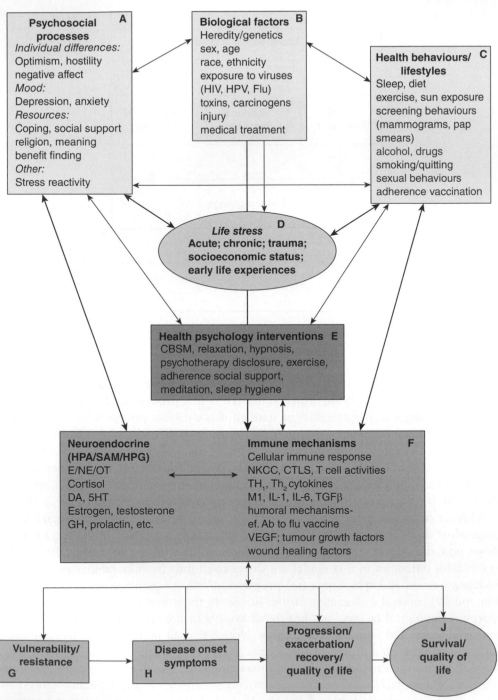

FIGURE 2.6 Conceptualization of the biopsychosocial model which integrates psychoneuroimmunology and health psychology

Source: Lutgendorf and Costanzo (2003).

So far I have focused on the factors labelled in this model as 'Psychosocial processes' (A) and 'Life stress' (D) in routes to health and illness outcomes. 'Health behaviours/lifestyles' (C) were also discussed in Chapter 1. The key to this model lists the various endocrine and immune factors involved in the biological routes through which stress influences health. Before continuing with psychobiological theories and notions of resilience, a more detailed explanation and definition of some of these 'Neuroendocrine and immune mechanisms' (F) is needed.

BIOLOGICAL RESPONSES TO STRESS

In Chapter 5, I take a more in-depth look at the effects of stress during childhood on physical health, but first, in this chapter, I consider what is meant by the stress response in

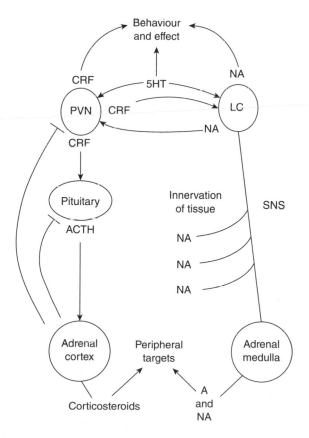

FIGURE 2.7   The stress response system

Key: A, adrenaline; ACTH, adrenocorticotrophic hormone; CRF, corticotrophin releasing factor; 5HT, 5-hydroxytryptamine; LC, locus coeruleus; NA, noradrenaline; PVN, paraventricular nucleus; SNS, sympathetic nervous system.

Source: Evans et al. (2000).

a physiological sense as well as the psychological triggers of this system. Importantly, it is essential to consider what is known about how and when this stress response develops and what may influence its development. Remember, though, that these are questions that keep many researchers busy for an entire academic career. There are still many unanswered questions and unexplored avenues, which are what makes this area so fascinating, yet more challenging, than areas where more factual or binary answers are readily available.

The stress response system in humans is the dual system of the sympathetic adrenomedullary (SAM) system and the hypothalamic-pituitary-adrenal (HPA) axis. These two arms are part of the same bipartite stress response system: the SAM system operating immediately a stress is perceived in the environment, and the HPA axis approximately 20 minutes later, after the initiation of a stress encounter. Figure 2.7 illustrates this stress response system in diagrammatic form.

In this diagram, the right arm illustrates the SAM system, resulting in production of adrenaline and noradrenaline (note that the US terms for these neurotransmitters are epinephrine and norepinephrine, respectively). The SAM system is the sympathetic arm of the autonomic nervous system and constitutes the neural pathway through which the brain exerts its influence on immune functioning. The left arm of the diagram represents the HPA axis, resulting in glucocortocoid production (corticosteroids such as cortisol), and is the endocrine or hormonal pathway through which the immune system is influenced.

Whilst both parts of the stress response system are vital, it is the activation of this second part of the stress response, the HPA axis, that has generated an exponentially large amount of research since the 1990s. The HPA axis operates via a negative feedback loop, which enables cortisol to be produced when needed. Information about hormone levels is fed back to the pituitary gland and hypothalamus of the brain and cortisol production reduced to return the system back to basal levels, all other things being equal. Under stress, a positive cascade of hormones swings into operation: the hypothalamus in the brain is triggered to release corticotrophin releasing factor (CRF), which stimulates the pituitary gland at the base of the brain to produce adrenocorticotrophic hormone (ACTH), which in turn stimulates the adrenal glands to produce corticosteroids, predominantly the hormone cortisol. This axis and hence the increased production of cortisol is then switched off via negative feedback to the hypothalamus and the pituitary gland which signals the end of the stressor, and adaptation back to pre-stress levels occurs. Figure 2.8 outlines the location of the components of the HPA axis, and Figure 2.9 illustrates the positive cascade and negative feedback loop of the HPA axis mechanism. Remember, this is under normal conditions, assuming the person has no underlying illness causing a physiological imbalance in neuroendocrine or immune functioning and assuming that once the stress has occurred the individual is able to return to pre-stress levels.

A normal circadian (24-hour) pattern for salivary cortisol, again all other factors being equal, reveals cortisol levels to be the lowest at late evening and night time, rising during the early hours of the morning, and peaking approximately 30 minutes after awakening. Levels then decline across the day, showing a relatively steep decline over the morning hours, and declining until late afternoon/early evening, before returning to a nadir during night-time hours. The typical diurnal (daytime) pattern of cortisol from awakening to

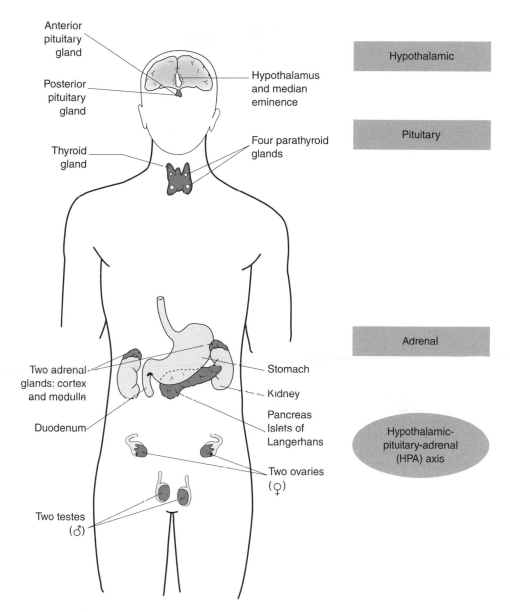

FIGURE 2.8 Sites of the principal endocrine glands highlighting the hypothalamic-pituitary-adrenal (HPA) axis

Source: Adapted from Brook and Marshall (2001).

evening is illustrated in Figure 2.10. These data are hypothetical but based on a range of studies which have examined salivary cortisol levels in children (see Jessop and Turner-Cobb, 2008, for a review of studies) and are also typical of the pattern found in adults.

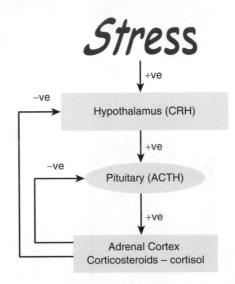

FIGURE 2.9   The hypothalamic-pituitary-adrenal (HPA) axis

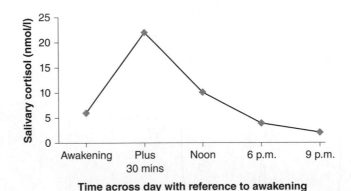

FIGURE 2.10   Typical diurnal pattern of salivary cortisol

Some of the early work on cortisol levels as measured in saliva revealed that newborn infants do not initially show the same circadian rhythm as adults, but instead exhibit two peaks of cortisol at 12-hour intervals, related to sleep–wake cycles rather than to clock time (Riad-Fahmy et al., 1982; Francis et al., 1987). It is not until approximately 3 months old that the morning peak in circadian rhythm appears, possibly linked to increased regulation of night-time sleep patterns, but the diurnal variation continues to peak and trough throughout the day depending on activities, napping schedules and feeding patterns (for a full review, see Gunnar and Quevedo, 2007). Newborns have also consistently been shown to be capable of responding to stressors, as observed in cortisol responses, including routine hospital examinations involving handling or mild restraint (e.g., discharge examination or height/weight measurement). Cortisol levels increase still further in response to mildly painful stimuli, such as the heel-prick blood sampling procedure, and minor surgical procedures, such as circumcision. Gunnar (1992) notes that, despite these increases in plasma cortisol sampled, healthy babies habituate to handling stressors and show sensitization to the heel prick, which implies a physiological learning element to the experience even at this youngest of ages. Reactivity of less healthy babies shows the greatest response and less adaptation in the form of habituation or sensitization to repeated stimuli.

In older infants and young children, attachment anxiety brought about by separation is one of the greatest stressors and, not surprisingly, good quality childcare and a high level of adult involvement in play activities have been found to alleviate such stress reactivity. In fact, a great deal of work has been conducted on the effects of high versus poorer quality childcare, a highly emotive subject that we discuss in depth in Chapter 5. Gunnar (1992) emphasizes that, in young children, HPA axis reactivity is not simply correlated with amount of crying or distress shown. Instead, it appears to be an adaptive function of the degree to which a child is attempting to cope with the stressful situation as well as deal with the expression of their own emotional responses to it. In other words, cortisol can be seen as a barometer of the internal coping process which children are learning to operationalize, and as such a greater cortisol response may not be harmful in itself, but could provide a measure of adaptability to the situation.

The biological circadian (24-hour) rhythmicity in cortisol production enables automatic preparation for the demands associated with daily living. In fact, cortisol is not only crucial in the stress response but essential for life, as well as being a crucial hormone for development (see Box 2.4 which describes the functions of cortisol).

BOX 2.4

Essential functions of cortisol

Development of brain, adrenal medulla, intestine and lung
Glucose production
Vascular responsiveness (blood pressure regulation)
Modulation of immune function, e.g., down-regulation of inflammatory responses

The increase in cortisol prior to awakening and the dramatic increase over the first 30 minutes after awakening constitute an automatic preparedness for the stressors of the daytime hours. Known as the cortisol awakening response (CAR), this natural increase is also subject to alteration depending on the prior stress levels of the previous day(s) and anticipation of impending events. As a point of semantics, this response was originally referred to in the literature as the 'awakening cortisol response' (ACR) but the recognized term is now the 'cortisol awakening response' (CAR). Under stressful conditions (e.g., when stress persists over time, is repeated or severe), if necessary psychosocial resources are not available when needed, or if there is alteration in night and day activity levels, then alterations occur in the levels of hormones produced at various stages of the hormonal cascade of the HPA axis and the system becomes disrupted. This relates to the concept of allostasis and allostatic load which are discussed below, the HPA axis being an allostatic system. Changes in cortisol, the end product of the HPA axis, are important as cortisol levels also have influence over the immune system, having a predominantly suppressing effect on the immune response, thus providing a major pathway for mind–body influence.

The over-production of cortisol in childhood (e.g., as a response to stress or infection) can lead to growth retardation, whilst insufficient cortisol can result in autoimmune disease due to immune overactivity; for example, type 1 diabetes. Examples of extreme cases of over- and under-production of cortisol in physical illness are seen in two specific types of condition: abnormally high levels of cortisol, termed *hyper*cortisolaemia, are seen in Cushing's disease, due to overactivity of the pituitary gland; abnormally low levels of cortisol, termed *hypo*cortisolaemia, are seen in Addison's disease, due to insufficient production from the adrenal glands (for more detail, see Widmaier et al., 2010). These conditions are highlighted here not as examples of stress-related conditions but as conditions which demonstrate two polar extremes of the effects of over- or under-production of cortisol, and hence the importance of this hormone in maintaining physiological health.

HOW CAN THE IMMUNE SYSTEM BE INFLUENCED BY HPA AXIS REGULATION?

Figure 2.11 gives a diagrammatic representation of the major components of the immune system and the connections between them (Sarafino and Smith, 2012). Two types of white blood cells (known collectively as leukocytes) are produced from the bone marrow: (i) lymphocytes (forming two distinct groups of T cells and B cells); and (ii) phagocytes (cells which attempt to engulf bodily invaders [antigens] and also play a key role in presenting antigens to the lymphocytes for further defence). B cells are capable of defence via the production of antibodies (immunoglobulins), and T cells, produced by the thymus gland, differentiate into different subcategories of cells, each with their own armoury (for a fuller description, see Sarafino and Smith, 2012). An important aspect in immune defence is the distinction between non-specific immunity, the generalized attack on antigens which the phagocytes are capable of, and specific immunity, which enables a more targeted attack on antigens via cell-mediated and antibody-mediated (humoral) immunity, based on their specificity.

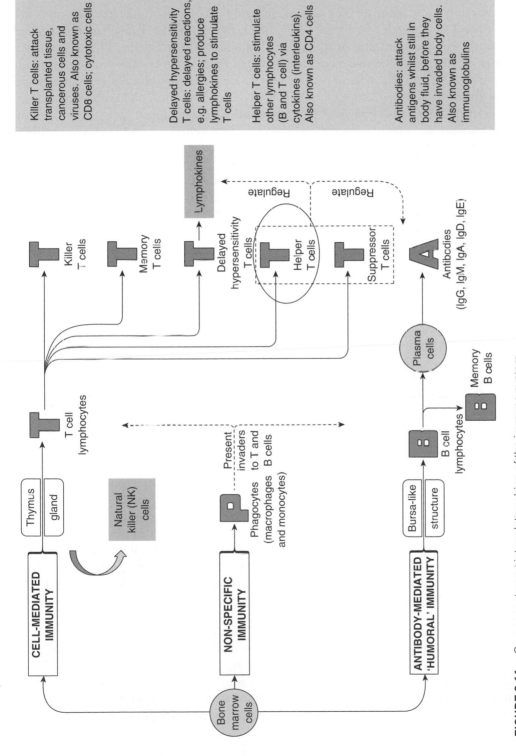

FIGURE 2.11 Components and interrelationships of the immune system

Source: Adapted from Sarafino and Smith (2012: 388).

Central to maintaining an immune defence and the balance of the immune system are the helper T cells (circled in Figure 2.11), one subgroup of the T-cell lymphocytes and part of the cell-mediated arm of the specific immunity. These T-helper (Th) cells form a number of subgroups: the two main ones that are of interest in considering stress and illness are the Th1 and Th2 subgroups. Th1 activity is associated with cellular immunity and Th2 with antibody-mediated (humoral) immunity. Both Th1 and Th2 have a characteristic profile of cytokines (also known as interleukins, IL), immune messengers which communicate between the immune system and the endocrine system. A Th1 cytokine profile is associated with the production of a range of interleukins including IL-2, gamma interferon (IFN-y), tumour necrosis factor (TNF) and IL-12, whilst a Th2 cytokine profile is associated with the production of interleukins, including IL-4, IL-5, IL-6, IL-10 and IL-13 (Evans et al., 2000). During the night time, a natural increase towards Th1 activity occurs, and during the day an increase in Th2 activity. Maintaining a balance between these two parts of the T-helper response is essential for health, within the natural fluctuations which occur between night time and day time. Chronic stress and a range of other psychosocial factors tend to shift the balance towards a Th2 response; acute stress shifts the balance towards Th1 activity. If the balance shifts too far and polarizes towards Th1 or Th2 activity, then over-activity in one arm of the immune balance or under-activity in the other can result in the onset or exacerbation of immune-related conditions. The examples given in Figure 2.12 are type 1 diabetes (over-activity of Th1 immune response) and asthma (over-activity of Th2 immune response). For a more detailed and fascinating description of Th1/Th2 immunity and its implications, see Evans et al. (2000).

As Figure 2.12 illustrates, in early childhood, there is a bias towards Th2-dominated immunity, which drives the antibody-mediated arm of the immune system. This is due to the absence of the hormone dehydroepiandrosterone (DHEA) prior to the maturational process of adrenarche, the maturation of the adrenal glands, which has an onset of approximately the age of 5 years and continues into puberty when DHEA stimulates sexual maturity (Evans et al., 2000). Evans et al. (2000) speculate that, from an evolutionary perspective, this represents an adaptive mechanism whereby children were most protected against the types of organisms that were of greatest threat to them and that they needed a greater Th2 polarization to survive these pathogens. Furthermore, they point out that fever, which is an essential part of Th1 immunity, is particularly harmful to young children due to the under-developed hypothalamic thermoregulation. This imbalance also leaves pre-adrenarche young children (under about 5 years) prey to pathogens against which Th1 immunity defends. Evans et al. (2000) illustrate the counter-regulatory effects of the Th1/Th2 balance with evidence that children who develop type 1 diabetes are less likely to develop asthma.

In terms of the cortisol awakening response (CAR), there is insufficient evidence to state conclusively when the CAR seen in adults appears in children. The handful of studies that have been conducted tend to be across a wide age range, often encompassing early childhood (pre-adrenarche) through to adolescence (see Pruessner et al., 1997; Rosmalen et al., 2005). Whilst there is evidence of the CAR in children, this effect is usually driven by the older children in the cohort, and without dedicated assessment of each age group, particularly of the

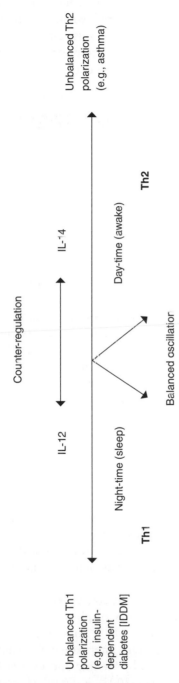

FIGURE 2.12   Th1/Th2 immune system balance and associated factors

Source: Adapted from Evans et al. (2000).

ages surrounding adrenarche, it is not possible to determine when the CAR develops (Jessop and Turner-Cobb, 2008). Some researchers would vehemently contest that the CAR does not fully emerge in children until after adrenarche has occurred, when DHEA enables the CAR to be triggered into action. The jury is still currently out on this issue, given the lack of data sufficient available on which to base firm conclusions and interpretations. I will return to the CAR debate in Chapter 3 when we consider cortisol assessment in children.

PSYCHOBIOLOGICAL THEORIES OF STRESS AND COPING

Prior to the conceptualization of stress as a transaction between a person and their environment, a much more physiological view of stress existed. Following on from William James's theory of emotion as far back as 1884 (James, 1884), which argued that emotions followed behaviour, the now well-known fight-or-flight theory of the stress response, recognizing the role of the hormones adrenaline and noradrenaline, was put forward by Walter Cannon (1929). Selye's general adaptation syndrome (GAS; Selye, 1956, 1976b) moved this work further towards what we recognize today in stress research, emphasizing adaptability to stressful events. Selye outlined three stages of the stress response: first, 'alarm'; followed by 'resistance', in which the body copes physiologically with the event by producing necessary stress hormones, particularly glucocorticoids; and, if the stress continues, then finally 'exhaustion' as the stress hormones become depleted. It was the inclusion of a third stage that caused subsequent stress researchers to think again.

A pioneering researcher who has advanced much of the thinking in this area is biologist and neurologist Robert Sapolsky of Stanford University. Based on discoveries in stress hormone research, Sapolsky (1994) has effectively reconceptualized this last part of Selye's theory by critically pointing out that, rather than vulnerability to illness being caused by the stress hormones running out, it is the damage that ensues when they continue to be produced at a high rate over a prolonged period of time that is the problem. As Sapolsky (1994: 13) puts it, 'the stress response itself can become damaging.' In other words, despite the news headlines and comments from medical doctors who should perhaps know better, it is the *response* to stress that can make you ill, rather than the stress itself. This is important as it puts the focus on the mechanism(s) behind the mind–body link, demystifying connections between stress and illness. On this basis, it is impossible for physical illness to be 'all in the mind' since psychological factors cannot be contained and result in triggering physical responses.

Current thinking in stress research has at its centre the concept of 'allostasis' and 'allostatic load'. The theory of *allostasis* is a biological theory of physiological regulation which extends homeostasis. Homeostasis is the process by which physiological systems are kept within a narrow range in order to maintain a constant internal environment; for example, blood oxygen, body temperature. Allostasis, coined by Sterling and Eyer (1988) and developed by McEwen (1998a, b; McEwen and Wingfield, 2003), is described as 'stability through

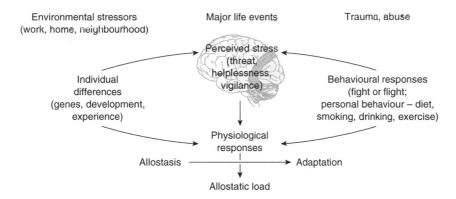

The perception of stress is influenced by one's experiences, genetics, and behaviour. When the brain perceives an experience as stressful, physiological and behavioural responses are initiated, leading to allostasis and adaptation. Over time, allostatic load can accumulate, and the over-exposure to mediators of neural, endocrine, and immune stress can have adverse effects on various organ systems, leading to disease.

FIGURE 2.13   The stress response and development of allostatic load
Source: McEwen (1998a: 172, fig. 1).

change' (Sterling and Eyer, 1988), and views the body's physiological systems as adaptive, enabling a person's responses to different physical states, to cope with noise, overcrowding, extremes of temperature, and physiological alterations necessitated by infection. Allostatic systems, which include those involved in the stress response, promote change and enable adaptation. This concept of adaptability fits well with the transactional theory of stress and coping, particularly when the associated concept of allostatic load is incorporated. *Allostatic load* represents the imbalance in allostatic systems, or accumulated lifetime stress (McEwen, 1998a). Figure 2.13 demonstrates how the stress response can generate allostatic load.

McEwen (1998a) presents three types of allostatic load which result from four conditions (Figure 2.14). The first type is where the physiological systems become overworked and the response continues as an acute reaction either as a result of multiple stressors or because the systems fail to adapt or, in psychological terms, to habituate to the stressor. The second type represents a failure of the physiological systems to shut off, thus continuing the high physiological output as in chronic stress conditions. The final type described is where physiological systems fail to respond to an initial challenge, a pattern sometimes seen in response to some severe prolonged stress following trauma.

Each type of allostatic load carries with it the history of the individual's stress experiences and responses, which can be thought of much like a fossil record, reflecting an individual's life experiences. The last type of allostatic load is perhaps the most fascinating in this respect as it is a relatively severe reaction and may follow as a consequence of other allostatic load patterns. In adults, this inadequate response pattern has been seen in people with post-traumatic stress disorder (PTSD), particularly those who have a history of sexual

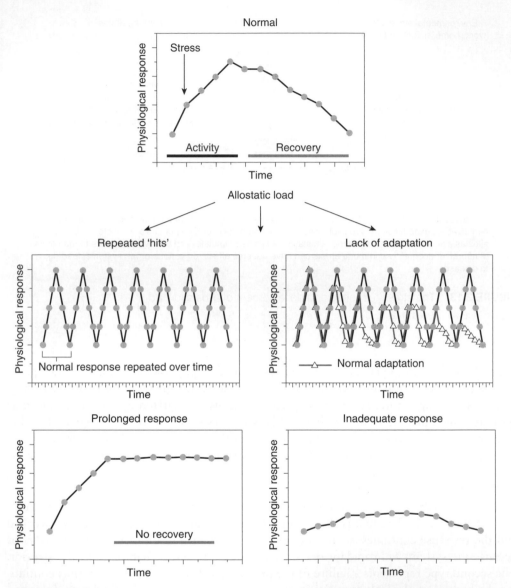

The top panel illustrates the normal allostatic response, in which a response is initiated by a stressor, sustained for an appropriate interval, and then turned off. The remaining panels illustrate four conditions that lead to allostatic load: repeated 'hits' from multiple stressors; lack of adaptation; prolonged response due to delayed shutdown; and inadequate response that leads to compensatory hyperactivity of other mediators (e.g., inadequate secretion of glucocorticoids, resulting in increased concentrations of cytokines that are normally counter-regulated by glucocorticoids).

FIGURE 2.14   Three types of allostatic load

Source: McEwen (1998a: 174, fig. 3).

trauma (Yehuda et al., 1995; Meewisse et al., 2007). In children, the pattern observed is slightly different. For example, in children with PTSD linked to sexual trauma, the associated allostatic pattern reflects the chronic stress pattern seen in the second type of allostatic load (Carrion et al., 2002). This implies a time trajectory in physiological responding to stress, borne out in allostatic load, in which an initial high level of cortisol following acute and chronic stress over time progresses to a hypocortisolaemic state. However, longitudinal research of this nature is virtually impossible to conduct directly. What is known is often inferred across several populations and generations but contributes to the overall picture of psychobiological stress responses. One of the earliest, and often overlooked, cross-sectional studies demonstrating allostatic load in children reported the chronic stressor of greater household density (measured by the number of people living per square foot of household space) as a predictor of poor health (Johnston-Brookes et al., 1998). In this study cardiovascular reactivity served as the allostatic load measure and was found to mediate the effect of household density on health outcome in boys aged 9–12 years. More recent studies, which will be covered in detail in Chapter 5, have examined the health effects of compound stressors, involving both acute and chronic stress in children (Marin et al., 2009) or cumulative stressors across childhood (Dube et al., 2009), both in line with the allostatic model of stress and health.

The concept of adaptation has also been referred to by physiologists as 'acclimatization', a process whereby the function of the homeostatic system becomes extended due to repeated or more extreme exposure – for example, to heat – and is reversible once the more normal range of exposure is restored (see Widmaier et al., 2010). However, if acclimatization occurs during childhood, at a critical phase of biological development (e.g., for nervous, endocrine or immune processes), then this may reset the system to varying degrees of permanency and is known as developmental acclimatization (Widmaier et al., 2010). The concept of allostasis advances these adaptation terms to incorporate exposure to psychosocial stress. In conjunction with the concept of allostatic load, the theory of allostasis enables greater understanding and potential for intervention in stress research with children.

RESILIENCY FACTORS AND INDIVIDUAL DIFFERENCES

Whilst cognitive and social ability may restrict the stress appraisal process in children and adolescents, individual differences in temperament and coping responses emerge across children of similar ages. Some of the greatest resources of resilience have also been seen in children. Since the 1970s, researchers have been interested in the qualities and characteristics of children who, despite adversity, demonstrate positive adaptation and thrive. Resilience has been defined as 'a dynamic developmental process encompassing the attainment of positive adaptation within the context of significant adversity' (see Cicchetti, 2010: 145). The development of resilience has been viewed as resulting from three domains: (i) personal qualities of the children, such as autonomy and high self-esteem; (ii) attributes of their family; and

(iii) characteristics of the broader social environment in which they live (Luthar et al., 2000; for a full review of this area and the mechanisms involved, including neurobiological and genetic correlates of resilience, see Cicchetti, 2010). Resiliency factors come up many times throughout this book: for example, when looking at stress during childhood (Chapter 5), and in Part II when we consider the experience of specific stressors such as parental bereavement and the experience of hospitalization and of pain in children.

CHAPTER SUMMARY

In this chapter, I have covered definitions, models and theories of stress and coping set within a health-related context. These are essential foundations for understanding the topics discussed throughout the rest of this book. Whilst much of the work presented here has focused on the adult literature, these ideas have been applied to child health, and differences and similarities have been highlighted. It should be obvious from the evidence cited that these theories and models not only enable observation of stress effects and coping ability, but also offer a challenge to develop interventions to reduce stress and improve health in children and consequently across the lifespan. A mix of research methods has been presented, within a biopsychosocial framework, to examine the underlying foundations of the link between psychosocial factors and health in children. It is to a more in-depth consideration of psychobiological research methods in child health that I turn in Chapter 3.

KEY CONCEPTS AND ISSUES

- Stress and coping
- Children's understanding of stress and illness
- The stress response system: SAM and HPA axis
- Classifications of stress
- Th1/Th2 immune balance
- Allostasis and allostatic load

FURTHER READING

Lazarus and colleagues' original transactional model of stress:

Lazarus, R.S. and Folkman, S. (1984) *Stress, Appraisal and Coping*. New York: Springer-Verlag.

The original children's concepts of illness article:

Bibace, R. and Walsh, M.E. (1980) Development of children's concepts of illness. *Pediatrics*, 66(6): 912–17.

Highly recommended, absolutely essential in understanding allostatic load:

McEwen, B.S. (1998) Protective and damaging effects of stress mediators. *New England Journal of Medicine*, 338(3): 171–9.

For a more detailed explanation of neuro-endocrine and immune processes, see:

Evans, P., Hucklebridge, F. and Clow, A. (2000) *Mind, Immunity and Health*. London: Free Association Books.

For more in-depth coverage of physiology, see *Vander's Physiology*:

Widmaier, E.P., Raff, H. and Strang, K.T. (2010) *Vander's Human Physiology: The Mechanisms of Body: Function*, 12th edn. New York: McGraw-Hill Higher Education.

For the best page-turner you will ever find in a biological text:

Sapolsky, R. (1998) *Why Zebras Don't Get Ulcers: An Updated Guide to Stress, Stress-related Diseases and Coping*. New York: W.H. Freeman.

USEFUL WEBSITE

National Scientific Council on the Developing Child (US): http://developingchild.harvard.edu/initiatives/council

RESEARCH METHODS AND ETHICAL ISSUES

3

Covered in this chapter

- Measurement of psychosocial factors
- Mixed methods
- Psychobiological research methods
- Immune markers of stress
- Neurotransmitter and endocrine markers of stress
- Measuring health outcome in children
- The laboratory/experimental research setting
- Naturalistic settings and field research
- Ethical issues and communication in health research with children

This chapter will outline psychobiological research methods and assessment tools relevant to child health psychology. The emphasis is on quantitative assessment, but the use of qualitative and mixed methods research techniques is also outlined. Attention is paid to practical issues, such as communication and compliance, in applying health psychology to child research. The importance of ethical considerations is also covered as a special issue within this area of work.

The concept of the biopsychosocial model was described in Chapter 1, and more recent encapsulations of this model were expanded upon in Chapter 2. In considering research methods and ethical issues in the context of the biopsychosocial model, it is necessary to be specific about exactly what is being measured and to use the most effective and appropriate tool to do this, within an optimal context for assessment. Stress can be measured by sampling either the basal levels of stress (baseline, underlying non-stimulated

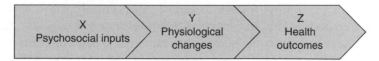

FIGURE 3.1   X-Y-Z model underlying the biopsychosocial concept

Source: Based on Elliott and Eisdorfer (1982).

levels), the magnitude of the stress response to a specific stressor (in the laboratory or natural environment), and the speed of adaptation to that stressor (the speed at which baseline levels are restored or fail to be restored). These are always challenges in research, and conducting research with children brings with it additional developmental challenges which affect understanding and experience as outlined in Chapters 1 and 2. Figure 3.1 represents the biopsychosocial approach at its simplest level, with three components ('X' representing psychosocial inputs, 'Y' physiological changes and 'Z' health outcomes). This basic X-Y-Z model is based on ideas put forward by Elliott and Eisdorfer (1982) who argued for the necessity of simultaneous investigation of all three concepts. The models of Cohen and Herbert (1996) and Lutgendorf and Costanzo (2003), described in Chapter 2, are also examples of X-Y-Z explanatory models of the biopsychosocial construct, albeit much more complex ones.

The theoretical rationale for this argument of simultaneous investigation of all three constructs is very sound, and such studies could be described as the 'gold standard' in biopsychosocial research. Yet, in reality, it is not always feasible or practical to implement simultaneous measurement for a variety of reasons, not least because of continued availability and willingness of participants or for financial reasons. For example, whilst an array of immune markers may be desirable, cost implications may determine that only psychosocial processes and health outcomes (X-Z) relationships are possible in a particular study. Similarly, the financial cost of conducting longitudinal research with children which allows for assessment of early life experience and impact on health in adulthood may be prohibitive, and, instead, studies of X-Y relationships with separate retrospective studies of Z-X are necessitated. In keeping with this broad X-Y-Z model, different components and their measurability in research with children and adolescents are considered below.

MEASUREMENT OF PSYCHOSOCIAL FACTORS

The measurement of psychosocial factors (X) includes the assessment of stress, coping responses, availability of resources such as social support, individual differences such as temperament, and demographic differences such as family socioeconomic status. In younger children, assessment of many of these variables cannot be conducted directly since age and maturity levels may require indirect assessment via a parent or caregiver to overcome pre-verbal or literacy constraints. The very status of being a child places the family, whether typical or atypical, and those in positions of supervision and authority over the child, as well as the child's peer or friendship groups, at the centre of their social world. It is essential, therefore, for assessment of psychosocial factors, such as stress or social support, to recognize this. In Chapter 2, I outlined types of stressor relevant to children, as well as some specific stress questionnaires, as just a handful of measures that are available. Questionnaire assessment needs to be age specific, in line with the developmental stage, reading age and relevant experience of the participants. Interview assessment may be more appropriate than questionnaire and there are various interview schedules available (e.g., the Children's Inventory of Social Support [CISS]: Wolchik et al., 1989). The field of developmental psychology has an impressive array of sophisticated experimental designs for use with young children, including those in the pre-verbal age groups, particularly in the area of attachment and temperament. Observational methods are also key in the assessment of stress and coping in children or indirect reporting of observations via parents or teachers (for examples of these, see Parke and Gauvain, 2009).

A further dimension in assessing stress involves the selection of groups of participants known to have experienced a specific stressor. At one end of the scale, this could be a minor life stress or eustress experience, as seen in children undergoing an expected life transition such as starting school (Turner-Cobb et al., 2008) or moving from junior to senior or high school. At the other end of the scale, this could feature a severe, potentially traumatic or toxic stressor such as childhood abuse, as exemplified by studies of children raised in Romanian orphanages (Gunnar et al., 2001). Chapter 5 looks specifically at different stressors experienced during childhood. In older children and adolescents, despite greater reading and verbal ability, the age appropriateness equally applies, with careful selection of questionnaires and interview style being key to accurate assessment and reliable data collection. For a review of research methods, including those specific to adolescence, see Tinson (2009).

Tables 3.1–3.3 list some examples of standardized questionnaires relevant to child and adolescent populations for the assessment of psychosocial factors of stress, coping and social support. This list is by no means exhaustive but gives a range of questionnaires in common usage, and a large range of other scales assessing domains such as emotion and behaviour in children is available (see Sclare, 1997). These tables reflect the greater availability of social support measures in children compared to those of stress and coping, although not in comparison with the availability of adult scales. The target age groups listed also highlight the difficulty of using the questionnaire form of assessment with younger children.

Despite the availability of such questionnaires, a common criticism of assessment in children is the lack of understanding of the child's perspective, with research taking an adult-centric view rather than attempting to perceive the psychosocial environment through child-centric eyes. Questionnaire-based methods may not by nature be very child-centric. This view is highlighted by Samuelsson and colleagues (1996) in their work to develop a map of social network support from the perspective of the child him/herself. They point out that, compared to measures available for the measurement of social support in adults, there is a lack of appropriate social support measures specifically designed for children. They specify three general requirements of a good measure in children: it must be (i) 'easy to understand'; (ii) 'not too time consuming'; and (iii) 'still useful in

TABLE 3.1 Stress: examples of standardized stress questionnaires used with children and adolescents

Target age group	Questionnaire	Description and example items
4–16 years	Life Events Scale (adapted for children by Coddington, 1972)	Occurrence of life events and an impact rating 30 items (0–3 scale) *'Your father or mother lost their job'* *'You were suspended from school'*
4–16 years	Children's Hassles Scale (Kanner et al., 1987)	Occurrence of events and rating impact by expressive faces 40 items (0–2 scale) *'You had to tidy your room'* *'You did something wrong at school'*
Adult populations, including students; applied in adolescents 14–18 years	Perceived Stress Scale (PSS; Cohen et al., 1983)	Overall measure of stress experience, not specific to life events or hassle stress *'In the last month, how often have you felt nervous and stressed?'*

TABLE 3.2 Coping: examples of standardized coping questionnaires used with children and adolescents

Target age group	Questionnaire	Description and example items
5 16 years	Kidcope (Spirito et al., 1988)	Younger children: 15 questions; older children: 10 questions (1–5 scale) Participants list problems they have experienced, then describe how they coped with them *'Did you blame someone else for causing the problem?'* *'I turned to my family, other adults or friends to help me feel better'*
12–19 years	Family Crisis Oriented Personal Evaluation Scale (F-COPES; McCubbin et al., 1985)	Includes subscales of reframing, passive appraisal, and social support 30 items (1–5 scale) *'When we face problems or difficulties in our family we respond by …* *… sharing our difficulties with relatives'* *… attending religious services'*
14–19 years	Coping Across Situations Questionnaire (CASQ; Seiffge-Krenke, 1995)	20 coping strategies assessed across eight hypothetical situations (0–9 scale) Participants asked which strategies they use in each situation *'I discuss the problem with my parents'* *'I try not to think about the problem'*

TABLE 3.3 Social support: examples of standardized social support questionnaires used with children and adolescents

Target age group	Questionnaire	Description and example items
8–10 years	Survey of Children's Social Support (SCSS; Dubow and Ullman, 1989); can be used in conjunction with the Appraised Support (APP)	SCSS: three questions assessing size of social network APP: 31 items; perceived emotional support and acceptance from various sources *'Who helps you when you need to talk about your feelings?'*
11–16 years	Wills Parental Support Scale (WPSS; Wills et al., 1992)	Emotional and instrumental support, parent–child conflict; 15 items *'When I feel bad about something, my parent will listen'* *'If I need help with my school work I can ask my parent about it'*
6–12 years	My Family and Friends Measure (Reid et al., 1989)	Emotional, instrumental and informational support, companionship; 11 items *'When you want to share your feelings ... '* ... followed by questions regarding the availability of social network members and satisfaction of this support'
12–16 years	Barrera Social Support Scale (BSSS; Barrera et al., 1993)	7 items (scale from 'little or none' to 'most possible'): alliance, worth, companionship, intimacy, guidance, affection Rates the support given by father, mother, sibling, friend
12–18 years	Newcomb Loneliness and Support Inventory (NLSI; Newcomb and Bentler, 1986)	Support, respect, inclusion (by parents, family members, other adults and peers) 16 items (1–4 scale)
14–19 years	Multidimensional Scale of Perceived Social Support (MSPSS; Zimet et al., 1988)	Perceived social support from family, friends, and a special person 12 items (0–5 scale)

research'. Building on earlier work using social mapping in adults (Antonucci, 1985; Tracy and Whittaker, 1990; Tracy and Abell, 1994) and clinical work with children and families (e.g., Gehring and Wyler, 1986), they developed the Five Field Map. This comprised a series of six concentric circles, with the child in the centre and social contacts mapped in circles radiating outwards. It is termed the 'Five Field Map' because it features five 'sectors' or social domains of family, relatives, formal contacts, school, and friends/neighbours. Social closeness of the individuals included in the network map is represented by their proximity to the central circle, from the perspective of the child. In this map, the outer ring represents 'negative contacts', meaning those that the child 'felt he/she was on

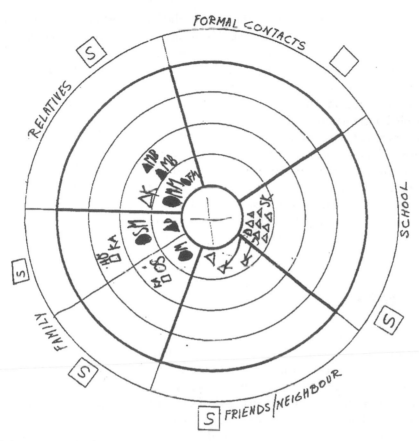

'Case 1: Robert, 9 years old. This map was drawn by a boy from the single-parent family control group. The mother has a good relationship with her ex-husband. There was a calm atmosphere in the home and the mother had great patience with her children. Robert placed both parents in the inner circle. The stepmother is also placed near himself. The relative, school, and friends/neighbours sectors all have many people placed close to the centre. Robert was satisfied with his network.'

Key: ▲, man; •, woman; △, boy; ○, girl; —/— = conflictual relationship; —//— = broken relationship; S, child's satisfaction with the sector (D, child's dissatisfaction).

FIGURE 3.2   Example of the Five Field Map

Source: Samuelsson et al. (1996: 335).

bad terms with', giving indication of negative support. An example of the Five Field Map is shown in Figure 3.2.

Visualization of social support in this way has generated good reliability and validity in children aged as young as 6–7 years and up to 16 years. It has been used in comparison studies differentiating between normal children living in single-parent families and those referred to a psychiatric clinic (Samuelsson et al., 1996). A range of scores can be calculated from such a map, including: positive support based on total and sector scores (calculating number of contacts and proximity to the child in the innermost circle); and negative support variables, such as negative contacts, dissatisfaction and conflicts (Samuelsson et al., 1996). A similar 'four field' map was used in a larger British sample of 258 children aged 4–7 years (omitting the infrequently used 'formal contacts' sector; Sturgess, 2001). This group formed a subsample of the Avon Longitudinal Study of Parents and Children (ALSPAC), a cohort study of children born between April 1991 and December 1992. This study enabled accurate and detailed inspection not only of networks but also the quality of relationships between children and parents/step-parents, siblings and friends. Studies using these social mapping techniques in children report the ease with which the child can understand the concept of support using this visual metaphor and that completing the map was intuitive and straightforward for them. There is enormous potential for developing these mapping techniques for use with children, particularly in relation to physical health outcome (Z), but as yet very few studies have used these techniques to look at these X-Z relationships or considered physiological assessments (Y) in relation to these mapping techniques.

MIXED METHODS

Being able to quantify relationships between psychological factors and health is important in predicting associations between variables and in developing interventions. The examples and references in this book draw largely from quantitative methodologies, making use of questionnaire assessment of psychological factors, of physiological assessment of endocrine and immune status, and of quantifiable measures of health outcome. Quantitative methods in the form of experimental laboratory methods, as well as field research, are also described in detail later in this chapter. A different type of methodology, which is also an extremely useful tool in health psychology research, particularly with children, is that of qualitative analysis. Qualitative methods involve words rather than numbers to make an assessment and evaluate experience, responses and behaviour. They are subjective in nature, rather than the more objective quantitative assessments. Qualitative methods involve a range of different types of analysis of individual interview and group discussion.

The point of view taken by my qualitative colleagues is that sometimes you simply need to ask the participant about their experience or what they think. There is often a visible readiness for a roll-up-your-shirt-sleeves brawl (metaphorically speaking) once quantitative and qualitative researchers get to comparing methodologies and the validity of their work. I wish to avoid this argument, not just for the sake of self-preservation but because, despite voicing a preference towards quantitative assessment, there is, of course, value and merit in both types of methodologies. The most important guide to choosing an appropriate methodology is the research question or hypothesis, with the aim of achieving the greatest concordance between the two. The best methodology to use is the one or ones that are the most appropriate to explore the research question most fully and to enable the fullest examination of the factors being investigated. In many cases, this may mean choosing between quantitative and qualitative assessment for a particular study, but in

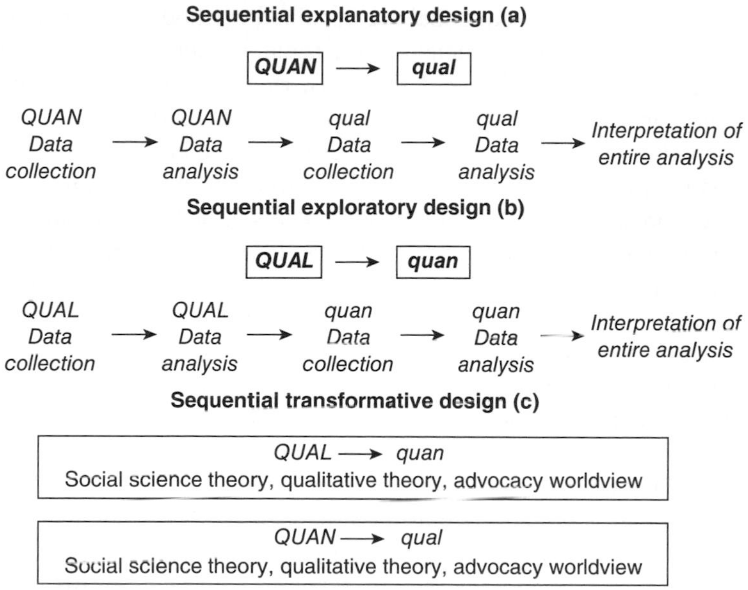

Sequential explanatory design (a)

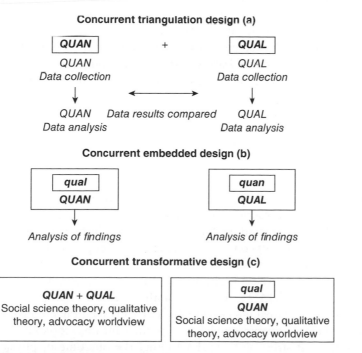

QUAN → qual

QUAN Data collection → QUAN Data analysis → qual Data collection → qual Data analysis → Interpretation of entire analysis

Sequential exploratory design (b)

QUAL → quan

QUAL Data collection → QUAL Data analysis → quan Data collection → quan Data analysis → Interpretation of entire analysis

Sequential transformative design (c)

QUAL → quan
Social science theory, qualitative theory, advocacy worldview

QUAN → qual
Social science theory, qualitative theory, advocacy worldview

FIGURE 3.3 Mixed methods: sequential designs

Source: Creswell (2009: 209).

Concurrent triangulation design (a)

QUAN   +   QUAL

QUAN Data collection   QUAL Data collection

QUAN Data analysis   Data results compared   QUAL Data analysis

Concurrent embedded design (b)

qual
QUAN

quan
QUAL

Analysis of findings   Analysis of findings

Concurrent transformative design (c)

QUAN + QUAL
Social science theory, qualitative theory, advocacy worldview

qual
QUAN
Social science theory, qualitative theory, advocacy worldview

FIGURE 3.4 Mixed methods: concurrent designs

Source: Creswell (2009: 210).

some cases the simultaneous or sequential use of mixed methodologies may result in a far better understanding and the advancement of the topic. For an in-depth description of the many combinations and uses of mixed methods, there are numerous texts available, although I would particularly recommend that by Creswell (2009).

Qualitative methodologies can be useful in research with children and adolescents for obvious reasons relating to verbal/literacy skills in younger children and to the need for emotional expression and peer discussion in adolescents. Combining quantitative methods and qualitative methods in the same study enables the researcher to gain a fuller understanding of the issue, and using questionnaire, interview, and physiological assessment enables a triangulation of ideas. Creswell (2009) describes six main types of mixed methods design, based on four features of data collection: (i) timing (one after the other, i.e., sequential, or both at the same time, i.e. concurrent); (ii) weighting (whether priority is given to one type of data collection or if both are equal in priority); (iii) mixing (whether fully integrated, separate but connected, or if one is embedded within the other); and (iv) the role that theorizing takes within the mixed methods study. This is not as complicated as it sounds (although that is not to say that the practicalities of conducting mixed methods research are by any means simple). The design of mixed methods comes down to deciding which type of data collection and analysis will take the major lead in the study, or if both types will contribute equally, and then deciding whether to employ both qualitative and quantitative methods at the same time or one after the other, and the order this needs to take in line with the research questions. The six types of design described by Cresswell (2009) involve three different types of sequential design and three different types of concurrent design. These design types are illustrated in Figures 3.3 and 3.4.

To give an example of a mixed methods design using the X-Y-Z model described above, variable X might represent perceived stress, variable Y the endocrine marker of cortisol sampled from saliva, and variable Z the incidence of acute illness such as headache in a sample of 11-year-olds. To investigate this using a sequential exploratory design, qualitative interviews may initially be conducted to explore the relationship between stress and descriptions of acute illness. Following qualitative analysis, a quantitative phase would follow, using a questionnaire measure of stress and a list of acute symptoms based on the findings of the interviews, thus building on the results of the initial qualitative exploration, in addition to the quantitative measure of cortisol. The final interpretation would use all the analyses, both qualitative and quantitative. Alternatively, a concurrent triangulation design might involve quantitative questionnaire assessment and biological measurement at the same time as qualitative interview. Quantitative and qualitative analysis would be performed separately and results compared. If mention of concurrent triangulation designs have not sent you running for the hills, take a look at a recent study by Sweet (2010) which examined associations between social status and physical health in a sample of African American students of low socioeconomic status, aged 14–18 years. The authors used a multi-phase mixed methods design composed of qualitative interviews which are analysed quantitatively. The findings were then used as a measure against which each participant was scored. In addition to questionnaire assessment of stress and social standing, the outcome of physical health was assessed via blood pressure measurement. This is a good example of the benefits of combining techniques of assessment and methodology, in this case in adolescent research.

PSYCHOBIOLOGICAL RESEARCH METHODS

Research methodologies which include assessment of biological factors (Y) in psychological research can be applied to both the laboratory/experimental and field setting. In order to understand why we might even be thinking about combining biological and psychological assessment and their inter-relationships or the predictive power of one over the other, it is worth taking a momentary meander back to a dominant research paradigm of the 1970s. Just briefly, we need to return to a concept which should be familiar to most psychology undergraduates, that of Pavlovian classical conditioning. Discovered by the Russian physiologist, Ivan Pavlov, in the 1920s, this paradigm is based on the process of associative learning. Traditionally using dogs in the laboratory, the unconditioned stimulus (e.g., food), known to elicit salivation, is paired with the conditioned stimulus (e.g., the sound of a bell). After multiple pairings between the unconditioned and the conditioned stimulus, the conditioned stimulus alone takes on the properties of the unconditioned stimulus as illustrated in Figure 3.5.

Many clinical interventions draw on classical conditioning, and elements of it may be present in the placebo effect. Taking this one (admittedly rather large) step further, the concept of conditioning can be applied to the immune system, aptly termed immune conditioning. This adaptation of the immune paradigm emerged in the 1970s and was pioneered by Robert Ader and his colleagues during study of the taste aversion paradigm in rats (for a fuller explanation, see Exton et al., 1999; Schedlowski and Pacheco-Lopez, 2010). Figure 3.6 gives a typical immune conditioning scenario in which the unconditioned stimulus is cyclophosphamide, an immuno-suppressant drug used in chemotherapy, with associated side-effects of nausea and vomiting. The conditioned stimulus is the saccharin solution (a sugary, non-toxic drink). Following multiple pairings of the drug with the saccharine solution during the training phase, in the test phase the saccharine solution takes on the immuno-suppressive effects of the drug. This effect is particularly strong due to the potency of the unconditioned stimulus (cyclophosphamide) used.

At this point, you would be forgiven for thinking I had side-tracked and ventured off along a seemingly unrelated avenue. On the contrary, immune conditioning not only shows the historical roots of powerful mind–body connections, it also has potential human applications. These are highly relevant, particularly to the clinical context in patients with immune-related conditions, with potential to offer therapeutic benefits. The basic idea is

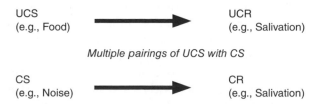

FIGURE 3.5 Basic principles of Pavlovian classical conditioning

Key: UCS, Unconditioned stimulus; UCR, Unconditioned response; CS, Conditioned stimulus; CR, Conditioned response.

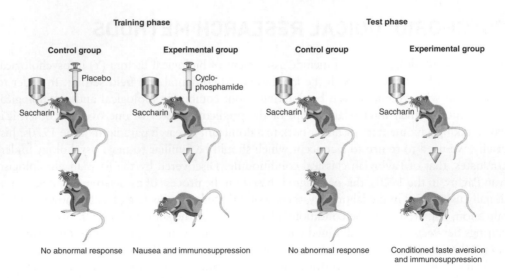

FIGURE 3.6   Immuno-conditioning via the taste aversion paradigm
Source: Schedlowski and Tewes (1999).

that in patients receiving chemotherapy drugs which, in addition to immune suppression, have the unpleasant side-effects of nausea and vomiting, the hospital environment may act as the conditioned stimulus, inducing these unpleasant side-effects as well as the immune suppression, due to association with the chemotherapy. When this happens, the experience of the hospital environment takes on the properties of the chemotherapy medication. Conditioning can occur not just through sound (e.g., noise) but through any of the senses (e.g., sight, taste, smell, touch) or a combination of senses. In terms of the hospital environment, this may be the characteristic smell of the hospital ward, the visual association of uniforms or colour of the décor, or the taste of food most recently eaten just prior to a chemotherapy session. Scientific studies examining this directly are few and far between, not least due to necessary ethical considerations, and results have been ambiguous, with some studies demonstrating immuno-suppression, immuno-enhancement or no effects at all. In a group of paediatric cancer patients (aged 4–18 years), the effects of two consecutive cycles of chemotherapy were examined, measuring symptoms and sampling blood for immune markers, including NK cell activity (known to increase following chemotherapy; Stockhorst et al., 2000; in Exton et al., 2000). One of the findings of this study was the increase in NK cell activity in anticipation of the second cycle of chemotherapy in patients who also experienced anticipatory nausea and/or vomiting prior to drug administration when exposed to the hospital environment. This is interpreted as support for immuno-enhancement since NK cell activity may slow tumour progression. Conditioned immuno-modulation remains both a challenge and a source of much potential (for clinical reviews, see Bovbjerg, 2003, 2006).

Immune conditioning (enhancement and suppression) is at the extreme end of the spectrum when it comes to influences on immune response. Whilst the immune conditioning paradigm is a powerful example of mind–body influences, most studies do not use nausea, vomiting and death as outcome variables when examining the effect of naturalistic influences or laboratory stressors on otherwise healthy participants. Immune conditioning not only shows the power of the mind–body relationship, its relevance is not to be underestimated. Whilst not all psychoneuroimmunology relationships are linked to conditioning, it is worth remembering that elements of the conditioning process may underlie some of the mind–body effects seen in humans. With this in mind, we move on to consider the utility of various biological markers which provide reliable evidence of alterations in endocrine and immune functioning associated with stressful environments and the presence or absence of various psychosocial resources, particularly that of social support.

IMMUNE MARKERS OF STRESS

Assessment of both *enumerative* and *functional* immune responses under stress have been used as immune markers in experimental and field research.

IN VITRO TESTS OF IMMUNITY: NK CELLS, T CELLS AND B CELLS

Enumerative immune markers are those which assess some aspect relating to the *number* of white blood cells. This includes *in vitro* (i.e., outside of the body; see Box 3.1) assessment of total white blood cell count or of lymphocyte subsets (e.g., CD4+, NK cell number) or proportions (CD4/CD8 cell ratios).

BOX 3.1

In vitro/in vivo

In vitro literally means 'in a glass' and 'refers to observations made outside the body'.

In vivo literally means 'within the living' and refers to 'biological events that take place inside the bodies of living organisms'.

(Macpherson, 1999)

Such assessments are made possible by advances in a technique known as flow cytometry, which uses laser beam technology to measure scattered light and the fluorescence of different types of cells. In addition to enumerative assessments of NK cell and cell-mediated immunity, *in vitro* antibody tests enable an enumerative assessment of humoral or antibody-mediated immunity. Assays enable assessment of antibodies against viruses which lay dormant or latent and are normally kept in check by Th1 immune processes. Since chronic stress can down-regulate cellular immune function, latent viruses again become active and stimulate an antibody-mediated immune response. A common example is that of the chickenpox virus or *Varicella zoster* virus (VZV). Once a child has been infected with this virus and experienced the symptoms of chickenpox, VZV then lays dormant and can reoccur in adulthood as the *Herpes zoster* virus or 'shingles'. Similarly, the *Herpes simplex* virus (HSV-1 associated with mouth sores or 'cold sores'; HSV-2 with genital sores) has an active phase when initially contracted, then becomes latent (inactive prior to symptoms) and can be reactivated following periods of stress. Other examples include the Epstein–Barr virus (EBV), contracted by the majority of Western populations at some point in their lives, often as children, with mild or unnoticeable symptoms. If first infected during adolescence or in early adulthood, symptoms of infectious mononucleosis occur (US 'mono'; UK 'glandular fever': often referred to as the 'kissing disease' due to its methods of transmission via saliva). The amount of antibody to these common viruses can be assessed in association with stress and psychosocial resources to obtain a measure of antibody-mediated/Th2 activity and down-regulation of cell-mediated immunity (for more detail, see Evans et al., 2000). Furthermore, cytokine analysis makes use of various enumerative techniques to assess numbers and proportions of a range of interleukins, in particular IL-2 and IL-6.

The role of cytokines to influence the Th1/Th2 balance, and consequently the number and function of T, B, and NK cells, makes them one of the most fascinating and potentially useful markers in stress research. Assessment of *functional* immune response measures the capacity of the cell to function effectively or to respond to an antigen (see Box 3.2). This can also be measured *in vitro* and includes assay assessment of T cell and NK cell cytotoxicity ('killing power'), lymphocyte proliferation (ability of lymphocytes to multiply) and cytokine release from white blood cells in response to an *in vitro* antigen challenge.

BOX 3.2

Enumerative/functional immune assessment

Enumerative immune assessment measures aspects relating to *number*; e.g., white blood cell count.

Functional immune assessment measures the capacity of the cell to function effectively or to respond to an antigen.

These *in vitro* immune assessments have frequently been used in psychoneuroimmune research, each with their own advantages and limitations (see Vedhara and Wang, in Vedhara and Irwin, 2005). Assessment of NK cell number and function has probably been used the most widely in research linking stress and health, due to the crucial role of NK cells in defending against malignant tumours and viral attack. The assessment of cytokines in psychosocial research has led to some enormous advances in the understanding of immune processes under stress and is still very much regarded as state of the art in psychoneuroimmunology.

So far, I have considered the assessment of immune markers which require the sampling of blood. This can be problematic, both ethically and practically, in the assessment of children. Box 3.3 addresses this issue and lists some immune markers available through saliva as an alternative fluid of assessment.

BOX 3.3

Blood versus saliva as a fluid of immune measurement *in vitro*

It is perfectly reasonable to be asking whether or not saliva could be used as an alternative bodily fluid for reliable immune assessment. Unless blood samples are already being taken as part of routine medical tests, the necessity of blood sampling can be intrusive and burdensome in children. Whilst the reliability for measurement of immune markers in general is not as robust when sampled from saliva compared to blood, the range of *in vitro* markers measurable from saliva is increasing rapidly, as new assay techniques are developed and reliability established. With these caveats in mind, the following are some of the salivary assays currently available for immune markers:

Th1 activity: for example, TNF alpha, neopterin, cytokines IL-1 and IL-6.

Th2 activity: for example, salivary IgA (SIgA).

IN VIVO TESTS OF IMMUNITY: T CELLS AND B CELLS

Another classification of immune assessment are the *in vivo* (literally meaning 'within the living') tests of immune function. These are relatively few and far between in human psychosocial research, for obvious ethical reasons. However, where they are possible, they provide an excellent measure of immune functioning. They reflect a more accurate picture of what is occurring in the body during an immune reaction, as opposed to one step removed as seen in the *in vitro* petri dish or assay.

The first of these is the *delayed-type hypersensitivity* (DTH) test, a functional measure of antigen-specific cell-mediated (Th1) immune response. There are different forms of this test with varying numbers and types of antigen used, the most common being tuberculin; others include tetanus or diphtheria, since these are antigens which individuals are commonly exposed to via infection or vaccination during childhood or adolescence. In the DTH test, antigens are usually administered subcutaneously on the volar surface of the forearm and a response to the antigen is indicated by reaction (area of redness, swelling) at the site of administration, measured 48 hours after the test has been applied, using specific criteria to assess the extent of the reaction. The underlying principle in this test is that a greater Th1 immune response is a 'healthier' or 'better' reaction to the antigen(s). Hence, those under greater amounts of chronic stress would be expected to show a poorer response. An interesting study of the DTH response was conducted by Shirakawa and colleagues (1997) in Japanese school children. They examined the delayed-type hypersensitivity associated with tuberculin vaccination and allergen type hypersensitivity (IgE) associated with hay fever and atopic disorders, such as asthma, in a sample of 867 children aged 12–13 years. An inverse relationship was found in which children recorded as having had a poorer DTH response (Th1) when they were between the ages of 6 and 12 years were more likely to develop asthma (associated with greater Th2 activity) by the age of 12 years. This fascinating study demonstrates how artificial engineering in order to protect children from cellular immune-related infections, as performed through childhood immunization programmes, may predispose towards a Th2-dominated balance, increasing atopic conditions such as asthma. I would argue that the benefits of immunization programmes far outweigh any such effects (see Chapter 1) but, as the reader, you must make up your own mind on the merits of vaccination. Whatever your views, this is an interesting phenomenon, as it sheds light on the Th1/Th2 balance and the changing face of disease epidemiology.

The other type of *in vivo* test, which in some respects has developed into its own testing paradigm within psychoimmune research, is that of *deliberate exposure* to a virus, or viral challenge. This involves one of two techniques: one is the use of vaccination with either a live but weakened or an inactivated form of a virus, such as influenza or pneumococcal virus; the other is exposure to a live virus. The *in vivo* antibody response to the first, a live but weakened or inactivated form of a virus, is measured usually by means of blood sampling. Studies in this area have focused on adult participants, looking, in particular, at associations between life events and social support in young adult university students (e.g., Marsland et al., 2001; Phillips et al., 2005; Gallagher et al., 2008), marital health and the experience of bereavement in older adults (Phillips et al., 2006), and the role of caregiving. In elderly spousal caregivers, poorer antibody response to vaccination has been reported quite extensively (e.g., see Kiecolt-Glaser et al., 1996; Vedhara et al., 1999).

This paradigm has rarely been used with children due to the ethics of blood sampling for experimental assessment but, given the vaccination programmes in the Western world, there is much potential for testing the antibody response in this way, particularly if alternative salivary assessment can be developed. The paradigm has recently been applied to the parental caregiving role, in a sample of 32 parents of children with developmental disabilities and 29 control parents of normally developing children, who received the pneumococcal vaccination (Gallagher et al., 2009). Significant associations were found between parental caregiving and parental antibody response at 1 month and at 6 months following vaccination. The parental caregiving group had a poorer antibody response to the vaccination than the control group of parents of typically developing children. Importantly, this effect was mediated by behavioural difficulties in the children, revealing that the relationship between parental caregiving and antibody status is not a simple one but accounted for by the behavioural challenges faced by the parent. It is particularly noteworthy that at 1 month post-vaccination, 20 per cent (one-fifth) of the caregiving parents did not mount an adequate antibody response to the vaccination (at the level of clinical protection) compared to 4 per cent of the control parents. At the 6-month assessment, the figure for caregiving parents with an inadequate response was approaching half (46 per cent).

Use of an *in vivo* hypersensitivity test or vaccination, in order to study the effects of psychosocial factors in children for research purposes only, is unlikely to receive ethical approval. If the testing can be combined with routine vaccinations that are already being administered, then the opportunity for research increases. The assessment of vaccine response following a childhood immunization programme is one possible method, if combined with a non-intrusive antibody assessment such as saliva measurement as discussed above. There are relatively few studies that have utilized school-aged vaccination programmes in the examination of psychosocial factors and immune response, but this is a fruitful area for future research.

The alternative *in vivo* viral challenge technique used is that of deliberate exposure to a live virus. This technique has been exemplified in a series of studies known as the 'common cold studies', originally conducted at the Common Cold Unit (CCU) in Salisbury, UK. The medical facility, composing a 600-bed hospital, was initially set up by funds from Harvard University in 1941, in order to contain the outbreak of epidemics predicted following the Second World War. Gifted to the Ministry of Health, it was run by the Medical Research Council (MRC) from 1946 onwards. Under the direction of virologist David Tyrrell, from 1957 until its closure in 1989, not only were many cold viruses isolated, but psychosocial factors were also considered in relation to disease susceptibility, with the collaboration of psychologists Sheldon Cohen and Andrew Smith. These are fascinating studies on many levels, not least because they required thousands of healthy participants to volunteer. Recruitment was through newspaper advertisements, inviting participants to take a 10-day holiday at the CCU during which time they might be infected with a cold virus. Strains of rhinovirus or coronavirus were administered to participants via nasal drops, after completing a battery of psychosocial questionnaires including stress measures. When participants became symptomatic, every detail of the symptoms was monitored, down to the amount of mucosal secretion via weighing of nasal tissues used. Although quarantined within the facility, participants were able to go outside and enjoy their surroundings and, when permitted, to interact with other volunteers, although at a distance if necessary. This was particularly good if symptom free, of course, when participants could enjoy an expenses-paid holiday. There are also reports of romances forming, honeymoons being taken and a variety of other social phenomena (for more detail on these incredible studies, see Tyrrell, 1970; Tyrrell and Fielder, 2002; or the many websites, newspaper articles and blogs that the CCU has generated).

Central to these studies is the notion that, despite known controlled exposure to a specific virus, not everyone exposed to the virus developed symptoms and became ill. In other words, exposure to the virus alone was not sufficient to cause illness. Psychosocial stress was found to be very firmly associated with the risk of becoming symptomatic following exposure. As Cohen and colleagues (1991) report, psychosocial stress was associated 'in a dose-response manner' (p. 609) with increased risk of becoming ill (i.e., the more stress reported, the greater the susceptibility to infection). Medical science may not yet have a cure for the common cold, but it seems that psychosocial factors are important ingredients in the likelihood of onset and the duration of symptoms following viral exposure.

NEUROTRANSMITTER AND ENDOCRINE MARKERS OF STRESS

In addition to the immune markers of stress, assessment of the levels of key neurotransmitters and hormones of the stress response, referred to in Chapter 2, have become a widely accepted tool in the toolbox of psychoneuroimmunology researchers. These include direct and indirect measures of the catecholamine neurotransmitters produced by the activation of the sympathetic adrenomedullary (SAM) system, adrenaline and noradrenaline (US terms, epinephrine and norepinephrine), and the hormones of the hypothalamic-pituitary-adrenal (HPA) axis, CRH (corticotrophin-releasing hormone), ACTH (adrenocorticotropic hormone) and cortisol. Measurement of the hormone cortisol, the end product of the HPA axis, has become widely used in human stress research. Initially through the assessment of blood and, to a lesser extent, urine samples, advances in the assessment of cortisol from saliva have opened up a wealth of research opportunities, and studies using salivary assessment of cortisol have grown exponentially over the past 20 years. The measurement of cortisol in saliva has earned its badge as a very reliable and non-invasive technique (Al-Ansari et al., 1982; Kirschbaum and Hellhammer, 1994). The assessment of cortisol in saliva is a particularly useful tool in biopsychosocial research with children (Woolston et al., 1983) from neonates to adolescents. Salivary sampling avoids the potentially stressful process of taking blood and allows repeated measurement over short time periods to assess reactivity in the laboratory or across days, weeks or months in longitudinal research, as well as enabling samples to be self-administered by the participant in their own home (for a detailed critique of the use of salivary cortisol measurement in children, see Jessop and Turner-Cobb, 2008).

TIME OF DAY AND SALIVARY CORTISOL SAMPLING

Sampling of cortisol from saliva has capitalized on the circadian and, in particular, the diurnal rhythm of cortisol (as described in Chapter 2), yielding specific time-of-day assessments. To capture the diurnal element of cortisol change, time of day is the single most important factor to consider in this assessment. Assessments of single time points can be indicative, but most useful are measures which incorporate a change across time effect. Measurements have included assessment of awakening levels, from immediately upon awakening and prior to rising, to assessment at timed intervals across the day. From these sampling times, calculations can be made which specify total amount of cortisol relative to the time elapsed and rate of change (decline) across the day (Pruessner et al., 1997; Sephton et al., 2000). Similarly, if repeated measures are taken over the first 45 minutes after awakening, measurement of the rate of increase across the first 30 minutes after awakening, known as the cortisol awakening response (CAR; see Chapter 2), can be assessed (Clow et al., 2004).

THE RELEVANCE OF GENDER, AGE AND COMPLIANCE IN SALIVARY CORTISOL TESTING

These measures of salivary cortisol collection have been used extensively with adults across a range of populations and increasingly with children from birth to 18 years. Of particular importance in the assessment of salivary cortisol in children are the factors of gender, age (including pubertal considerations) and compliance (Jessop and Turner-Cobb, 2008). There is a lack of consensus in the literature concerning gender-related cortisol differences in children for both basal levels and during experimental laboratory challenge. With respect to age, we know that the age at which the circadian pattern of cortisol production emerges is usually between 2 and 20 weeks after birth (Santiago et al., 1996; Groschl et al., 2003). Considerable variability in the cortisol rhythm exists across the first 4 years whilst the circadian rhythm establishes itself (Gunnar and Donzella, 2002; Groschl et al., 2003; Watamura et al., 2004). Assessment of the CAR is less well documented in children than in adults and, as mentioned in Chapter 2, in many respects the jury is still out with regard to the developmental stage at which the CAR becomes established. Studies of the CAR have often drawn from cohorts containing a wide age range without sufficient focus on specific age groups of younger children, but, in general, results suggest that the CAR is present in normally developing children, albeit reduced compared to adults (Pruessner et al., 1997; Rosmalen et al., 2005).

Crucial to assessment of the CAR is the accurate measurement of the awakening sample (Federenko et al., 2004) as this forms the baseline measure of the CAR. Compliance in children is particularly relevant here as obtaining a true awakening assessment is fraught with difficulties. For example, children may wake before the parent or caregiver has time to administer the sample, and early morning sampling may be more likely to meet with refusal to participate for numerous reasons. Even 5 minutes of concerted effort to persuade a 4-year-old to provide a saliva sample could induce stress and artificially inflate the CAR, not to mention the ethical issues this implies (see below). This is not to say that reliable morning samples cannot be obtained, but careful consideration and protocol design are essential if meaningful results are to be obtained, and it may explain the paucity and sometimes the ambiguity of work of this kind.

PRACTICALITIES IN SAMPLING SALIVA

In terms of practicalities, you may be wondering how saliva can be sampled. The type of sampling device and procedure used, as well as the precautions and considerations necessary, will vary depending on the type of marker being assessed. For assessment of cortisol, there are a number of devices now available, all based on the cotton swab or compressed dental roll which the participant leaves in the mouth for 1–3 minutes to soak up saliva, upon which it is returned to a test tube with a plastic inner tube, centrifuged to draw out the saliva, and the sample assayed. Flow rate is not relevant to the assessment of cortisol in saliva but can be for other measures, such as IgA, where a timed sample is essential. Commercial companies have produced various sampling devices designed specifically for younger children. As well as flavoured swabs (which met with mixed reviews due to the possible assay interference of the flavouring), swabs have been developed which are longer but smaller in diameter for children under 6 years of age, and cottontip-like devices for infants and toddlers. Figure 3.7 shows some of the sampling devices available.

Collection devices and reliable assays for assessment of salivary cortisol are readily available, but what can be problematic is designing an appropriate protocol which enables collection of meaningful data. Important considerations and restrictions for the sampling of salivary cortisol include: medication (those taking some types of steroid medication, for example, should be excluded); consumption of food and drink (needs restricting for between 30 and 60 minutes prior to sampling); and lifestyle factors, such as diet, exercise, sleep and smoking, which should be recorded (Kirschbaum and Hellhammer, 1994; Jessop and Turner-Cobb, 2008).

Before we leave the topic of salivary assessment of the stress response, it is important to remember that, although it is the most reliable and widely used salivary measure, an increasing number of other stress hormones can now be assessed in saliva. These include DHEA and DHEA-S (adrenal hormones with opposite effects to cortisol), melatonin (anterior pituitary hormone which decreases with puberty onset; Brook and Marshall, 2001: 410), and oxytocin (posterior pituitary hormone necessary for labour and delivery, but also known as the hormone of affiliation; Evans et al., 2000; Taylor et al., 2000; Brook and Marshall, 2001; Detillion et al., 2004). A stress marker of increasing interest is that of salivary alpha amylase (sAA) as a proxy or surrogate marker of SAM activity (Granger et al., 2007; Stroud et al., 2009; Susman et al., 2010). It is a 'surrogate' marker as it is not directly measuring adrenaline as produced from the SAM system, but the amount produced is a reflection of the activity of the sympathetic nervous system (Davis and Granger, 2009). Using simultaneous assessment of both HPA axis and SAM system functioning, Davis and Granger (2009) examined mother–infant dyads attending for 'well-baby' clinic visits which included receiving routine vaccinations. Using four groups of dyads, with infants aged 2, 6, 12 and 24 months, they found sAA to increase reliably in response to the stress of vaccination by 6 months of age onwards. Unlike the recognized 20-minute response time and 20-minute recovery for cortisol, the sAA response was observed 5 minutes post-stressor, and recovery took place at 10 minutes poststressor. Interestingly, this study also found synchrony in pre-test levels of sAA between mothers and infants from 6 months to 24 months but not at 2 months old (Davis and Granger, 2009). Cortisol reactivity was observed at 2 and 6 months but not at 12 and 24 months, in line with other studies that report a reduced ability to induce a stress

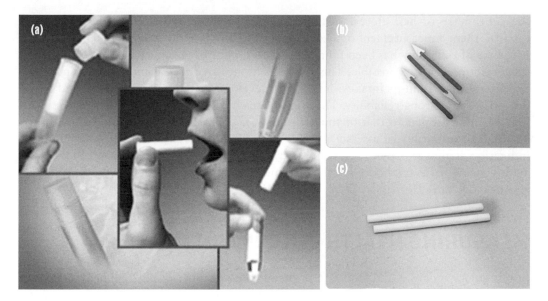

FIGURE 3.7 Saliva sampling devices: (a) the Salivette® (Sarstedt) and equivalent oral swab (Salimetrics) for use by children from 6 years through to adults; (b) Sorbette (small children and infants); (c) children's swab (children under 6 years)

response in this age group (Gunnar and Donzella, 2002). As Davis and Granger (2009) point out, the differences in cortisol and sAA findings strongly indicate the need for the timing of samples to correspond closely with the measure being used, as a study protocol based on the broader timing necessary for cortisol sampling could completely miss the reactivity and recovery associated with sAA reactivity and recovery.

Whilst blood and saliva are the most widely used bodily fluids for the assessment of cortisol, they are not the only ones. Urine samples were frequently used for cortisol assessment long before saliva was established as a reliable marker. Most recently, psychosocial research has branched into the measurement of cortisol from hair, mainly in adults. There is a small body of work using hair cortisol assessment in neonates (e.g., Koren et al., 2003; Yamada et al., 2003, 2007), but to date there are no published psychosocial studies which sample cortisol from hair in young children. A very appropriate population for cortisol assessment from hair is that of pregnant women as it enables a retrospective assessment of chronic stress during pregnancy (Kalra et al., 2005, 2007). The effect of pregnancy stress on birth outcome and on child health is covered in Chapter 4, where several studies using hair cortisol in pregnant women are highlighted. For the sake of methodology, the key element to grasp is the beauty of hair cortisol assessment as a 'retrospective calendar' or marker of chronic stress (Sauve et al., 2007; Kirschbaum et al., 2009). Since hair grows on average about 1 centimetre per month and cortisol is excreted into hair, each centimetre of hair represents the amount of stress the person experienced during the previous month. So, to assess stress during the previous month, the centimetre of hair closest to the scalp can be measured; during the previous 3 months, then, a measurement of 3 centimetres of hair from the scalp would be required. Evidence of reliability has been found for up to 6 months (i.e., 6 centimetres), although longer periods may be possible. This method has intuitive appeal and, despite an emerging interest, is still in its infancy in terms of developing collection protocols and assays demonstrating strong reliability. The stage of scientific development of research in this area is rather similar to that of the early days of salivary assessment of cortisol in the 1990s. The full utility of assessment of cortisol from hair remains to be seen, but early indication is that it provides a 'valid and useful tool' to measure chronic stress, and avoids many of the methodological problems associated with sampling fluids in human research (D'Anna Hernandez et al., 2011: 348).

MEASURING HEALTH OUTCOME IN CHILDREN

In our gold standard X-Y-Z model, Z is the outcome measure of physical health status. A variety of assessments can be made in this respect, broadly divided into (i) disease aetiology or onset; (ii) disease progression; and (iii) ultimate recovery or length of survival. This last category is somewhat controversial as the quality of life may, of course, be as, or more, important as length of life. Both survival and quality of life are considered here as important outcome measures. Onset of acute illness and progression in chronic illness are perhaps the most applicable of these outcomes. The ultimate assessment of the effect of psychosocial factors on outcome is perhaps the intervention study, implemented as a randomized controlled trial. Interventions are referred to throughout the book.

In terms of acute illness, upper respiratory infection (URI) provides one of the most useful paradigms in which to measure links between stress and illness. Even in the field setting, outside of the laboratory, where exposure to a virus cannot be controlled, the common cold and flu in many ways offer the ultimate example in the study of immune resistance versus susceptibility. For example, if you take a group of otherwise healthy children and follow them over a period of approximately 6 months, it is highly likely that the majority will exhibit common cold symptoms. Using a carefully selected set of criteria (see Cobb and Steptoe, 1996; Turner-Cobb and Steptoe 1998), these can be verified and objectively measured, in conjunction with psychosocial variables and physiological markers. In this way, onset, duration, severity and a range of other health outcomes can be assessed. In Chapters 5 and 6, we look in depth at some of these studies as applied to healthy children and the implications of the findings for child health. In particular, we consider the differences between acute and chronic stress on URI health outcomes in naturalistic studies (Turner-Cobb et al., 2011). Other studies have measured acute health outcomes in otherwise healthy individuals by assessment of minor acute symptoms such as headache, stomach ache, or feeling faint or dizzy. A range of scales exist which assess health outcome specific to certain chronic illnesses, functional ability, pain and quality of life, palliative care and survivorship in children and adolescents, and these are mentioned throughout the chapters of this book.

THE LABORATORY/EXPERIMENTAL RESEARCH SETTING

The laboratory or experimental research setting was mentioned in Chapter 2 when look-ing at acute stress reactions. There has been considerable work since the 1960s utilizing developmental psychology laboratory designs particularly to explore attachment and cog-nition paradigms in children. Some of the classic examples include distraction techniques and quality of interaction when the infant's mother leaves the room, the depth perception experiment in toddlers, and Piaget's cognitive stages of development using children from 4 to 12 years old (e.g., see Parke and Gauvain, 2009). These types of experiment and some rather complex variations on them are well recognized in the developmental psy-chology literature. Some of these laboratory methods have been adapted to encompass themes relating to health, for use in paediatric illness, or in healthy children who have experienced chronic stress, as detailed in subsequent chapters.

In the laboratory setting, acute stress responses can be assessed using experimental paradigms, such as the social stress test, to measure pre- and post-test responses or reactiv-ity to stress. Individual characteristics, measures of support, coping ability and any range of psychosocial factors can be compared between participants. The Trier Social Stress Test, reviewed as amongst the best laboratory tests of social stress (Dickerson and Kemeny, 2004), has been adapted for children (TSST-C) and validated in the 9–15-year age group (Buske-Kirschbaum et al., 1997; Kudielka et al., 2004). In the TSST-C, children are told the beginning of a story and given 5 minutes to prepare an exciting ending to the story which they are asked to present to the panel in the 5-minute public-speaking task. They also receive a 5-minute maths task consisting of times tables sufficiently appropriate and challenging for their age group and ability. The TSST-C has been applied to children with atopic disorders which are largely Th2-driven responses, such as atopic dermatitis (AD) and allergic asthma (AA). Measured by salivary cortisol taken at 10-minute intervals throughout the stress test, a hypo-responsiveness or dampening of the HPA axis response compared to controls has been reported in AD children aged 9–14 years and in AA chil-dren aged 7–12 years (Buske-Kirschbaum et al., 1997, 2003).

NATURALISTIC SETTINGS AND FIELD RESEARCH

In addition to the experimental laboratory, the naturalistic field setting has often been the setting of choice for cross-sectional and longitudinal assessment in health research with children and adolescents. A number of assessments, including the use of questionnaire and interview, self-administered saliva sampling for cortisol, and the common cold and flu as an outcome measure in these settings, have already been described above. In addition to these, the diary method of assessment has much potential utility in health research, whether recording quantitative data, qualitative data or a combined approach (for an excellent text on this, see Alaszewski, 2006). Many of the questionnaire and health assessment measures described above, for example, can be presented in diary format, and have proved to be a popular methodology with children and particularly with adolescents (Turner-Cobb et al., 2008).

Perhaps the ultimate research study, particularly apt in child research, is that of the large, longitudinal cohort study. Such research follows large numbers of children across several years or decades in order prospectively to assess influences on health and well-being or educational provision. There have been several large-scale birth cohort studies of this kind in the UK which include assessments of child health. The ALSPAC cohort, mentioned above, examined over 19,000 mothers who gave birth in the early 1990s and followed up the children to date in order to examine environmental influences on health and development (see www.bristol.ac.uk/alspac/sci-com/Avon). The most recent UK cohort study is the Millennium Cohort Study, funded by the Economic and Social Research Council (ESRC) and consisting of approximately 19,000 children born in 2000–2001, followed at regular intervals from birth, including assessment of child and parental health, and receiving their fifth survey 'sweep' in 2012. On a different scale, but similarly interesting for the in-depth longitudinal nature of the study, is the UK BBC television series *Child of Our Time* which documents 25 children born in the year 2000, and their families, over the course of 20 years. This study introduces some interesting ethical issues in terms of the degree of research testing the children are subjected to as they grow up, the issue of consent, and the effects of being under the watchful eye of a TV camera. This conveniently brings us onto the subject of ethical issues in child research.

ETHICAL ISSUES AND COMMUNICATION IN HEALTH RESEARCH WITH CHILDREN

When considering biological methods, such as blood sampling for endocrine and immune measurement, additional ethical issues carry a high priority in research with children, as with other vulnerable populations. This calls for careful consideration of the methodology and assessment used over and above the considerations that already exist for research with adult participants. It is necessary to consider ethical issues right from the start, at design stage, and to adhere to the appropriate research ethics code of conduct for the type of study and context in which the research is being conducted. Whilst this may seem obvious, special consideration of ethical standards has not always been the case in biomedical and biopsychosocial research, and ethical standards and requirements change over time. If you take a look along the corridors of scientific and medical history, you will find a catalogue of what we would now consider outrageously, unbelievably unethical practices.

Lederer and Grodin (1994) conclude in their historical overview of the use of children as research subjects that 'the history of pediatric experimentation is largely one of child abuse' (1994: 19). These are strong words, but the authors give some chilling examples of the exploitation of children at the hands of researchers and scientists which fully support their assertion. These examples include the trialling of vaccinations on vulnerable children such as those with what would now be termed severe learning difficulties or those from disadvantaged backgrounds living in almshouses and orphanages, without consent. Interestingly, they document the extensive use of children of the researchers themselves. Needless to say, the outcome of vaccine trials was frequently unsuccessful and, in many cases, resulted in side-effects, or even death, in otherwise healthy children.

Such practices were not only conducted back in the eighteenth and nineteenth centuries but persisted and, indeed, were advanced well into the twentieth century. One highly cited experiment of this kind was that of the controversial research conducted at the Willowbrook State School for the 'mentally retarded' in New York as late as the 1970s. In order better to understand contagious hepatitis and to develop more targeted vaccines, children were deliberately exposed to the hepatitis virus, then their immune response to the virus was monitored (Nicolson, 1986; Lederer and Grodin, 1994). Parents who gave consent for their children to be in the study were given preference in admission to the school (Lederer and Grodin, 1994). At the time, justification for deliberate viral exposure was on the basis that most children entering the institution would develop infectious hepatitis within the first 6 months of being there anyway, and that deliberate exposure on an isolation ward resulting in preclinical symptoms was better than natural exposure which might lead to greater severity of the condition (Nicolson, 1986). This study raises ethical objections and differences of opinion on a number of levels, including consent issues, and whether the research should be considered as therapeutic or non-therapeutic. Such practice and justification would, of course, not be acceptable by modern ethical standards.

Similarly, throughout history, children were frequently the experimental choice for the use of new procedures and surgical techniques, such as X-rays in pregnant women and infants, and the use of the stomach tube in gastrointestinal research in young children including newborns. Psychologists were not exempt from this behaviour. Far from it: in fact, psychological research and practice from the 1920s to the 1970s abounds with examples of incredibly unethical research. For example, take a look at some of the chilling practices conducted under the auspices of psychological research on topics related to childhood, such as attachment (Harlow's monkey experiments); the nature–nurture debate and sexual identity (the sex-change story of David Reimer); fear responses in young children (Watson's Little Albert experiments); or Johnson's 'Monster Study' which induced stuttering in orphan children (see the web link to these experiments at the end of this chapter).

Why did scientists such as psychologists and medics behave in this way? You can imagine the excitement of researchers who, for the first time, had the use of a new procedure, a novel piece of apparatus, or whose theory was new and exciting in its explanation of human behaviour. Naturally, they wanted to test it out – discover its capabilities and its limitations, its capacity to improve the human condition perhaps. Yet, the combination of these new discoveries with the lack of formal ethical constraints was rather like test driving a rather fast car on a road with no speed limits before installing the brakes. This is not to say that the researchers were without moral codes, but it may have been the lure of medical advance, the promise of treatment and cure, perhaps the status associated with publication of their often biased and not fully reported findings, that bred a research culture that permitted them to underestimate or to 'turn a blind eye' to the human risks involved. Indeed, many scientists appear to have convinced themselves that their experiments were for the good of their subjects or that the benefits outweighed the risks.

There are many issues in this historical catalogue of unethical research practices, one of the most notable being that of informed consent, as well as issues of confidentiality, coercion and deception. Whilst these are key issues for research with human participants of any age, there are special considerations necessary when conducting research with participants under the age of 18 years. Below is a brief outline of each of these, with reference to the most salient aspects for research with this population.

INFORMED CONSENT

It is now common ethical practice for research participants to provide informed consent prior to taking part in a research trial, whether that involves administering medication, physiological procedures, a psychosocial intervention, answering questionnaires or being interviewed. In research with children and adolescents, parental consent, as well as consent from the child as participant, are essential to consider. Lederer and Grodin (1994: 17) describe parental consent as being 'the exception rather than the rule' for research on children in the 1950s and 1960s. The value and status of children in the twenty-first century is reflected in the laws and ethical practices that now safeguard them. Alderson and Morrow (2004) point out that, following the UK Family Law Reform Act (1969), children over 16 years can legally provide consent for medical treatment, but the guidelines for medical research require parental consent for those aged under 18 years. Much psychological research is non-medical, yet there is frequent overlap with medical research if physiological samples are being taken or if participants are recruited based on their status as patients. In non-medical psychological research, parental consent is usually required up to the age of 16 years, but issues of competency, vulnerability, harm and benefit also determine the consenting format.

In addition to informed parental consent, the issue of informed assent (a willingness to take part in the research), following an age-appropriate description of the research, is important to obtain in children of verbal age. Some exceptions and grey areas exist, however. In cases of research conducted with schools, head teachers may agree to act *in loco parentis*; that is, to take responsibility on behalf of the parent, providing consent for classes or groups of children. Even then, written information is required to be sent out to parents who should, at minimum, have the opportunity to 'opt out' of the research study on behalf of their child. This 'opt out' method may be acceptable when, for example, non-intrusive questionnaires are being used with children aged 7 years plus. The 'opt in' method of recruitment is usually essential when taking biological samples. This requires parents specifically to provide written consent to the researcher before the child can take part in the study. Online studies (e.g., chat rooms, questionnaires) raise further grey area issues in terms of obtaining research consent with children, and a distinct lack of guidance currently exists in the literature. Age-related competence, health status, patient status, and project methodology all need careful consideration. Children with special needs fall into a further category of vulnerability which places greater emphasis on parental or legal guardian consent.

CONFIDENTIALITY

Maintaining confidentiality of participants and the data they provide is of utmost importance in research, and the assurance of confidentiality is a part of consent/assent. The exception to this, which applies to children, is when the participant indicates that they may harm themselves or others. In such cases, it may be necessary to take action to inform relevant parties – parents, teachers, health or legal professionals – and such arrangements need to be made clear in the consent agreement. Confidentiality (retaining participant data within the remit of the study) is not synonymous with anonymity (being unable to link data back to the participant). Confidentiality is fundamental to good ethical research practice, whereas anonymity, on the other hand, may in some situations be a useful strategy for data collection; for example, it may be beneficial to collecting more accurate reports if the data are of a sensitive nature, such as sexual practices in adolescents. Yet, in situations when concern for the participant or those around them arises, data collected anonymously cannot be directly traced back to the individual, thus potentially creating an ethical dilemma. So, as a rule of thumb: confidentiality always (disclosure caveat as above), and anonymity if the study requires it and there is sufficient justification.

COERCION

In obtaining research consent, two related issues require consideration: coercion and deception. In the examples given above, prior to the 1970s, children were not only frequently omitted from the process of consent/assent, but they were also frequently deceived and often coerced or exploited, or their parents were coerced into consenting for them. Current laws and ethical guidelines require that no form of coercion is used in research and this is particularly pertinent to children, who may be more easily coerced and enticed into participation by the offer of even a small reward. Coercion is viewed as a form of power imbalance which detracts from making an unbiased, informed decision about the research and needs to be avoided in both overt ways (e.g., giving gifts as rewards for taking part or using threats as punishment for declining participation) and more subtle ways (e.g., the phrasing of invitations to participate; Weithorn and Scherer, 1994).

There is much debate about the issue of whether or not to pay research participants a nominal fee. In research with children, the use of payment, whether monetary or in the form of confectionary, is not considered good ethical practice, and is best avoided, especially in younger children. Yet another grey area exists here and this is the use of lottery-style incentives, in which participants are given the opportunity to be entered into a prize draw. The value of the reward is a major factor in determining the ethics of this style of incentive. For adolescents, such incentives are often very useful in encouraging participants as it appeals to a sense of healthy competition, as well as to the enjoyment of the research and an identity with the study. For more details on the general issue of research payment, although not specific to children, see Francis (2009) who also notes that the offer to cover participant expenses (e.g., travel and car parking) poses no ethical problems and is to be encouraged. It may feel rather patronizing to tell participants that what they will get out of a study is finding out about a particular topic of interest or that their contribution will benefit others in the future, but in research that is not immediately directly therapeutic to the individual, this is often the best incentive. In my experience, in instances where a nominal fee has been offered to parents for participation, it is more often than not declined and taking part in research for the sake of others is often cited as the reason. The important point here is that, as for consent, it is not only the child participant for whom the avoidance of coercion needs consideration, it is also the parent(s), teachers, or others involved in authorizing research recruitment and participation.

DECEPTION AND DEBRIEFING

The use of deception or the withholding of information may be necessary in some experiments. It should, however, particularly in the case of children, be carefully considered (and avoided if any degree of harm may result), kept to a minimum, and followed by debriefing as soon as possible after testing. Understanding of deception and debriefing is illustrated well in a study by Hurley and Underwood (2002). In this experiment, using 178 children aged 8–12 years, the researchers conducted a laboratory test in which it was necessary to deceive children by having a stooge ('actor') pretend to win a computer game. They questioned the children about their understanding of the concepts used in the research, such as confidentiality, assent and how they had been deceived, as well as of the research goal. They interviewed them after they had agreed to take part and following a debriefing session. Most children understood the concept of assent in relation to their participant rights in the study, and the older children understood how they had been deceived. Yet the researchers report that only 45 per cent of the 8-year-olds understood from the debriefing what they had been told about the deception employed in the experiment. They call for researchers to take into account the developmental level of children in the use of debriefing, and suggest that if children do not understand, then 'debriefing could do more harm than good' (Hurley and Underwood, 2002: 139; see Box 3.4).

BOX 3.4

Applying research ethics within an X-Y-Z framework

Design a study to assess the effect of stress on physical health in 11-year-old children.

Considerations:

What is the health status of the population to be recruited: patients or healthy children?

What are the aims, objectives and hypotheses or research questions being addressed?

What combination of measures will be used: questionnaires, biological measures (endocrine or immune markers), interview, observation, laboratory experimentation?

How and where will the subjects be recruited?

How will you gain informed consent?

What procedures can be put in place to maintain confidentiality?

Is it necessary to include deception and, if so, how will the children be debriefed?

In what way(s) will the parents be involved in the study?

What are the main ethical issues involved and which ethics committees or review boards will need to be approached for approval prior to the start of the study?

The key concepts and general guidelines outlined above form some of the fundamentals of research, particularly pertinent to work with children. They are based on the ethical codes, legal requirements and professional practices which have emerged since the 1940s to safeguard individuals participating in research. These include the Nuremberg Code (1947), cited as the 'first international guidelines on ethical research', and the Declaration of Helsinki (1989), which is referred to as the 'first international code on research written by doctors' (Alderson and Morrow, 2004: 26). In addition to these codes, each country and profession have their own set of ethical standards which set the boundaries for the *types* of research which can and cannot be conducted and *how* data are collected. There are distinctions between the ethics involved in conducting medical procedures, doing medical research and conducting research on healthy participants. In health psychology, there is frequently an overlap of research ethics and medical research. Ethical requirements of both frequently need to be adhered to, and relevant approval sought from both research and medical/health-related review boards. Research in the UK is also subject to the Data Protection Act (1998) which serves to protect the rights and privacy of individuals.

For psychology in the UK, the professional standard is the Code of Ethics and Conduct of the British Psychological Society (BPS), last updated August 2009, and their Code of

Human Research Ethics (2011). The BPS Code of Ethics and Conduct is based on four ethical principles: respect, competence, responsibility, and integrity; each with a statement of values and set of standards. These principles apply across all psychology professions, client or patient/practitioner based as well as for research. The BPS also provides Generic Professional Practice Guidelines and Division Specific Guidelines, including the Division of Educational and Child Psychology. Approval for research involving National Health Service (NHS) staff, patients or relatives of patients is through the NHS National Research Ethics Service. In the US, the American Psychological Society (APA) code is the equivalent reference for psychologists. The APA Ethical Principles of Psychologists and Code of Conduct (2010) list five ethical principles and ten ethical standards. The US Society for Research in Child Development (SRCD) also lists 16 principles specifically for research with children (latest version March 2007), including three relating to consent. The approving authority in the US is the Institutional Review Board (IRB). Websites from which these ethics codes and guidelines can be accessed are provided at the end of this chapter.

As you can see from this brief review, research ethics is, to put it mildly, a rather thorny subject. It is also not static but constantly evolving, changing over time to keep up with technological advances in recruitment methods and data collection, as well as with medical developments and current cultural, social and political trends. Attention to the latest guidelines is essential, as is compliance with legal requirements defined by legislation, such as the UK's Human Tissue Act (2004), which these ethical requirements also work within. Importantly, it is not just how the research is conducted and the protocol that are subject to scrutiny before data can be collected. *Who* can collect the data is another vital consideration in research, particularly when collecting data from children, as for vulnerable adults. Legal requirements, such as the UK's Criminal Records Bureau (CRB) disclosure, are in place to ensure that researchers satisfy background checks prior to being permitted to collect data, in order to safeguard child participants. To conclude with a quote from the ethics and standards web pages of the BPS, which is worthy of adopting as a mantra: 'Ethics is central to everything we do whether in research or practice.'

CHAPTER SUMMARY

This chapter has covered a lot of ground, from the basics of biopsychosocial assessment, including standardized measures of psychosocial factors used in research with children and adolescents, to a whistle-stop tour of biological assessments available for such research. The background of immune conditioning has been introduced as a shining example of mind–body interaction, and the intriguing possibilities of its application have been discussed. Health outcome measurement has been highlighted with regard to different research settings with examples of a range of quantitative, qualitative and mixed methods research. Finally, the thorny subject of research ethics was approached from the perspective of learning from past horror stories, of which there are many, and covered current professional ethical codes of conduct and requirements in health-related research with children. This chapter is intended to serve as a resource for the research presented throughout the rest of the book. We now move on in Chapter 4 to examine the effects of psychosocial factors during pregnancy and early childhood on subsequent health outcomes.

KEY CONCEPTS AND ISSUES

- Assessment in biopsychosocial research
- Immune conditioning: immuno-suppression and immuno-enhancement
- Social stress testing
- Stress reactivity and adaptation
- *In vitro* and *in vivo* measures of assessment
- Enumerative and functional immune responses
- Viral exposure and the common cold paradigm
- Research ethics: informed consent, confidentiality, coercion, deception and debriefing

FURTHER READING

For an extensive account of the common cold studies at the CCU:

Tyrrell, D. and Fielder, M. (2002) *Cold Wars: The Fight against the Common Cold*. Oxford: Oxford University Press.

For a particularly good chapter on immune conditioning:

Exton, M.S., King, M.G. and Husband, A.J. (1999) Behavioral conditioning of immunity. In M. Schedlowski and U. Tewes (eds), *Psychoneuroimmunology: An Interdisciplinary Introduction*. New York: Kluwer Academic/Plenum. pp. 443–52.

And an updated journal review on this topic:

Schedlowski, M. and Pacheco-Lopez, G. (2010) The learned immune response: Pavlov and beyond. *Brain, Behavior, and Immunity*, 24(2): 176–85.

A useful research methods text giving examples of how to conduct mixed methods research:

Creswell, J.W. (2009) *Research Design: Qualitative, Quantitative, and Mixed Methods Approaches*. London: Sage.

One of the original papers on social support mapping in children:

Samuelsson, M., Thernlund, G. and Ringstrom, J. (1996) Using the five field map to describe the social network of children: a methodological study. *International Journal of Behavioral Development*, 19(2): 327–45.

For a useful collection of child psychology scales, including those relevant to health:

Sclare, I. (1997) *Child Psychology Portfolio*. Windsor: NFER-Nelson.

For more detail on ethical issues, there are two particularly good texts, one with a UK focus:

Alderson, A. and Morrow, V. (2004) *Ethics, Social Research and Consulting with Children and Young People*. Ilford, Essex: Barnardo's.

And one from the US perspective, which includes an excellent historical overview and a chapter dedicated to scientific issues in psychosocial and educational research with children:

Grodin, M.A. and Glantz, L.H. (1994) *Children as Research Subjects: Science, Ethics and Law*. Oxford: Oxford University Press.

USEFUL WEBSITES

COHORT STUDIES

The Avon Longitudinal Study of Parents and Children (ALSPAC): www.bristol.ac.uk/alspac

The Millennium Cohort Study: UK study funded by the Economic and Social Research Council (ESRC) and housed by the Centre for Longitudinal Studies (CLS): www.cls.ioe.ac.uk

ETHICS, ETHICAL CODES AND GUIDANCE

For a lay account of the top ten *unethical* experiments in psychology, including some of the chilling experiments done in the name of psychological research on topics related to childhood: http://listverse.com/2008/09/07/top-10-unethical-psychological-experiments

The British Psychological Society (BPS) website gives access to the BPS Code of Ethics and Conduct (2009) and Code of Human Research Ethics, as well as a whole host of ethics information for research and practice, including a questions and answers page: www.bps.org.uk

The American Psychological Association (APA) Ethical Principles and Code of Conduct: www.apa.org

The Society for Research in Child Development (SRCD) Ethical Standards for Research with Children: www.srcd.org

The UK Data Protection Act (1998): www.legislation.gov.uk/ukpga/1998/29/contents

Details of the UK Human Tissue Act (2004) can be accessed from: www.legislation.gov.uk

The UK Criminal Records Bureau (CRB): www.homeoffice.gov.uk/agencies-public-bodies/crb

THE INFLUENCE OF PRENATAL EXPOSURE TO STRESS

4

Covered in this chapter

- Terms, definitions and developmental periods in pregnancy
- The normal basal maternal endocrine environment during pregnancy
- The stress response during pregnancy
- Effects of prenatal stress on the fetus *in utero*
- Effects of prenatal stress on birth outcome
- Effects of prenatal stress on infant and child development
- Prenatal stress effects in the adolescent years and into adulthood
- Interventions to reduce prenatal stress and subsequent effects
- The maternal perspective and a link to immune effects

To examine the effect of psychosocial factors on child health, I take a chronological perspective, starting with experiences before birth in this chapter, then moving on to consider psychosocial influences during childhood itself in Chapter 5. This chapter explores prenatal exposure to psychosocial stress, and the effect on birth outcome, including preterm or early birth, low birth weight, and other indicators of newborn health, as well as neonatal health during the first month of life. In this chapter, I also consider the effects of prenatal exposure to stress and other psychosocial factors during pregnancy upon subsequent development in respect to physical health during childhood. I would be short-changing you, however, if this chapter stopped there. I also consider what is, perhaps, one of the most exciting ideas in developmental psychoneuroimmunology today: that the prenatal psychosocial experience may have the potential to influence physical health into adulthood.

I begin by giving some terms and definitions, then outline the normal endocrine response to pregnancy and the potentially disruptive effect of psychosocial stress on the endocrine milieu during pregnancy. In other words, we are still looking at stress hormones with respect to basal levels, reactivity to and recovery from stress, but we are now considering how the condition of pregnancy changes the starting point of this relationship. Importantly, we examine the altered plasticity or allostatic range of the maternal stress response and what this means for the long-term effect on the developing fetus and the subsequent health trajectory throughout the lifespan. Both short-term (birth outcomes) and long-term (infancy through adulthood) effects of stress during pregnancy beautifully illustrate biopsychosocial theory in action.

TERMS, DEFINITIONS AND DEVELOPMENTAL PERIODS IN PREGNANCY

Before we embark on the details of psychosocial influences during pregnancy, it is first necessary to become familiar with some often misused terms. From the perspective of the unborn child, there are three periods of prenatal development: (i) the germinal period (first 2 weeks after conception) when it is termed a zygote or blastocyst; (ii) the embryonic period (weeks 3–8 of pregnancy) when it is termed the embryo; and (iii) the fetal period (after week 8 of pregnancy until birth) when it is known as the fetus (see Sigelman and Rider, 2009). For clarity, I will avoid using the somewhat emotive term of 'unborn baby' and instead will use the term which is most relevant to the developmental stage we are considering, which in most cases will be 'fetus' since the fetal stage is where psychosocial effects appear to have most effect. The term 'baby' will be reserved for post-birth or post-natal descriptions (with the term 'neonatal' referring to the first month of life).

From the maternal perspective, there are three trimesters of pregnancy, each of which constitute approximately 3 months, albeit of unequal lengths given the 40 weeks of pregnancy. The first trimester consists of pregnancy weeks 1–12; the second trimester, weeks 13–27; and the third trimester, weeks 28–40. It is worth noting a couple of points here to save confusion later on. First, be aware that the usual 40 weeks of pregnancy cited is calculated from the first day of the mother's last menstrual period. The terms 'pregnancy' and 'gestation' are used synonymously. Yet conceptional age or fetal age is measured from the first day of conception, approximately 2 weeks later, so based on a 38-week development. Essentially, these are the same, but they incorporate different parts of the process, and I will refer to gestation or pregnancy meaning the full 40 weeks since last menstrual period. Secondly, babies born from 37 weeks of gestation onwards are considered full term and not premature, given the final stage of lung development which has occurred by this point, enabling normal survival outside of the uterus. This brings me to the use of the term 'uterus' as opposed to the older (rather more 'biblical' sounding) term 'womb'. For some reason, I have noticed that the term 'womb' when used in lectures often causes a nervous shuffling or a pre-emptive momentary silence, and students get very anxious

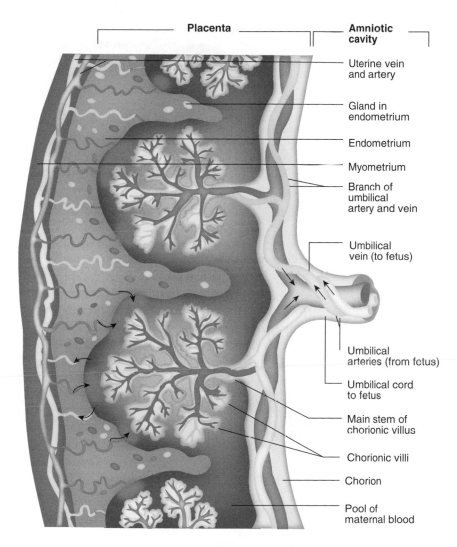

FIGURE 4.1   Interrelations of fetal and maternal tissues in the formation of the placenta

Source: E.P. Widmaier, H. Raff and K.T. Strang (2010) *Vander's Human Physiology: The Mechanisms of Body Function*, 12th edn. New York: McGraw-Hill Higher Education, p. 618. Reproduced with the kind permission of the McGraw-Hill Companies.

about knowing which term to use. So, to save awkward silences, anxiety and shuffling during the reading of this book, out of preference I will use the more medical term 'uterus', but also be aware that both are used interchangeably in the literature and that there is sometimes a US bias towards the term 'womb'.

It is during the embryonic period that the placenta develops. Connected to the embryo/fetus via the umbilical cord, this lifeline provides a two-way system transporting oxygen

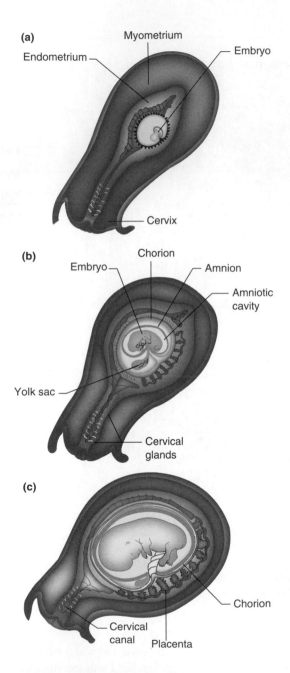

FIGURE 4.2 Placental attachment within uterus showing development of the embryo at 3, 5, and 8 weeks after fertilization

Source: E.P. Widmaier, H. Raff and K.T. Strang (2010) *Vander's Human Physiology: The Mechanisms of Body Function*, 12th edn. New York: McGraw-Hill Higher Education, p. 618. Reproduced with the kind permission of the McGraw-Hill Companies

and nutrients from the mother's bloodstream *to* the embryo/fetus and carbon dioxide and metabolic waste *away from* the embryo/fetus into the mother's bloodstream. The placental barrier, a semi-permeable membrane within the placenta, is responsible for enabling small molecules to pass through, whilst preventing the passing of large blood cells between mother and embryo/fetus and providing protection from toxins (see Sigelman and Rider, 2009). Figures 4.1 and 4.2 illustrate the placenta and attachment to the uterus during development. The placenta is essentially an endocrine organ, described as a 'transient endocrine unit' (Wadhwa et al., 1996: 433) and a 'stress sensitive organ' (Mastorakos and Ilias, 2000: 101). The reasons for this powerful terminology should become apparent throughout the rest of this chapter.

But what has pregnancy got to do with stress hormones? As discussed in Chapter 2, the effect of psychosocial stress on physiological functioning triggers activation of the sympathetic adrenomedullary (SAM) system and the hypothalamic-pituitary-adrenal (HPA) axis, leading to increases in stress hormones available to deal with the stressor. However, if these responses are frequent or maintained, then continued excess production of these hormones can be harmful to normal functioning and, ultimately, to physical health. Based on this line of reasoning, stress can be seen as a potential environmental teratogen (i.e., something that may have a harmful influence on an embryo or fetus), just as some pathogens (e.g., chickenpox virus or toxoplasmosis parasite) and chemicals (alcohol or prescribed drugs such as thalidomide) are teratogens (for more on teratogens, see Sigelman and Rider, 2009). What is of interest here is the impact on the fetus when the mother perceives an event as stressful, and how this maternal experience gets translated into physical health effects for the child. Can stress really be seen as a 'teratogen' or are we over-exaggerating our claims to put it in the same league as drugs and environmental hazards? To explore this idea, we need to examine the evidence for what the immediate and longer-term consequences of maternal stress during pregnancy really are. In order to do this, I first consider the normal maternal endocrine and immune environment during pregnancy, and, in particular, the relationship of the HPA axis to fetal functioning. We will then go on to examine the response to stress during pregnancy and the impact of extremes of this response on the fetus, birth outcomes, neonatal and subsequent child development and beyond.

THE NORMAL BASAL MATERNAL ENDOCRINE ENVIRONMENT DURING PREGNANCY

To understand both the normal maternal endocrine response to pregnancy and the response to stress during pregnancy, it is necessary to go back to the description of the normal endocrine environment in non-pregnant states (reviewed in Chapters 2 and 3). In the absence of pre-eclampsia (pregnancy-induced hypertension), there is no consensus in the literature with regard to changes in basal levels of adrenaline and noradrenaline during pregnancy, although a diurnal decline representing higher morning and lower evening levels in both these SAM system hormones has been noted (de Weerth and Buitelaar,

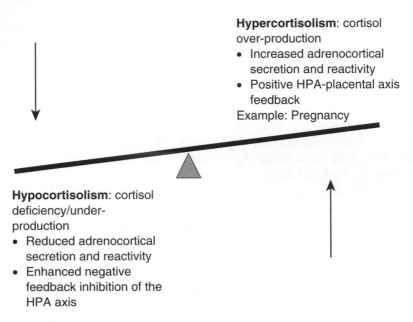

Hypercortisolism: cortisol over-production
- Increased adrenocortical secretion and reactivity
- Positive HPA-placental axis feedback

Example: Pregnancy

Hypocortisolism: cortisol deficiency/under-production
- Reduced adrenocortical secretion and reactivity
- Enhanced negative feedback inhibition of the HPA axis

FIGURE 4.3   Fulcrum showing hypo/hypercortisolism

2005). In addition, blood volume and cardiac output increase during pregnancy (de Weerth and Buitelaar, 2005). The part of the stress response system to undergo the most major change during pregnancy is the HPA axis, and cortisol plays a crucial part in this. In contrast to the *hypo*cortisolaemic (low cortisol) states sometimes seen in autoimmune disease or in some subpopulations of individuals with post-traumatic stress disorder, pregnancy has been described as 'a transient ... period of relative *hyper*cortisolism' (i.e., high cortisol levels; Mastorakos and Ilias, 2000: 98; see Figure 4.3). Now, if such phrases fail to have you signing up for a postgraduate qualification in the psychoendocrinology of pregnancy or a career in psycho-obstetrics, then I am not sure what will. But read on, there is even more to get excited about.

So, for a comparatively short window of time, during the three trimesters of pregnancy, cortisol, the end-product of the HPA-axis, is produced at a comparatively high rate or increased basal level. This increase in cortisol is not equally distributed across the three trimesters but increases as pregnancy progresses, culminating in delivery. In fact, cortisol levels rise throughout pregnancy and peak at two to three times non-pregnant levels during the third trimester, and the adrenal glands hypertrophy (enlarge) due to the increased demands upon them (Mastorakos and Ilias, 2000). In other words, the state of pregnancy provides a perfect playground for the researcher wanting to look at hypercortisolaemic states, since the baseline levels of cortisol and other hormones of the HPA axis are temporarily raised. Yet the HPA axis, operating as it does on a negative feedback loop in the maternal circulation, is not the whole story when it comes to understanding stress hormones in pregnancy. The maternal HPA axis feeds into the placental axis of the fetus, generating a second feedback loop, but this time a *positive feedback* or hormonal cascade with the fetus (Wadhwa et al., 1996). These two feedback loops (one negative, one positive) operate in conjunction with each other to form what is known as the HPA-placental axis. Box 4.1 outlines the normal endocrine response of the HPA axis hormones during pregnancy and the development of the HPA-placental axis. A further hormone is introduced here, beta endorphin (βE), an opioid (naturally occurring pain reliever), produced by the hypothalamus and the pituitary.

BOX 4.1

The normal endocrine response to pregnancy

1 A progressive increase in hormones of the HPA axis (e.g., CRH, ACTH, cortisol) and beta endorphin (βE) throughout pregnancy which culminates at labour and delivery.
2 HPA-placental axis development resulting in a positive placental adrenal feedback loop in combination with the negative feedback of the HPA axis:

   i cortisol inhibits CRH expression in the hypothalamus; leads to *negative feedback*;
   ii cortisol stimulates expression of the placental CRH gene resulting in an increase in CRH messenger RNA (CRHmRNA). Increased placental CRH, ACTH, and βE lead to maternal pituitary-adrenal axis stimulation and result in increased cortisol production from the adrenal cortex; leads to *positive feedback*.

See Wadhwa et al. (1996).

Central to the HPA-placental axis is the production of placental CRH (corticotropin-releasing hormone) which is the driving force in stimulating the *positive* feedback loop which leads to increased CRH, ACTH (adrenocorticotropin hormone), cortisol and beta endorphin during pregnancy. This CRH system is increasingly activated over the course of pregnancy (gestation), peaking prior to delivery as CRH levels are vital to the onset of labour (Mastorakos and Ilias, 2000). CRH levels are reported to be suppressed between 3 and 6 weeks following delivery, but to return to normal levels by 12 weeks after delivery (Mastorakos and Ilias, 2000). It is interesting, by contrast, that cortisol levels return to normal pre-pregnant states soon after delivery (Mastorakos and Ilias, 2000).

THE STRESS RESPONSE DURING PREGNANCY

So we have looked at the normal endocrine state during pregnancy and the development of the HPA-placental axis. If the normal state of pregnancy is to raise basal levels of crucial stress hormones, this begs the question of what happens at the level of stress reactivity. In other words, what happens when the mother, in this already heightened hormonal state of pregnancy, experiences stress? The hormonal mechanisms and milieu created by the

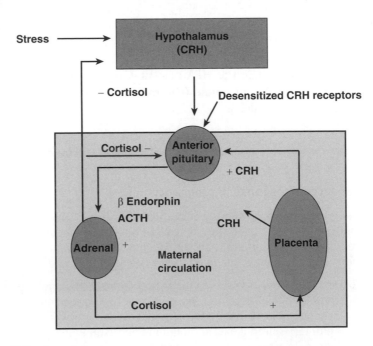

FIGURE 4.4   HPA-placental axis

Source: Sandman et al. (1997: 268).

HPA-placental axis have important implications for stress reactivity during pregnancy, particularly in the third trimester, when HPA axis and placental hormone levels are at their highest. Whilst in the maternal circulation, increases in cortisol activate the negative feedback control over the HPA axis via the hypothalamus; the effect of cortisol on the placenta stimulates production of placental CRH (Sandman et al., 1997). As pregnancy proceeds, this potentially leads to a situation where the HPA axis response to stress reduces (due to enhanced negative feedback), effectively immunizing the mother to the CRH effects of stress. Yet, at the same time, the effect of cortisol on the placenta stimulates the production of CRH and amplifies the stress response. Figure 4.4 shows a model of the HPA-placental axis, illustrating concurrent placental CRH stress amplification and maternal pituitary desensitization or stress immunization (Sandman et al., 1997), and Table 4.1 outlines these concepts.

There is good evidence for the coexistence of maternal stress immunization and fetal stress amplification during pregnancy. A review by de Weerth and Buitelaar (2005) summarizes the results of studies investigating stress reactivity during pregnancy based on stress tests involving pain and discomfort as the stressor or psychological stress created through cognitive tasks. They conclude that physiological activation in response to stress, as assessed by blood pressure, heart-rate reactivity and cortisol reactivity to laboratory stressors, has been found to be diminished during pregnancy compared to non-pregnant women and pregnant controls (for review, see de Weerth and Buitelaar, 2005). Yet, as these researchers point out, whilst dampened SAM and HPA axis reactivity is important in

TABLE 4.1 Stress effects on the HPA-placental axis

Stress *immunization*

Normal maternal response to stress is reduced as pregnancy proceeds.
Mechanism: increased threshold for stress-induced pituitary release of ACTH and β endorphin by hypothalamic CRH (ability to stimulate pituitary decreases). Thus, HPA response to stress lessens as pregnancy proceeds

Stress *amplification*

Placenta amplifies the stress signal resulting in CRH rise → risk of preterm delivery.
Mechanism: pituitary ACTH stimulates adrenal cortisol, resulting in increased placental CRH, i.e., placental CRH stimulated by adrenal cortisol

---

Source: Sandman et al. (1997: 000).

terms of pregnancy outcomes, speed of recovery (i.e., return to baseline) following the termination of the stressor, or habituation and recovery to repeated or ongoing stressors, is equally important but an often neglected area in stress research. This is particularly so in relation to pregnancy. The evidence for stress amplification in the fetus is seen from examining the immediate and long-term effects of maternal stress during pregnancy on postnatal health outcome. This brings us to the topic of prenatal programming.

Prenatal or fetal programming, sometimes called 'fetal imprinting' (Merlot et al., 2008), is the term given to the manner in which development of the nervous, endocrine and immune systems are shaped during gestation. In a review of fetal programming, Sandman and colleagues (2011: 9) describe the placenta as the vehicle conveying information from the 'maternal host environment into the fetal developmental program'. Prenatal stress is a key source of these fetal programming effects, and there are several ways in which they can influence health outcome. In order to summarize the literature in this area, it is easiest to conceptualize effects along a developmental trajectory. Remember, however, that research is a lot more arduous than it is often given credit for and, of course, findings on prenatal stress influences have not always been made in such a logical order. However, the beauty of a textbook is having all this complex literature summarized for you. So, the effects of prenatal stress on child health can be divided into (i) effects on the fetus *in utero*; (ii) effects on birth outcome; (iii) effects on infant and child development; and (iv) influences in the adolescent years and into adulthood. Each are now considered in turn.

EFFECTS OF PRENATAL STRESS ON THE FETUS *IN UTERO*

First, we start with the effects of maternal stress on fetal behaviour *in utero*. Such effects have included fetal hyperactivity and a range of cardiovascular responses, such as increased fetal heart rate, increased motor activity, and reduced fetal responsiveness to novel stimuli if the mother had higher placental CRH in the third trimester (for review, see Sandman et al., 2011). These early responses are interesting since, as Sandman and colleagues (2011) argue, they enable us to see the effects of prenatal programming on the developing nervous system, independent of the effect of the birth experience and subsequent influences of parenting and socialization. Of course, this early environment might alternatively be viewed as prenatal parenting. Box 4.2 asks what you think about this issue.

BOX 4.2

What do *you* think?

With regard to the influence of psychosocial factors, when does parenting begin? At birth? At conception? Prior to conception?

In 1994, research by Professor Peter Hepper at Queen's University, Belfast, made headlines in the national newspapers when it was reported that babies who had been exposed to the theme tune of the Australian TV soap opera *Neighbours* whilst *in utero* were soothed by the music after birth. This was put forward as evidence of fetal learning and memory (Hepper, 1996, 1997). This idea of external stimuli being able to influence the fetus has become widely accepted, and it is not unusual to find expectant parents attempting to enrich the intellectual potential of their offspring during fetal development (Figure 4.5). This is a good example of using the influence of prenatal exposure to positive effect.

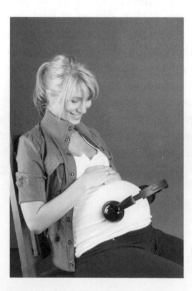

FIGURE 4.5   Pregnant woman with headphones

Source: www.istockphoto.com/file_closeup/?id=7074192&refnum=541096&source=sxchu04&source=sxchu04.

EFFECTS OF PRENATAL STRESS ON BIRTH OUTCOME

Continuing with our chronological perspective, although admittedly we have diverted slightly from this path in Box 4.2, one of the most significant outcomes in the stress and development literature of the past decade relates to the findings of prenatal stress on birth outcome – preterm birth, reduced birth weight or reduced growth (i.e., being 'short for gestational age'). Preterm birth (see Figure 4.6) may be associated with reduced birth weight or reduced length, but these features may also be independent of length of gestation (i.e., the baby may be born at or after 37 weeks but still have reduced weight or growth).

What evidence is there to support the notion of stress during pregnancy influencing birth outcome? Human studies have linked prenatal stress to premature birth (i.e., being born preterm, before 37 weeks of pregnancy), being small for gestational age, and having a low birth weight. In a recent review of this literature, Class and colleagues (2011) point out that the consequences of preterm birth can lead to increased infant mortality (death) and lifetime morbidity (physical and psychological ill health). Rates of preterm birth are increasing throughout the UK, with an incidence in England and Wales of 8 percent, which equates to 1 in 13 of all live births (Tommy's charity website; Office for National Statistics [ONS] 2007 report). In the US, preterm birth rates have been reported as climbing towards a figure of 13 per cent of live births in 2005, which is a 20 per cent increase since the 1990s, but showing a decline between 2006 and 2008 (latest statistics available) to 12.3 per cent (March of Dimes: www.marchofdimes.com website based on natality

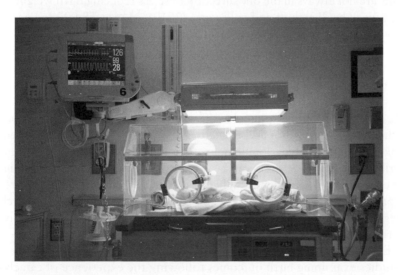

FIGURE 4.6   Premature baby

Source: iStock photo 13198333 (www.istockphoto.com/search/text/premature%20baby/source/basic).

data from the National Center for Health Statistics). These figures represent an average across the UK or the US, but there is variation by county or state as well as by age and race. It is estimated that a proportion of preterm deliveries may be due to better medical care resulting in elective preterm delivery for medical reasons, a quarter to other risk factors such as infection, and about a third due to multiple births (see Tommy's charity website; ONS). A further third is estimated to be due to 'unexplained and spontaneous' reasons, including social factors such as socioeconomic status (see Tommy's charity website; ONS). Stress is an obvious contender within this last category, whether directly (experiencing a major life event) or indirectly (experiencing adverse life events as a consequence of low socioeconomic status).

In a Swedish study using population registries, an impressive 2.6 million individuals who had been born between 1973 and 2004 were retrospectively identified and it was assessed whether or not the mother had experienced the death of the baby's father or of a first-degree relative during pregnancy (Class et al., 2011). The researchers conclude that it is during months five and six of pregnancy, during the second trimester, that exposure to life-event stress can have the greatest impact on preterm birth or reduced birth weight or size (Class et al., 2011). A Danish study of 1.38 million mothers examined stress experienced from the death or serious illness of a close relative not just during pregnancy but also during what they term the 'periconceptional period', up to 6 months before conception (Khashan et al., 2008). They report significantly reduced birth weight in babies whose mothers had experienced death of a first-degree relative either periconceptionally or across any of the three trimesters of pregnancy, and the offspring were at increased risk for being small or very small for gestational age. Similarly, they report that the impact of stress on fetal growth was greatest when exposure was during the second trimester (Khashan et al., 2008).

Yet results are not always in the one direction of stress reducing birth weight and growth. Interestingly, work by Tegethoff and colleagues (2010), in over 78,000 women at approximately 30 weeks of pregnancy, provides evidence for major life stress (e.g., associated with home, work, finance, relationships, pregnancy and health), at any point during those 30 weeks, to be associated with shorter gestation and with *greater* body weight and length. Emotional stress (e.g., fear, nervousness, hopelessness) in the mother during pregnancy was associated with shorter gestation and with smaller body length in the baby at birth (Tegethoff et al., 2010). The authors argue that this is evidence of fetal regulation and adaptation to environmental stress or 'adversity' *in utero*, which demonstrates fetal resilience and the ability to take an alternative developmental path as shaped by the fetal environment.

As described in Chapter 2, stress can be categorized using various taxonomies to reflect the degree or severity of experience. When it comes to trying to evaluate birth outcome following prenatal stress experiences, this is equally pertinent. Some researchers in the area of pregnancy outcome have distinguished between life stress which could in some cases be termed 'ordinary life experiences' and the more severe experience of 'trauma' (Mulherin Engel et al., 2005). Whilst there is a comparatively small amount of work in this area, studies examining birth outcomes following the experience of cataclysmic acute stressors have reported effects after a range of natural or human disasters: for example, hurricanes such as Hurricane Katrina (Xiong et al., 2008), earthquakes such as China's

Wenchuan earthquake (Tan et al., 2009), or terrorist attacks, including that on the World Trade Center (Mulherin Engel et al., 2005). For a review of the effects of prenatal stress from disasters and their effect on birth outcomes, see Harville and co-workers (2010), who conclude that the impact of prenatal stress is on fetal growth rather than on gestational age. Harville et al. (2010) argue for the importance of the effect on maternal mental health in influencing childhood outcomes. Findings from studies of natural disasters are generally in line with the notion that stress can cause detrimental effects on birth outcome. Yet, as Tan et al. (2009) point out, such events, and hence the effects seen in these cohorts, can be viewed as 'outliers' as they are examples of extremes. However, these extremes serve as a useful barometer of stressful experiences on birth outcomes so it is useful to take a look at some examples before moving on.

In a sample of over 13,000 newborns, approximately half born before the Wenchuan earthquake and half afterwards, researchers report significantly greater numbers of low birth weight babies and poorer Apgar scores (health assessment given at birth) in those whose mothers experienced the earthquake (Tan et al., 2009). Significantly more birth defects were also found (e.g., ear malformations), particularly if exposure to the earthquake was during the first trimester of pregnancy rather than the second or third trimester. Similarly, women who experienced Hurricane Katrina and who were exposed to a greater number of traumatic stressors related to the hurricane (e.g., those who believed their life to be threatened or experienced a close bereavement) had a higher incidence of preterm birth than those exposed to fewer hurricane-related stressors (Xiong et al., 2008). Interestingly, in a study of the 9/11 attacks in New York, post-traumatic stress symptoms (PTSS) and moderate scores on depression were both linked to *longer* rather than shorter gestations (Mulherin Engel et al., 2005). Additionally, head circumference at birth was smaller in babies of mothers who reported PTSS, and the authors point out that this could influence infant neurocognitive development (Mulherin Engel et al., 2005). Of particular note in this study is the idea that PTSS may indicate a low level of maternal cortisol production, in the same way that paradoxical hypocortisolaemic (low cortisol) states have been reported in some of the literature on adults with PTSD. They argue that since high levels of cortisol increase the chances of early birth, then low cortisol levels and a generally 'hypo' response in these severely stressed women may explain why gestation is increased rather than reduced in this population (Mulherin Engel et al., 2005). This fits with the third type of allostatic load described in Chapter 2, and may be interpreted as providing further evidence of adaptability as described above. It also brings us neatly to the role of stress hormones in shaping birth outcome.

THE ROLE OF STRESS HORMONES LINKING PRENATAL EXPERIENCES WITH BIRTH OUTCOME

As outlined above, during pregnancy the normal state is to have raised levels of a range of hormones, each with their own purpose in bringing about healthy development of the fetus. Whilst stress reactivity may be dulled in the mother, it appears that stress may be amplified in the fetus, and substantially increased stress hormone levels may influence

birth outcome. Hormones of the HPA axis, in particular CRH and cortisol, are implicated, and highlight the relevance and crucial importance of considering psychosocial
factors in birth outcomes, most notably that of preterm delivery. Whilst a rise in CRH is
essential to bring about labour and delivery, if levels of this hormone increase too rapidly,
too early in pregnancy, then this may induce premature delivery. Metaphorically speaking,
during pregnancy the hormone party is in full swing, everyone is having a good time, but
if a couple of people have a few too many drinks and start getting out of hand, fun turns
to disruption and before you know it, the party is over. We are back to the idea of physiological balance: pregnancy is a state of heightened physiological balance or allostasis
with the potential for allostatic load consequences observable in the form of birth outcomes (for a full explanation of allostasis and allostatic load, see Chapter 2).

The role of CRH

An increasing amount of evidence has been found to support a link between stress and
CRH as indicators of birth outcome. For example, maternal stress in weeks 28–30 of
pregnancy has been linked to birth outcome, gestational age at birth and birth weight
(Wadhwa et al., 1996), and maternal stress during the third trimester has also been associated with increased maternal plasma levels of ACTH (adrenocorticotropin hormone)
and cortisol (Sandman et al., 1997). Hobel and colleagues (1999) investigated stress and
CRH in a longitudinal study using three gestational stages of 18–20 weeks, 28–30
weeks, and 35–36 weeks of pregnancy. They examined demographic and medical factors, perceived stress and state anxiety in the mothers and found preterm delivery to be
associated with higher CRH levels than controls at all three gestational stages. Maternal
stress levels and age at 18–20 weeks of pregnancy were linked to CRH levels at 28–30
weeks. Similarly, elevated ACTH at all three stages and elevated cortisol at the earlier
two stages of pregnancy were associated with preterm delivery. Research suggests stress
and CRH levels as potential preterm birth markers, with CRH serving as an early indicator for preterm birth.

Studies in the past few years have become increasingly interested in this notion of *timing of stress exposure* during pregnancy to delineate any specific critical periods where the
effect of maternal stress on birth outcome is most detrimental. For example, in a sample
of 158 mothers and their newborn babies, Ellman et al. (2008) assessed maternal cortisol
and placental CRH levels via maternal blood plasma in relation to newborn neuromuscular (e.g., muscle tone and flexibility) and physical maturation (e.g., of skin, eyes, ears,
genitalia). They identified higher maternal cortisol levels at 15, 19, and 25 weeks of pregnancy (trimester 2), and CRH levels at 31 weeks (trimester 3), as being associated with
poorer maturational outcomes in male but not in female neonates, when assessed independently of gestational age. Their findings support the idea of placental priming via
cortisol early in the second trimester to influence CRH production and premature birth
(Ellman et al., 2008). Most studies point to this second trimester as the crucial time for
stress exposure influencing birth outcomes. I will come back to this issue of timing when
we look at the effects of pregnancy stress on development later in this chapter.

The role of cortisol

A study by Entringer and colleagues (2011) assessed diurnal salivary cortisol by sampling seven times across the day over a period of 4 days in a group of 39 women of varying gestational stages of pregnancy (between 10 and 35 weeks). This protocol enabled them to assess a more detailed cortisol profile than some previous studies have done, using fewer sampling days or times across the day and including both the cortisol awakening response (CAR) and diurnal change measurement. Controlling for gestational age at sampling time, they found a higher level of cortisol at awakening, a smaller CAR and greater cortisol across the day to be associated with a shorter length of gestation (Entringer et al., 2011). By way of comparison, this study also sampled single plasma and salivary cortisol levels at the start of the four-day sampling but these unitary assessments were not associated with length of gestation which highlights the value of taking detailed cortisol measurements. Compliance was also monitored and increased in this study with the use of EMA (Ecological Momentary Assessment). EMA is a tool which enables participants to report events, feelings, or behaviours in real time, using reminders or prompts, via mobile devices, to respond to or record certain events (for more detail see Moskowitz and Young, 2006). In the Entringer et al (2011) study, EMA served as a reminder and recording device for cortisol assessment. Interestingly, using EMA for recording negative affect, Entringer et al. (2011) report that it was not correlated with gestational length although associated with higher diurnal cortisol. Therefore, this indicates that predicting the effects of stress on birth outcome is a better indicator than subjective mood reporting.

In another study, Bolten et al. (2011) found higher cortisol levels during pregnancy in a sample of 81 women with healthy singleton pregnancies to be associated with lower birth weight and being short for gestational age. However, self-reported levels of distress and perceived stress during pregnancy were not related to cortisol levels or birth outcomes. Like Entringer et al. (2011), the authors argue for levels of cortisol in pregnancy providing a more accurate indicator of intrauterine growth and birth outcome than self-reports of stress. Yet other studies (Goedhart et al., 2010) report high maternal depressive symptoms to be linked to the baby being small for gestational age and having a low Apgar score, although they do not not report any association between depressive symptoms and preterm birth. Goedhart et al. (2010) suggest cortisol as a mediating mechanism between maternal depression and birth outcomes, as well as maternal risk behaviours such as alcohol consumption and smoking during pregnancy.

As discussed in Chapter 3, a relatively new sampling procedure in the human stress arena is that of sampling hair for the assessment of cortisol. This technique is particularly appropriate for the sampling of cortisol levels during pregnancy as it provides a retrospective measure of chronic stress on a month-by-month or three-monthly trimester assessment. In just the past 5 years, published work has reported human studies using this technique to assess stress during pregnancy, with some promising results. For example, Kalra and co-workers (2007) report a significant correlation between perceived stress and hair cortisol (taken from hair 1–1.5 cm closest to the scalp) in a group of 25 healthy pregnant women who were at the border of their first and second trimester. Kirschbaum and colleagues (2009) sampled hair cortisol in a total of 142 women, the majority of whom (n = 103) had given birth 2–4 days previously, as well as those who had given birth 3–9 months previously (n = 19) and a control group of 20 slightly younger women who were not pregnant and who had no previous children (nulliparous). You can clearly see in this study how hair cortisol is a useful tool for measuring chronic stress that has occurred at specific retrospective periods of time, as hair was sampled based on the pregnancy trimesters, being divided by the researchers into 3-cm segments. This enabled many different and useful comparisons across trimesters and across groups (for full details see Kirschbaum et al., 2009) but, most importantly for what we are considering here, they found cortisol in the third trimester of pregnancy to be significantly and reliably twofold higher than in the control women.

Another study provides further confirmation of the reliable assessment of the detectability of increasing cortisol levels across pregnancy trimesters comparing saliva (sampled three times a day at weeks 14, 18, 23, 29 and 34 of pregnancy and 6 weeks postpartum) and hair cortisol (D'Anna-Hernandez et al., 2011). The researchers successfully utilized a novel protocol of repeated hair cutting in order to isolate cortisol from hair in each trimester (cut at 15, 26 and 36 weeks and 3 months postpartum) and further compared the samples with segmenting a single sample of full trimester length hair (D'Anna-Hernandez et al., 2011).

Yet the first and only study to date which reports the use of hair cortisol in relation to birth outcome or preterm birth is that by Kramer et al. (2009) (however, bearing in mind the growing interest in this area, I suspect more will have been published by the time this book goes to press). These researchers included the measurement of hair cortisol amongst an impressively wide range of other biological and questionnaire measures of stress and medically related factors in a Canadian study of over 5,000 preterm births. These authors found a *positive* association between hair cortisol and preterm birth in a subsample of 207 preterm mothers (delivered before 37 weeks) and 444 controls, based on a segment of 9 cm of hair. In this study, higher cortisol levels during pregnancy were associated with longer gestation since cortisol levels were higher in women who delivered at term compared to those who delivered before 34 weeks of gestation (Kramer et al., 2009). Now, if you have been following this train of thought and hanging on my every word, you will have realized (and not just because I placed it in *italic*) that this positive association runs contrary to expectations. If greater stress triggers more cortisol production, and higher levels of stress are associated with preterm delivery, then, you maybe asking, what is going on in this study and is measurement of hair cortisol really worth pursuing? You will see from my descriptions of these hair studies that I have been quite fanatical about stating the length of hair segment assayed (important because it reflects a period of time where 1 centimetre equates to 1 month, see Chapter 3). In the study by Kramer et al. (2009), note that a 9-cm segment of hair, covering at least the full gestational period, is analysed, as one segment reflecting cortisol levels over the whole pregnancy. As the authors acknowledge, stress effects may be 'obscured' by assessing all three trimesters at once, and studies isolating different trimesters are needed. With growing evidence of the utility of hair cortisol assessment and its special relevance to testing in pregnancy, it would be fair to say that the writing is on the wall for the next big wave of research in prenatal stress.

Before we leave this topic of cortisol assessment in hair, this all begs one further question: can prenatal stress exposure be measured in neonates using the retrospective sampling procedure of hair cortisol? Quite possibly, is the answer, although the logistics of hair collection (including variable hair growth in newborns) present obvious difficulties. There is only one study to date which has looked at human neonatal hair cortisol in relation to psychosocial stress. Work by Yamada et al. (2007) reports a higher level of hair cortisol in hospitalized infants receiving neonatal intensive care (via the NICU) compared to healthy term infants, and of the NICU infants, a greater number of days on the ventilator predicted higher cortisol levels. We return to the subject of hospitalization during childhood in Chapters 6 and 7 and pick up on this theme again there.

MECHANISMS UNDERLYING EFFECTS OF PRENATAL STRESS ON BIRTH OUTCOME AND DEVELOPMENT

As with associations linking psychosocial factors and physical health outcomes, an explanatory mechanism is needed. How can stress influence gestation age, birth outcomes and development? We have looked at various hormones of the HPA axis which are implicated, predominantly cortisol and CRH, but what is their mechanism of action? How can maternal stress, as observed in cortisol responses, transmit across the placenta to influence fetal development and birth outcome, potentially programming development with life-long consequences? The exact mechanisms are yet to be uncovered but research suggests that there are at least two mechanisms which may be in operation. In an excellent review of this literature, Van den Bergh (2005) details work relating to these two mechanisms. The first is that of hormone transfer across the placenta, whereby high levels of stress hormones such as cortisol in the mother directly influence the fetus via exposure in the uterus. Whilst the protective barrier of the placenta restricts the amount of glucocorticoids passing through to the uterus, there is evidence that under stressful maternal conditions one of the protective enzymes responsible for this protection is reduced. This enzyme is known as 11-beta-hydroxysteroid dehydrogenase type 2 (11beta-HSD2), and has the function of converting cortisol to its inactive form, cortisone, in the placenta. If levels of this enzyme are reduced, then a greater amount of active cortisol is able to pass through the placenta to the fetal environment. Whilst levels of cortisol are substantially higher in the mother than the fetus, a strong correlation does appear to exist between maternal plasma cortisol and amniotic fluid cortisol (Sarkar et al., 2007). The correlation between these cortisol levels has been related to maternal anxiety, providing evidence for this placental enzyme reduction mechanism (Glover et al., 2009). Furthermore, evidence from several sources also implicates reductions of this enzyme in cases of intrauterine growth restriction (for example, Kajantie et al., 2003; McTernan et al., in Van den Bergh, 2005; Dy et al., in Glover et al., 2009). For a review of the role of this placental barrier enzyme, see O'Donnell et al. (2009).

The second mechanism is that of impaired or abnormal blood flow within the uterus. Van den Bergh (2005) cites evidence to suggest that maternal stress and anxiety are associated with greater resistance to blood flow in the uterine arteries, lack of oxygen to the fetus, and effects on cerebral circulation in the fetus. As de Weerth and Buitelaar (2005) suggest, it is most likely that a combination of mechanisms is in operation linking prenatal stress to fetal health outcome, but from a theoretical perspective mothers who show the greatest stress reactivity and the poorest adaptation or recovery to stress experiences are the ones most at risk in terms of effects on the fetus.

EFFECTS OF PRENATAL STRESS ON INFANT AND CHILD DEVELOPMENT

What evidence is there to support the notion of prenatal or fetal programming linking physical health in childhood and of health effects on those children into adulthood? The longer-term effect of prenatal exposure to stress hormones in humans is not a simple or easy affair to study. Work in this area originated in rodent and primate models where gestation and lifespan developmental stages are relatively brief (e.g., compared to guinea pigs who have a gestation of approximately 65 days, an average lifespan of 3–4 years, and adolescence within a few months of life). Work in humans brings different challenges to the study of lifetime prenatal stress effects. The majority of human studies have focused on birth outcomes and neonatal health, and much research calls for more longitudinal work to be conducted, particularly in mapping critical weeks of gestation with subsequent outcome at specific months, years, or stage of life.

Studies which have demonstrated the effects of prenatal stress on postnatal outcomes are listed in Table 4.2, divided into outcomes observed during infancy (first year of life), childhood (from age 1 to 10 years), and the very limited research which has so far examined the outcome of prenatal stress into adolescence. Research of a sufficient longitudinal nature to examine effects of prenatal stress or birth outcomes in adulthood is sparse for obvious reasons. A notable study in this area, although restrospective, is that by Wust and colleagues (2005) who linked birth weight to cortisol stress responses in adulthood, and we come back to this below.

The majority of studies have found effects in the direction of stress being associated with poorer developmental outcomes, including behavioural, cognitive and temperament difficulties. There are, however, a handful of studies that have reported opposite effects. For example, in a study of 104 mothers and infants, Rothenberger et al. (2011) found mid-pregnancy stress and depressive feelings, as assessed by questionnaire, to be associated with less infant affective reactivity (crying, fussing) at age 3 and 5 months. They argue that mild prenatal stress may have positive outcomes for infants rather than negative ones, and their findings support the evolutionary model mentioned above. Interestingly, the effects in this study were also not mediated by cortisol. Effects found by Davis and Sandman (2007) again show the relevance of *timing* effects of prenatal exposure to cortisol (see Table 4.2) since elevated cortisol early in pregnancy was found to have detrimental effects on development, but elevated levels late in pregnancy appear to have

TABLE 4.2 Effects of prenatal stress on postnatal outcomes observed during infancy, childhood, and adolescence

Study	Prenatal period of stress exposure	Nature of stressor or stress measure	Sample size (mother–child dyads)	Type of postnatal outcome	Age at postnatal outcome
Infancy					
Davis et al. (2011)	15, 19, 25, 31, 36 weeks	Infant cortisol response to heel-prick test	$n = 116$	Larger cortisol response to heel prick if mother had greater stress in late 2nd or 3rd trimester; slower behavioural recovery to heel prick if mothers had higher cortisol in early pregnancy or more psychosocial stress throughout pregnancy	24 hours after birth
Huizink et al. (2003)	(i) Early pregnancy, weeks 15–17; (ii) Mid-pregnancy, weeks 27–28	(i) Maternal daily hassles (ii) Pregnancy-specific anxiety; fear of giving birth	$n = 170$	Poorer mental and motor development	8 months
de Weerth et al. (2003)	Late pregnancy, weeks 30–35	Stress defined as high or low based on maternal cortisol levels	$n = 17$	Behavioural (more crying, fussing and negative facial expressions); temperament (more 'difficult' behaviour), higher scores on emotion and activity	First 5 months: weeks 1, 3, 5, 7, 18, 20; effects strongest for weeks 1–7
Davis et al. (2007)	30–32 weeks	Maternal anxiety and depression; perceived stress	$n = 247$	Infant temperament: increased negative reactivity	2 months
Bosquet Enlow et al. (2009)	6 months post-delivery	Lifetime maternal stress exposure and perinatal trauma; laboratory stressor	$n = 23$	Poorer recovery from behavioural distress and cardiorespiratory activation following laboratory stressor in infants of mothers reporting greater trauma	6 months

(Continued)

TABLE 4.2 (Continued)

Study	Prenatal period of stress exposure	Nature of stressor or stress measure	Sample size (mother–child dyads)	Type of postnatal outcome	Age at postnatal outcome
Buitelaar et al. (2003)	Early pregnancy 15–17 weeks Mid-pregnancy 27–28 weeks	Maternal daily hassles; pregnancy-related anxiety	$n = 170$	Mental and psychomotor development	8 months and to a lesser extent at 3 months
Yehuda et al. (2005)	Third trimester effects most pronounced	PTSD during third trimester following direct exposure to World Trade Center collapse on 9/11	$n = 38$	Low cortisol levels in mothers and children	1 year
Brand et al. (2006)	Recruited across all stages of pregnancy	PTSD following direct exposure to World Trade Center collapse on 9/11	$n = 98$	Temperament: more distressed by novelty	9 months
Davis and Sandman (2010)	15, 19, 25, 31, 36 weeks	Salivary cortisol; pregnancy-specific anxiety	$n = 125$	Elevated early pregnancy cortisol linked to slower rate of development and poorer mental development; elevated late pregnancy cortisol linked to *accelerated* cognitive development and *higher* mental development scores' early pregnancy-specific anxiety related to lower mental development scores	During and at 12-month assessment
Childhood					
Gutteling, de Weerth, Willemsen-Swinkels et al. (2005)	15–17, 27–28, 37–38 weeks	Perceived pregnancy stress	$n = 119$	Perceived stress and fear of giving birth to handicapped child predicted behavioural and temperament problems	27 months

Study	Timing	Measure	n	Outcome	Age of child
Gutteling, de Weerth and Buitelaar (2005)	Sampled in all three trimesters	Maternal salivary cortisol and pregnancy anxiety	n = 29	Cortisol reaction to first day of school	5 years
Gutteling et al. (2006)	Early pregnancy	Maternal life events		Learning and memory	6 years
Buss et al. (2010)	19, 25, 31 weeks	Pregnancy anxiety	n = 35	Pregnancy anxiety at 19 weeks associated with reductions in volume of grey matter of brain on MRI scans, indicating vulnerability for neurodevelopmental and cognitive impairment	6–9 years
Adolescence					
O'Connor et al. (2005)	Across trimesters	Prenatal maternal anxiety	n = 74	Awakening levels and response, afternoon and evening cortisol in child	10 years (pre-adolescent)
Van den Bergh et al. (2008)	12–22, 23–32, 32–40 weeks	Maternal anxiety	n = 58	Anxiety at 12–22 weeks associated with high, flattened cortisol profile in adolescents and in girls additionally with depressive symptoms	14–15 years (adolescents)

positive effects. The effects on temperament and cognitive development are relevant to our consideration of child health and important in relation to subsequent risk for adult psychopathology. What is of particular interest to us here, though, is the physical health outcome. As summarized in Table 4.2, Bosquet Enlow et al. (2009) in their study of 23 infants (6 months old) and their mothers, found a combined effect of perinatal trauma (defined as trauma surrounding the last few weeks of pregnancy, delivery and the first two neonatal weeks) and maternal lifetime trauma. Infants whose mothers had experienced high perinatal and lifetime trauma were slower to recover from the increased behavioural and cardiorespiratory responses induced during a laboratory stressor. This double effect of perinatal stress and accumulated lifetime stress brings us back to the allostatic load models described in Chapter 2.

PRENATAL STRESS EFFECTS IN THE ADOLESCENT YEARS AND INTO ADULTHOOD

As Table 4.2 makes clear, there is currently very little literature on the effects of prenatal stress exposure on physical health outcomes in the teenage years. The first study to examine the longer-term effects of pregnancy experience on cortisol levels was conducted by O'Connor et al. (2005) using data from the Avon Longitudinal Study of Parents and Children (ALSPAC), a research cohort mentioned in Chapter 3. In this study, they assessed cortisol at awakening, 30 minutes after awakening, and towards the end of the day at 4 p.m. and 9 p.m. Interestingly, they found no statistically significant rise from awakening to plus 30 minutes after awakening, but both awakening levels and afternoon levels (4 p.m.) were each separately correlated with anxiety at 32 weeks of pregnancy. The effect for awakening cortisol was the most robust, even when controlling for obstetric factors (e.g., birth weight for gestation age, smoking and alcohol consumption) and socioeconomic factors (e.g., household crowding and mothers' education) as illustrated in Figure 4.7 (O'Connor et al., 2005).

The absence of the CAR in this sample is not highlighted by the authors (O'Connor et al., 2005), but if you are interested in this topic, you might want to consider the relevance in light of the discussion about the CAR in Chapter 3. Absence of this phenomenon in a group of 10-year-olds could be due to pre-adrenarche or pre-puberty effects or it might be that pregnancy anxiety has the effect of flattening this response: either way, it is an interesting finding which might have implications for future work and a rather large 'watch this space' hint that work in this area is only just gaining momentum. The only other work to date which has specifically examined pregnancy stress and cortisol in adolescence comes from a similarly well-controlled, prospective, longitudinal study by Van den Bergh and colleagues (2008). The authors report a significant association between pregnancy anxiety experienced between 12 and 22 weeks of pregnancy in the mothers and a high, yet flattened, diurnal cortisol profile in the children at 14–15 years old ($n = 58$). This effect was found for both male and female

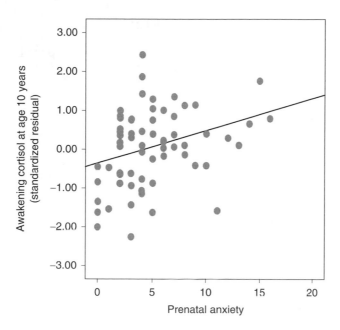

FIGURE 4.7   Prenatal anxiety (at 32 weeks of pregnancy) and awakening cortisol in pre-adolescent children

Source: O'Connor et al (2005: 214, fig. 2).

adolescents, and for girls only, the additional finding emerged that the diurnal profile acted as a mediator of depressive symptoms. Both these studies are evidence of prenatal stress or anxiety having a longitudinal effect on altered HPA axis functioning to the point of pre-adolescence/adolescence.

Of course, these studies beg the question of how far into the future it is possible to predict health outcomes based on prenatal psychosocial experiences. Such longitudinal studies have yet to be conducted. Interestingly, a pioneering study by Wust and colleagues (2005) looked at reactivity to stress in a laboratory setting in a sample of 102 young adults (twin males with a mean age 18.57 years). As illustrated in Figure 4.8, the authors found low birth weight but not gestational age to be associated with significantly greater stress reactivity. This study only looks retrospectively, but it is tantalizing since it projects into late adolescence/early adulthood. The scope for future studies combining assessments across the lifespan is enormous.

Whilst most of the studies reported here do not look specifically at physical health outcomes, most examine intervening physiological mechanisms that have in other studies been found to alter susceptibility to illness or, conversely, give insight into factors to be avoided in order to encourage a better long-term health outcome. As a result of such work, there is an increasing interest in interventions to reduce pregnancy stress or prenatal adversity with the goal of improving health outcomes.

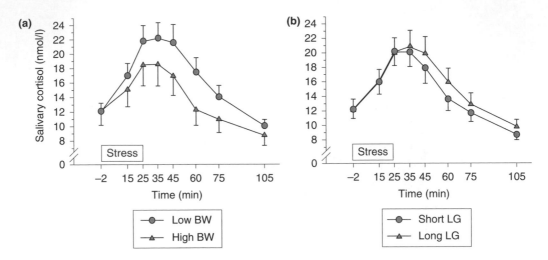

FIGURE 4.8 Birth weight and salivary cortisol responses to stress in adult life: mean salivary cortisol responses (g.s.e.m.) to psychosocial stress (Trier Social Stress Test) in subjects differing in their birth weight (BW) and their length of gestation (LG), respectively. In order to represent the effects of continuous measures graphically, variables BW (a) and LG (b) were dichotomized by median split (BW: mdZ2700 g; LG: mdZ38 wk)

Source: Wust et al. (2005: 594, fig. 1).

INTERVENTIONS TO REDUCE PRENATAL STRESS AND SUBSEQUENT EFFECTS

You need only look at the range of antenatal support groups and birth plan options available in developed countries to glean that there is a lot of interest in reducing anxiety during pregnancy, improving the maternal birth experience, and optimizing physical health outcomes for the baby. There have been major advances in this area in the past quarter of a century. As well as improved scientific knowledge and technology informing medical practice, much of the improvement in psychological care has maternal anxiety reduction at its core. In reducing stress in this way, birth outcomes and subsequent developmental effects may be improved. Yet, as we have seen above, it is still relatively early days in understanding how the stress mechanisms operate in pregnancy and in being able to map prenatal stressors and their timing to specific ages and outcomes, especially into adulthood.

There are a small but growing number of studies that have included assessment of physiological measures, such as cortisol, in order to understand better the mechanisms in operation. For example, lower levels of morning salivary cortisol have been reported in a group of low-income Latina women (*n* = 41) implementing brief self-guided stress reduction instructions over the course of a day (Urizar et al., 2004). Two studies have also found cortisol reductions following stress-reduction programmes (Urizar and Munoz, 2011; Ventura et al., 2012). Urizar and Munoz (2011) implemented cognitive behavioural stress management (CBSM) in a group of low-income Spanish women in their second trimester of pregnancy who were at high risk for depression, compared to a control group of low-risk mothers and those receiving standard care. Looking at cortisol outcomes in both the mothers and their babies, at 6 months after delivery salivary cortisol was significantly lower in the infants whose mothers had received CBSM or whose mothers were in the low-risk control group than those in the standard care group. At 18 months after delivery, the CBSM mothers themselves had significantly lower cortisol levels than the usual care group (Urizar and Muñoz, 2011). The procedures associated with medical advances, whether amniocentesis testing or *in vitro* fertilization (IVF), whilst greatly beneficial, can create their own brand of stressors. In the second of the studies mentioned above, using a randomized controlled design, Ventura et al. (2012) assigned 154 women undergoing an amniocentesis test to one of three 30-minute conditions whilst in the waiting room: (i) listening to music; (ii) sitting and reading; (iii) sitting and waiting. They report the greatest reduction in plasma cortisol following the music condition and also noted a reduction in anxiety scores (Ventura et al., 2012).

Other studies have assessed maternal relaxation interventions on the infant. For example, Fink and colleagues (2011) report relaxation benefits in terms of fetal heart rate in response to mothers receiving guided imagery or progressive muscle relaxation, with guided imagery having most effect. The ultimate question is perhaps not just whether prenatal intervention can reduce stress, but whether or not prenatal stress effects on birth outcome and development are reversible. Evidence suggests some degree of adaptability or plasticity yet, as outlined earlier in this chapter, some adaptations may not be undesirable and it is worth bearing in mind that, at some level, stress may induce evolutionary changes which enable us to cope with the stressor environment. This is more food for thought but, in the meantime, we turn just briefly to the maternal perspective.

THE MATERNAL PERSPECTIVE AND A LINK TO IMMUNE EFFECTS

I simply cannot leave this topic without mention of the effects of pregnancy on maternal health outcome, particularly because of the spiral of effects the implications may have for child health. Sandman and colleagues (2011) refer to 'maternal programming' as the process by which the brain and behaviour of the mother are remodelled during pregnancy. They describe both direct effects associated with caregiving, such as those related to attachment processes, and indirect effects associated with memory and stress reactivity (Sandman et al., 2011). This links with the stress immunization during pregnancy mentioned above, and includes affective and cognitive programming and psychopathology particularly in relation to postnatal depression. The notion that pregnancy creates changes in cognition and behaviour is not a new one, and the personal stories of many mothers might concur with these research findings. This is not to say that effects are long lasting or that the influences are all negative. However, that the hormone alterations of pregnancy act as maternal programming, in a parallel fashion to prenatal programming, is an interesting concept to consider and promotes a greater understanding of the dyadic relationship contributing to child health outcome. There is also increasing recognition that the birth experience itself is inherently stressful and that, at one end of the spectrum, can result in post-traumatic stress disorder (for review, see Ayers et al., 2008).

In connection with the maternal perspective, there is another missing link that we need to consider before summarizing this chapter. That is the effect of stress hormones on the immune system during pregnancy and the postpartum period, since it is important to understand what is happening at the maternal endocrine and immune level in order to understand the experience of the fetus. Changes in the hormonal milieu (in particular CRH) during pregnancy orchestrate the necessary environment for healthy development and, ultimately, the safe delivery of the baby. In addition, the influence of steroid hormones (e.g., cortisol) appears to drive changes in the balance of the Th1/Th2 immune profile pre- to postpartum. With reference to Figure 2.1 in Chapter 2, this means that, during pregnancy, there is a shift towards the Th2 type of immunity, with the associated anti-inflammatory cytokine profile of antibody-mediated immunity, and away from the cell-mediated Th1 pro-inflammatory cytokine profile. The reason for this is most likely that it facilitates the state of pregnancy since the Th2 cytokine environment is more conducive to implantation and cell growth (Wilder, 1998). If you are still paying attention and have not drifted into Th1/Th2 confusion (if you have, please refer back to Chapter 2), you may have noticed that this shift is a pattern similar to that seen under conditions of chronic stress.

As a result of the shift in favour of a Th2 cytokine profile during pregnancy, the mother is protected against autoimmune conditions associated with cell-mediated immunity or Th1 immune activity (e.g., rheumatoid arthritis and autoimmune thyroid disease), but is more susceptible to autoimmune conditions associated with Th2 immune activity or antibody-mediated immune diseases (e.g., systemic lupus erythematosus; Wilder, 1998). Incidentally, the effect of this shift is also evidenced by increased susceptibility to parasites requiring a Th1 immune response to eliminate them and exacerbations of viruses associated with Th2 activity (Wilder, 1998). In the postpartum period, when the immune balance swings back to the pre-pregnancy state of relative hypocortisolism, the situation is reversed and there is greater likelihood of a flare-up of a pre-existing autoimmune condition, such as rheumatoid arthritis, or onset where the condition did not previously exist (Wilder, 1998). Similarly, Th2 autoimmune conditions which develop during pregnancy tend to improve postpartum (Wilder, 1998).

CHAPTER SUMMARY

In this chapter, I have considered the effect of the developmental environment – prenatal to postnatal – on health outcome and the concept of prenatal programming. As well as contributing to a greater understanding of the theory and processes involved, research in this area enables development of interventions to reduce stress and improve birth outcome. We have looked at psychosocial stress effects during pregnancy on birth outcome and child health, with a peek, as far as the literature enables, into early adulthood. We have considered the implications of the work to date and the enormous amount of research yet to be done. In keeping with the allostatic model described in Chapter 2, prenatal stress is only one contributor, albeit an important one, in the mosaic of stresses that influence physical health outcomes in childhood and subsequent life stages. In the next chapter, we continue to examine the developmental stress environment by considering the effects of stress during childhood itself.

KEY CONCEPTS AND ISSUES

- Pregnancy stages, placental development, embryonic/fetal development
- Placental barrier enzyme 11-beta-hydroxysteroid dehydrogenase type 2 (11beta-HSD2)
- The placental-HPA axis
- Prenatal stress
- Hypercortisolism
- Stress amplification/stress immunization
- Prenatal programming/maternal programming

FURTHER READING

An excellent text for more background information on gestational development and teratogens:

Sigelman, C.K. and Rider, E.A. (2009) *Life-Span Human Development*, 6th edn. Belmont, CA: Thomson/Wadsworth.

Some incredible photography which will fill you with awe and wonder, but not for the faint-hearted:

Jirasek, J.E. (2001) *An Atlas of the Human Embryo and Fetus: A Photographic Review of Human Prenatal Development*. New York: Parthenon.

An excellent review of laboratory stress responses in pregnancy:

de Weerth, C. and Buitelaar, J.K. (2005) Physiological stress reactivity in human pregnancy: a review. *Neuroscience and Biobehavioral Reviews*, 29(2): 295–312.

This article gives a good description of the placental-HPA axis:

Sandman, C.A., Wadhwa, P.D., Chicz-DeMet, A., Dunkel-Schetter, C. and Porto, M. (1997) Maternal stress, HPA activity, and fetal/infant outcome. *Annals of the New York Academy of Sciences*, 814: 266–75.

This paper gives an excellent review of this laboratory's work across multiple studies and longitudinal work covering both fetal and maternal programming:

Sandman, C.A., Davis, E.P., Buss, C. and Glynn, L.M. (2011) Exposure to prenatal psychobiological stress exerts programming influences on the mother and her fetus. *Neuroendocrinology*, 95(1): 8–21.

An excellent review article – as good as its title suggests:

Van den Bergh, B.R. (2005) Antenatal maternal anxiety and stress and the neurobehavioural development of the fetus and child: links and possible mechanisms. A review. *Neuroscience and Biobehavioral Reviews*, 29: 237–58.

USEFUL WEBSITES

UK statistics:

Office of National Statistics: www.statistics.gov.uk/

Tommy's charity (after St Thomas's Hospital, London): www.tommys.org

US statistics:

US preterm birth data, including an excellent interactive map for comparison across states: www.marchofdimes.com

THE EXPERIENCE OF STRESS DURING CHILDHOOD

5

Covered in this chapter

- The experience of stress in healthy children
- The contributions of temperament, individual difference and quality of childcare
- Effects of severe or toxic stress, including post-traumatic stress disorder
- Family environment and intergenerational transmission of stress
- Health in adulthood and across the lifespan
- Communicating stress
- The longer-term outlook and opportunities for intervention

In tandem with Chapter 4, which examined the influence of the prenatal environment, including stress during pregnancy, on birth outcome and subsequent child health, this chapter considers the effect of stress during childhood on health during childhood and beyond. Whilst the focus of this chapter is on health in early childhood, as this is where the majority of research has been conducted, as with pregnancy effects I also go on to consider the longer-term effects on subsequent health into adolescence and adulthood. The theories put forward in Chapter 2 are applied here in considering these longer-term effects, including intergenerational impacts, of early life adversity. Both episodic (acute) and enduring (chronic) stress experiences are addressed in the context of implications for intervention and normalization of the hypothalamic-pituitary-adrenal (HPA) axis.

THE EXPERIENCE OF STRESS IN HEALTHY CHILDREN

In Chapter 2, I covered the concepts of stress and coping. Our working definition of stress is an interaction between the external stimulus of the environment and the internal resources to cope with it, which determines the response. There, I noted the difference between acute (or episodic) and chronic (or enduring) stress, which is based on duration and severity of the stressor. An acute stress may generate a series of further acute insults or challenges and lead to the more enduring effects of chronic stress. Such a combination of stressful events or mix of acute and chronic stress experiences, whether initially related or not, has been aptly described as a 'stressor mosaic' (Miller et al., 2007: 190). Severe or traumatic stress may be experienced by individuals who have suffered a particularly extreme form of stressful experience, such as a major road traffic accident or severe childhood maltreatment. Illness itself is inevitably a stressor, and in Part II of this book I will go on to consider the experience of illness during childhood, including chronic illness, terminal conditions, and the experience of pain. Before that, however, in this chapter, I conclude Part I of this book by focusing on the stress response in healthy children undergoing acute, chronic and severe stressors and evidence for the physical impact this may have on physical health in the short term and in the longer term. This forms a basis for understanding the more complex issues associated with children who are coping with the stress of chronic or life-threatening conditions, covered in later chapters.

In Chapter 2, as well as using the terms acute and chronic stress, I referred to a taxonomy of the National Scientific Council on the Developing Child ([NSCDC] 2005) which classifies stress into three levels: positive, tolerable, and toxic. Given the magnitude of impact, it is tempting to jump straight into exploring the effects of toxic levels of stress, such as that experienced following severe childhood maltreatment or deprivation. Yet, for reasons that I hope will become obvious by the end of this chapter, if not already, I will start with the more mild forms of stress, those which, using the NSCDC terminology, are defined as 'positive' stress or 'tolerable' stress.

POSITIVE STRESS AND TOLERABLE STRESS

The question of whether or not stress during childhood has any significant effects on the developing stress response system may seem straightforward. Surely, there is a simple answer: that the greater amount of stress experienced, the more 'damage' (psychological and physical) is bestowed upon the child, in a simple dose–response manner. If this is the case, then the best approach to parenting would be to protect your child from all known stress exposure during childhood: whether physical (pain) or psychosocial (including maternal separation and meeting new people) or at least keep it to a bare minimum (the 'wrapping up in cotton wool' approach). Yet most people would agree that such an approach would undoubtedly be harmful, if not impossible, and that anyone who suggests this is perhaps a little unhinged. I am certainly not advocating this approach. Whilst maternal attachment and adequate parenting are important, and their lack can result in developmental delays associated with severe deprivation or maltreatment (see below), evidence would suggest that, in fact, some exposure to mild forms of psychosocial stress is not only desirable but essential. As you may imagine, there is something of a hot debate within the field over this issue.

Surprisingly, there is comparatively little research looking at the physical impact of everyday stressors or minor life stresses and stress reactivity in otherwise healthy children, although interest in this area is growing. However, it is important to have an understanding of the responses and processes involved in more minor stresses before attempting to understand the effects of more severe forms of stress.

BASAL CORTISOL AND STRESS REACTIVITY

To get to grips with this area, what we need to know is twofold: first, information relating to the basal (underlying) cortisol levels and the diurnal cortisol profile; second, we need an accurate assessment of cortisol reactivity when faced with a challenge (naturalistic or laboratory induced). Using data from both these sources, we can further assess the combined effect of the presence or absence of early life stress coupled with the outcome of subsequent stress challenge, which is where it all begins to get interesting. We know that the diurnal cortisol profile starts to establish itself somewhere between 1 month and 5 months of age, usually by about 3 months of age (see Chapter 2), for both girls and boys (Santiago et al., 1996; Groschl et al., 2003; Gunnar and Quevedo, 2007), although defining absolute levels of cortisol in children is difficult due to a range of factors including sampling techniques (for review, see Jessop and Turner-Cobb, 2008). We also know that cortisol levels in children can vary according to lifestyle factors such as maternal consumption of alcohol or smoking (see Hunter et al., 2011), as well as demographic factors (socioeconomic conditions, age and sex). Low socioeconomic status has been associated with higher basal cortisol levels in children, at least up until the point of starting senior school at the age of about 12 years (Lupien et al., 2001). Indeed, poverty is considered an important underlying factor in the stress–health link and early childhood economic disadvantage a major cause of stress on a number of levels (see Chapters 1 and 2). Whilst findings are inconsistent with regard to sex effects, age effects have been consistently reported (Jessop and Turner-Cobb, 2008).

Yet there appears to be much variability or 'plasticity' in the underlying rhythm of the HPA axis up until the age of about 3–4 years, which has important implications not only for the effects of early life adversity but also for early intervention. There is growing evidence that younger infants, up to 6 months of age, respond to acute mild stressors with a physiological cortisol response similar to the magnitude seen in adults. However, although findings are mixed, by the end of the first year of life, there is considerable evidence that this response diminishes (Gunnar and Donzella, 2002), until around puberty when the type of response we would expect to see in adults begins to emerge once again, and this occurs at an earlier age in girls than in boys (Gunnar, Wewerka, et al., 2009; see also references to the role of adrenarche on cortisol levels pre-puberty discussed in Chapter 2). There is debate, however, over the degree to which the cortisol response diminishes during the childhood years, although by comparison such a stress hyporesponsive period is clearly documented in rodents, possibly as an evolutionary mechanism to protect the brain from overexposure to glucocorticoids during development (Lupien et al., 2009). For excellent reviews of the stress response in children, see Gunnar and Quevedo (2007), Jansen et al. (2010), and Hunter et al. (2011).

CORTISOL IN INFANTS AND TODDLERS

In their review of cortisol reactivity in children up to 24 months old, Jansen and colleagues (2010) distinguish between painful physical stressors (e.g., vaccination or heel-prick procedure) and mild physical stressors (e.g., examination, bathing, nappy change), both of which result in a greater stress reaction than the psychological stress caused by separation from the maternal caregiver or evoked emotions such as fear, novelty or anxiety. However, they make a very important point which highlights the need for further work in this area across a wider age range. This is that the assessment of cortisol responses to these various categories of stress have been unequally distributed, so that much of the research on physical and painful stressors has been conducted on infants up to 6 months of age, whilst work looking at the stress of maternal separation has focused on young children 9–18 months old (Jansen et al., 2010). They also point to several crucial caveats to the findings so far in this area, including the importance of considering individual differences in temperament (e.g., levels of fearfulness and attachment strength) rather than drawing conclusions from whole group data where there is likely to be variation in temperament. One reason for reduced stress reactivity by 12 months of age, which has been alluded to by several researchers, is the developmental increase in the range of behaviours available to cope with the stressor, including language and communication, and increased levels of cognitive understanding. The findings in this area are tantalizing but, as Jansen et al. (2010) note, there are two important directions for future work which both relate to a more in-depth mapping of stress reactivity in children:

1   The need for age-specific studies to include different types of stressors across all age ranges to the extent that adequate age-specific comparisons can be made.
2   The assessment of multiple stress response systems: in addition to cortisol as a measure of the HPA axis, assessment of the sympathetic adrenomedullary (SAM) system, e.g., via salivary alpha amylase measurement, may provide a useful assessment of more immediate stress reactions.

CORTISOL BEYOND THE INFANT AND TODDLER YEARS

But what about stress reactivity in children beyond the infant and toddler years, when stress takes on more of a social dimension? Moving on from the stress of bathing, heel-prick tests or maternal separation anxiety, psychosocial stress linked to performance and expectations becomes increasingly appropriate with age. Set against the context of low basal cortisol in children pre-puberty, what is sufficient to generate a stress response in children between about 18 months and up to 11 years old? In addition to unpredictability and uncontrollability of the stressor, the third key component for a stress-inducing paradigm, at any age, recommended by Dickerson and Kemeny (2004), is the concept of social evaluative threat (SET) mentioned in Chapters 2 and 3. Social evaluation is part of everyday life interactions

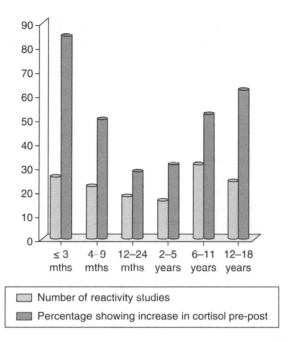

FIGURE 5.1 Successful cortisol reactivity studies by age group (up to 2012)

Source: Based on table 1 in Gunnar, Talge and Herrera (2009. 954), with additonal studies published between 2008 and 2012 accessed via Pubmed (search terms including reactivity, cortisol, children, stress test).

for adults and children, but is particularly poignant in children who may not yet have learnt useful ways of coping with a challenging experience. Children may be more likely to experience social evaluation as a threat to the self, possibly with long-lasting effects. Response to SET can be investigated under controlled laboratory conditions by exposing participants to social stress paradigms. We have already established that there are underlying developmentally driven influences on the diurnal pattern of cortisol, so given that the starting line naturally varies, we should not expect to have the same reactivity response across all ages of development. In an excellent review of stressor paradigm studies in children, Gunnar and colleagues (Gunnar, Talge and Herrera, 2009) identify a pattern in cortisol whereby the success of the stress test declines rapidly from infancy through to children of about 5 years of age. As Figure 5.1 demonstrates, in children 6–11 years old, the likelihood of being able to generate a cortisol response to a stressor starts to increase and continues to do so throughout adolescence (Gunnar, Talge and Herrera, 2009).

As Gunnar, Talge and Herrera (2009) point out, the reason for these age-related differences goes beyond the underlying developmental changes or dip in cortisol levels occurring in childhood. Some of the differences in findings may be attributable to the type of laboratory test or paradigm used and whether or not it is sufficiently meaningful to elicit a stress response (Gunnar, Talge and Herrera, 2009; Hunter et al., 2011). There are, of course, many practical and ethical considerations in conducting stress testing with children (see Chapter 3), including the practical importance of being able to obtain an accurate baseline cortisol response at the start of testing (Gunnar, Talge and Herrera, 2009). This is not an easy task, as sitting still and listening to the instructions of the researcher is unlikely to come naturally to children. Similarly, creating stress paradigms which are sufficient to elicit a response, yet are ethically sound, is a challenge to research with children. Most researchers agree that SET is an important element of a social stress test in eliciting cortisol and is increasingly so with older children (Gunnar, Talge and Herrera, 2009; Quesada et al., 2012). Threat to the child's social support system or closest attachments such as a parent are key stress-eliciting features of SET in children (Gunnar, Talge and Herrera, 2009). In many respects, the race is on to develop a reliable, ethically sound stressor paradigm for children that is developmentally appropriate yet equivalent in its ability to initiate the stress response across different age groups from early childhood through to adolescence and adulthood.

To make sure we are not attempting to reinvent the wheel on the subject of stress reactivity in children, let us look at what has been found, the components of different stress paradigms and some recent advances in this area. Some recent laboratory work has found cortisol reactivity in children pre-puberty, with a pattern similar to that found in adults. For example, cortisol reactivity has been elicited in children as young as 3 years old using a stress task adapted to include key social elements which elicit stress in adults. One such study, designed around a matching game, played at home under the watch of the experimenter, applied social comparison techniques (e.g., 'It's an easy task, even little children can do it') and reward incentives in the form of a toy prize (Kryski et al., 2011). As can be seen in Figure 5.2, these researchers found the typical quadratic effect for cortisol reactivity and recovery typically seen in adult responses to laboratory stress paradigms. This consists of an initial steep increase from baseline to 10 minutes after the start of the stress test, followed by a continued but smaller increase from 10 to 20 minutes, a minimal decline from 20 to 30 minutes, then a steeper decline from 30 to 40 minutes post-stressor.

Whilst social comparison and social evaluation overlap as concepts, they are not the same. The component of social evaluation itself has, however, for ethical and developmental reasons, been incorporated into stress tests only with children from the age of 7 years upwards. What constitutes SET in children is far from straightforward, and finding a meaningful child equivalent of the adult paradigm, which effectively elicits stress responses in children, has not proved to be a simple task. Innovative work by Yim and colleagues (2010) has directly compared acute stress responses in children aged 9–12 years with that of young adults (18–25 years) using a modified version of the adult Trier Social Stress Test (TSST-M) which contained the same tasks for both adults and children. Remember that the TSST is conducted in front of a panel of at least two experimenters and a video camera, and participants are required to perform a number task and to give a speech (see Chapter 2). In this study, they manipulated the speech task to incorporate SET relevant for both children and adults by asking them to talk about a school-based scenario in which they had to introduce themselves to a new class of students and, amongst other things, say why they would be liked. In doing so, they were able to elicit a similar, significant salivary cortisol response in children and adults with no significant difference between the two age groups, although the cortisol values for adults were higher overall than for the children. Also, as would be expected, sex differences in cortisol were observed in the adult group but not in the children. These researchers also separated out the children's group into younger children (9–10 years) and older children (11–12 years) in order to assess the effectiveness of the TSST-M across these different ages.

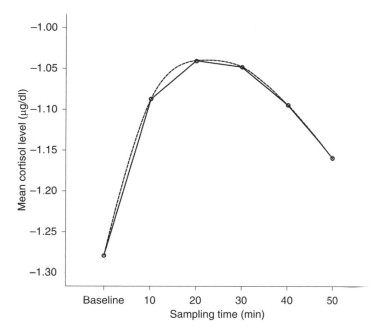

FIGURE 5.2   Mean child cortisol level as a function of cortisol sampling time

Source: Kryski et al. (2011:1132).

They found that both older and younger children independently elicited a significant cortisol response as shown in Figure 5.3 (Yim et al., 2010). This figure illustrates lower cortisol levels and responses in the younger children, rising with age towards puberty, as discussed earlier, although pubertal development was not directly assessed in this study.

Applications of children's versions of stressor paradigms have also been applied to combinations of stress experience. Of note are studies which have incorporated the impact of prior life stress in the naturalistic or real world environment (in other words, a measure of allostatic load or stress burden) on the ability to elicit the acute stress response in the laboratory. For example, work by Gunnar and colleagues (Gunnar, Frenn, et al., 2009) report evidence for stress hyporesponsivity to the TSST-C in 10–12-year-old adopted children in the US. However, this effect was only for those children who had previously experienced moderate amounts of early life stress as a result of overseas foster care who were then adopted before 8 months of age. This effect was not found for children who had experienced more severe early life stress either as a result of being adopted at the later age of one year or for older children following the experience of institutionalized orphanage care. Neither was the effect found in the non-adopted control children living with their birth parents and matched on their educational level and income (Gunnar, Frenn, et al., 2009). This implies that there is no simple dose–response relationship between life stress and response to subsequent stress. The authors suggest the interaction of individual factors and point to the plasticity of psychophysiological systems, the recognition of resiliency in the face of moderate adversity, and, equally, the negative effects of overprotective environments where minimal stress is experienced (Gunnar, Frenn, et al., 2009).

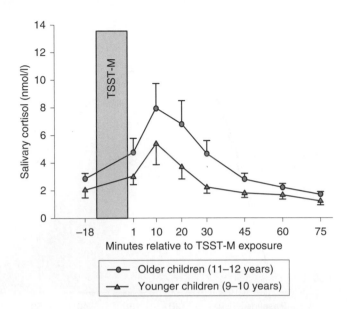

FIGURE 5.3   Older and younger children's salivary cortisol responses to the TSST-M

Source: Yim et al. (2010: 245)

Cortisol responses to acute laboratory stress in children have also been linked to memory. In a group of 8–10-year-olds, half of whom were exposed to stress using the TSST-C paradigm and half were not subjected to stress, Queseda and colleagues report poorer memory retrieval in those exposed to stress when the children were subsequently tested in a matching-pairs memory card game (Quesada et al., 2012). Yet effects are not always in the direction of high stress and poorer memory. Using the TSST-M, Quas and co-researchers (2011) cleverly assessed memory recall for events related to the test itself in a group of 9–12-year-old girls, by recalling participants to the laboratory 2 weeks after the stress test. They found that those who produced the greatest cortisol increases to the original test performed better on the memory test, indicating important links between emotion and memory for events (Quas et al., 2011). The TSST-C has also been applied to chronic illness populations in children. Comparing HPA axis responsivity between children with atopic inflammatory conditions, such as atopic dermatitis (aged 8–14 years) or allergic asthma (aged 7–12 years), and healthy age- and sex-matched controls, a blunted response has been reported for children with the inflammatory atopic condition compared to controls (Buske-Kirschbaum et al., 1997, 2003). These studies point to an underlying HPA axis dysregulation in children with allergic atopic conditions, a range of conditions whereby Th2 pro-inflammatory responses are overactivated and exacerbated by stress due to a dampened cortisol response or inability to mount a sufficient response to an acute stress challenge (see Buske-Kirschbaum, 2009).

STRESS REACTIVITY DURING ADOLESCENCE

Before concluding this section on stress reactivity to laboratory stressors and focusing on naturalistic stressors and stress paradigms, we need to consider the period of adolescence. During the teenage years, there is effectively a double or even a triple hit on the stress response system, since basal cortisol levels and stress reactivity show a marked increase, whilst, in addition, this is the period when the effects of early life stress or adversity may emerge. As clearly illustrated in their review of the life-cycle model of stress (Figure 5.4), Lupien et al. (2009) emphasize the vulnerability of the frontal cortex of the brain during adolescence as this brain region is still developing during these years. By way of contrast, the hippocampal region of the brain develops during the first couple of years of life, so whilst it may not be affected by stress during the adolescent years, early life stress may have already influenced development of this area of the brain, increasing stress vulnerability (Lupien et al., 2009).

In other words, adolescence is a critical, stress-sensitive period in which past and present exposure to life adversity are illuminated. Adolescence can be seen as a naked demonstration of the psychophysiological stress response in all its glory and, as such, provides a porthole for observation of the effects of accumulated childhood stress and state of HPA axis reactivity as well as some indication of future health outcomes. So what causes this change from a relatively stress-protected state of hypocortisolism in the childhood years to the state of hypercortisol reactivity in adolescence? One obvious candidate is adrenarche (see Chapter 2) and pubertal development, but whether this switch is due solely to the hormone-fuelled physiological changes occurring (e.g., surges in oestrogen and testosterone, DHEA and cortisol) or in part due to other age-related factors is under debate in the literature. Work by Hankin and colleagues (2010) provides a good example of this 'switch' in stress reactivity in a sample of children and adolescents aged 4–14 years, who were at risk for depression (as defined by subclinical behavioural symptoms). They report cortisol hyporeactivity in response to a stress task in the children aged 4–8 years, but a 'switch' to cortisol hyperreactivity in mid-adolescent children at aged 14 years, and attribute this to pubertal development (Hankin et al., 2010). Other work using the TSST-C or similar social stress tasks has also reported an increase in cortisol reactivity in adolescents aged 13–17 years compared to children in the age range 7–12 years (Gunnar, Wewerka, et al., 2009; Stroud et al., 2009; Sumter et al., 2010). Whilst some of this work suggests evidence of pubertal development being the agent of increased reactivity, only rarely is pubertal stage measured directly rather than assumed from age. In Gunnar's study (Gunnar, Wewerka, et al., 2009), pubertal maturation was directly measured in a sub-sample of the population and, interestingly, only a marginal correlation was reported with cortisol reactivity. In Sumter et al.'s study (2010), pubertal status and age were both associated with stress reactivity, but the relative contribution of one over the other could not be determined.

So the debate continues, but evidence weighs on the side of pubertal development (for review, see Dahl and Gunnar, 2009) with age as its proxy marker. Research which includes pubertal development as a variable has often lacked an accurate yet suitable measure of puberty staging acceptable to both participants and parents. Whilst self-report may for obvious reasons be the most suitable option, questions may be perceived as intrusive (e.g.,

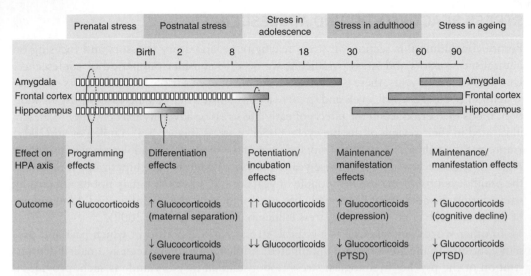

How the effects of chronic or repeated exposure to stress (or a single exposure to severe stress) at different stages in life depend on the brain areas that are developing or declining at the time of the exposure. Stress in the prenatal period affects the development of many of the brain regions that are involved in regulating the hypothalamus-pituitary-adrenal (HPA) axis – that is, the hippocampus, the frontal cortex and the amygdala (programming effects). Postnatal stress has varying effects: exposure to maternal separation during childhood leads to increased secretion of glucocorticoids, whereas exposure to severe abuse is associated with decreased levels of glucocorticoids. Thus, glucocorticoid production during childhood differentiates as a function of the environment (differentiation effects). From the prenatal period onwards, all developing brain areas are sensitive to the effects of stress hormones (broken white bars); however, some areas undergo rapid growth during a particular period (solid white bars). From birth to 2 years of age the hippocampus is developing; it might therefore be the brain area that is most vulnerable to the effects of stress at this time. By contrast, exposure to stress from birth to late childhood might lead to changes in amygdala volume, as this brain region continues to develop until the late 20s. During adolescence the hippocampus is fully organized, the amygdala is still developing and there is an important increase in frontal volume. Consequently, stress exposure during this period should have major effects on the frontal cortex. Studies show that adolescents are highly vulnerable to stress, possibly because of a protracted glucocorticoid response to stress that persists into adulthood (potentiation/incubation effects). In adulthood and during ageing the brain regions that undergo the most rapid decline as a result of ageing (tinted bars) are highly vulnerable to the effects of stress hormones. Stress during these periods can lead to the manifestation of incubated effects of early adversity on the brain (manifestation effects) or to maintenance of chronic effects of stress (maintenance effects). PTSD, post-traumatic stress disorder.

FIGURE 5.4   Life cycle of stress

Source: Lupien et al. (2009: 440, fig. 2).

asking about presence of pubertal hair). Advances in non-intrusive measurement of pubertal staging have emerged from the sports performance literature (Khamis and Roche, 1994) but have not as yet been used in the developmental psychobiological literature of the type examined above. In addition to the HPA axis response, two studies in this area (Stroud et al., 2009; Sumter et al., 2010) have also assessed SAM responses by measuring salivary alpha amylase (sAA). They have also manipulated the stress testing paradigm to incorporate aspects of social rejection (Stroud et al., 2009) or stress anticipation (Sumter et al., 2010) as these represent socially meaningful aspects of adolescence. Social exclusion was found to increase sAA response in adolescents compared to children (Stroud et al., 2009), but effects found by Sumter et al. (2010) for sAA during the stress task or in anticipation were less convincing. The notion of stress anticipation being of particular social relevance to adolescence was strongly supported, however, by the significant relationships found for cortisol reactivity during the anticipation phase of the task (Sumter et al., 2010). This provides evidence for meaningful SET in adolescence since anticipation of social evaluation was particularly salient in this age group.

Importantly, one point that these studies all agree on is the lack of gender effects in cortisol stress reactivity during adolescence. Stress reactivity using the TSST has been cleverly applied to adolescents aged 10–13 years who were assessed not only on their physical health symptoms but also on the degree of bullying they had received from their peers (Knack et al., 2011). Those who had been the victim of bullying responded to the stress test by showing a higher cortisol level immediately after the test and a faster drop during recovery 30 minutes later (Knack et al., 2011). In addition, those who had been bullied revealed a flatter cortisol awakening response (CAR) and poorer physical health (Knack et al., 2011). This study neatly combines laboratory stress reactivity to examine the effect of a naturalistic stressor in adolescence.

THE CONTRIBUTIONS OF TEMPERAMENT, INDIVIDUAL DIFFERENCE AND QUALITY OF CHILDCARE

THE NATURALISTIC ENVIRONMENT AND STRESS RESPONSIVITY IN CHILDREN

Work that has been conducted into the normal response to stress in otherwise healthy children has consistently made use of the experience of two types of environment which are both considered potential sources of stress in the naturalistic domain (i.e., experienced in the real world as opposed to experimentally induced in a laboratory). These are (i) childcare/daycare/preschool; and (ii) the transition to school (starting primary school/kindergarten) as well as changing schools (transitioning to senior or high school in the preteen years and adolescence). Both of these types of events have been used as examples of naturally occurring stressors which children in developed countries will experience as part of their daily life and which are expected to produce at least a temporary shift in the profile of stress hormones. This increase in stress hormones is expected as a natural response produced in order to cope with the new experiences and challenges brought about by the change in the physical and social environment. As detailed in Chapter 2, the important factor in relation to health outcome is the ability to adapt to the new environment within a relatively short space of time. A profile of reactivity followed by adaptability, as shown by a return to baseline or near baseline levels, means that stress hormones are produced when needed and return to 'normal' levels for that individual following adaptation. If you are really following this, then I hope you will have realized that what I have just described is somewhat of an oversimplification.

Nevertheless, I hope you are bursting with questions such as: How long after the event does the stress response switch off? Can the response switch off and on again and does this matter? What happens if the stress response continues? These are important questions which relate to the concepts of allostasis and allostatic load described in Chapter 2. To explore such questions, we need to look in depth at research findings from studies that have been conducted in two areas: the experience of childcare and the transition to school.

The experience of childcare

The notion of non-maternal care of a child seems to have the power to generate a range of diverse yet equally passionate views and opinions from couples with and without children, those who are single and those in partnered relationships, and cutting across different age groups of the population. You do not have to search far to find a media story which documents the untold psychobiological damage caused by the experience of childcare. With the increased demand for childcare, such stories were rife back in the 1980s and 1990s, and the quandary

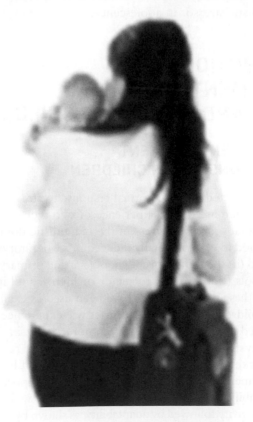

FIGURE 5.5   Working mother

Source: www.istockphoto.com/stock-photo-5920760-off-to-work.php?st=a13e6c3

over childcare continues today. There is no shortage of advice and discussion on parenting from a number of sources: I have noted two major, national radio programmes dedicated to discussion of whether or not mums should work and the issue of childcare quality in the past week alone, and dedicated Internet forums and resources abound on this topic (e.g., Mumsnet; see Figure 5.5). Apart from anything else, this tells us that, set amongst our economic, social and cultural needs, there is a biological and psychological drive towards rearing children in the best way possible, and that inadequate care of children creates fear, a natural fear that is easily provoked and often played upon by social media and product marketing.

Stepping aside from this fear-fuelled public image of childcare, what does research really indicate about the effects of childcare on the health and well-being of children? In line with the Lazarus and Folkman (1984) model of stress and coping described in Chapter 2, two interacting components are central to understanding the effects of the childcare experience. The first is the quality of care provided (conditions of the external environment) and the second is the temperament of the child (internal resources available). These two factors and their interaction account for the majority of the findings of both positive and negative effects of childcare and have been investigated by a number of researchers, most extensively by Gunnar and colleagues in the US. Rather than a decline in cortisol in the afternoon period, increases from morning to evening have been observed in children attending out-of-home-based childcare or home-based care of low quality compared to those receiving home-based care of high quality or no out-of-home care (Dettling et al., 2000; Watamura et al., 2003), as can be seen in Figure 5.6. This figure represents data from 61 children in the age range 0.5–14 years (average age 5.1 years). The steepest decline in cortisol across the day, usually associated with better health outcomes, is observed in home-based care of high quality. Interestingly, these effects appear not to be explained by family characteristics (Dettling et al., 2000).

Similarly, evidence has been found for the sensitivity of care across a range of different childcare contexts to be associated with the antibody-mediated immune response immunoglobulin A (IgA) measured in saliva (Vermeer et al., 2012). Regardless of whether the care context was in large or small groups of childrens, and the number of hours spent in childcare, it was the sensitivity of the caregiver(s) that influenced the immune response in this group of 68 toddlers. As shown in Figure 5.7, children receiving care which was rated lower on sensitivity (based on the emotional support provided by the carer) had lower levels of salivary IgA throughout the day compared with those whose carers provided more emotional support or sensitivity.

A combination of low-quality childcare interacting with child temperaments of negative affectivity (greater fear, anger, discomfort) and lower effortful control (less control over impulses, less able to sit quietly, more likely to call out inappropriately) has been associated with increases in cortisol across the day (Dettling et al., 2000). The temperament story is not a simple one, though, and far from being only the shy or more introverted children who show greater reactivity to attending childcare, cortisol increases have also been observed in the more exuberant or extroverted children (Watamura et al., 2003; Zimmermann and Stansbury, 2004). Gunnar and colleagues (2003) conceptualize the effect of temperament as having both direct and indirect effects on cortisol levels, as illustrated in Figure 5.8, based

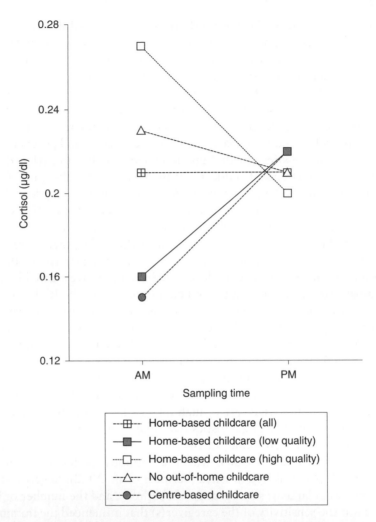

FIGURE 5.6 Morning to afternoon cortisol in children attending childcare
Source: Dettling et al. (2000: 831, fig. 2).

on a sample of 82 preschool-aged children (3–5-year-olds). In particular, the temperament combination of surgency, coupled with poorer ability to control impulses, seems to elicit negative behavioural consequences which increase the stressful experience for the child. The indirect effects are conceptualized as being mediated via behavioural factors, such as aggression shown by the child, which may lead to peer rejection towards the child (Gunnar et al., 2003). Thus, a scenario can be envisaged in which a more outgoing or surgent temperament is perceived as aggression by other children who, in turn, respond with social rejection which leads to an increase in the cortisol response of the child who is rejected, despite their attempts to be included. Equally, it could be explained that a shy child may find the social experience of childcare more stressful initially, but their less exuberant

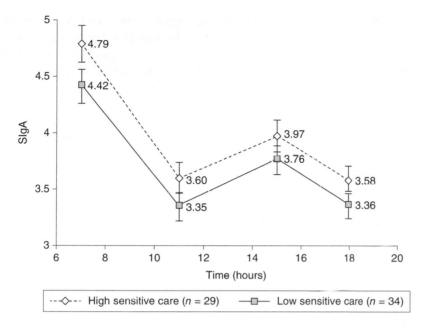

FIGURE 5.7   Salivary immunoglobulin A (sIgA) and childcare

Source: Vermeer et al. (2012: 165, fig. 2).

style of interaction may be more conducive towards acceptance by other children, and cortisol levels decrease with acceptance as a positive experience of the environment.

So, the simple answer to the complex question concerning the effects of childcare on physiological functioning is that good-quality childcare, matched to the temperament of the child, or at least accommodating of a range of temperaments and able to build social

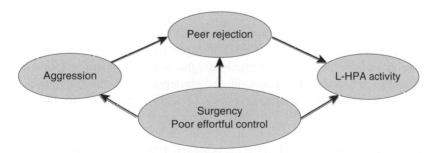

FIGURE 5.8   Conceptual model of the direct and indirect pathways from temperament (surgency and poor effortful control) to children's levels of cortisol in the classroom

Key: Surgency = impulsivity, exuberance, extroversion, sensation-seeking; effortful control = regulatory competence or impulse control.

Source: Gunnar et al. (2003).

competence, is not damaging. Given the obvious cognitive and social skills that group care offers, it may confer positive opportunities for child development. Few studies have measured the SAM system or cardiovascular activity in the preschool or daycare setting in order to assess the effect of this environment. Of note is a study which furthers this idea of positive childcare experiences and which was ahead of its time in this respect (Lundberg et al., 1993). These researchers compared SAM system indices of blood pressure, heart rate and adrenaline/ noradrenaline, as well as the HPA axis marker of cortisol, in a Swedish sample of 60 children assessed at the age of 3.5 years and 5.5 years. Quality of care was not directly assessed, but based on the socioeconomic status of the geographical areas sampled, the researchers assumed a high level of quality of care. They report a higher heart rate, greater levels of adrenaline and noradrenaline, and lower levels of cortisol on daycare days than at home weekend days for both age groups (Lundberg et al., 1993). They interpret these findings as daycare providing more challenge and social interaction for children in the context of an environment where they felt in control and, as a result, were able to experience stimulation and pleasure at day-care. Consistent with other studies in this area, sex differences were not found.

The transition to school

The other key life event for children that has been used as a marker for understanding stress responses is the experience of the transition to school (Figure 5.9), since this is a potential social stressor for the majority of children in developed countries, albeit at slightly different ages (e.g., the age of 4 years plus in the UK, and the age of 5 years plus in the US). In fact, entering school has been described as representing 'a useful and accessible model for study-ing stress effects in normal children' (Boyce, Adams, et al., 1995: 1014). Just as in the social stress laboratory experiments, the experience of starting school represents a social stressor fully armed with social evaluation experiences from peers and teachers and novel social, cognitive and physical challenges. Starting school is a child's first formal experience of edu-cation, and may present a range of unpredictable and uncontrollable demands. What hap-pens at a physiological level during the school transition is of interest theoretically as a window on early stress reactivity in the natural environment. It also has practical utility in assessing whether the responses are normal and, indeed, necessary or if there is sufficient disruption of the cardiovascular, endocrine or immune response to warrant health concerns.

Work conducted in the 1990s identified upregulation and downregulation of different immune processes in 5-year-olds transitioning to kindergarten (in the US), but all within the normal range expected for that age group (Boyce, Chesney, et al., 1995; see Box 5.1 for more detail about this study). In parallel with the childcare literature, temperament and individual differences have been reported as key variables in understanding the stress experience of starting school and cortisol as an important biomarker of this experience. Other work by Boyce and colleagues (Boyce, Adams, et al., 1995) examined cortisol as a predictor of immune changes in the transition to kindergarten. They found cortisol increases at school transition to be consistent with a shift away from cell-mediated immunity (Th1) towards antibody-medi-ated immunity (Th2), and children whose mothers were more highly educated showed greater cortisol reactivity. Other factors influencing the extent of the stress response at school transition include the related factors of degree of similarity between preschool and school

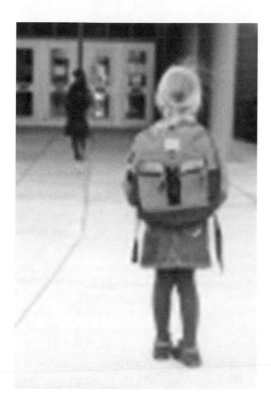

FIGURE 5.9   Child starting school

Source: www.istockphoto.com/stock-photo-6114929-first-day-of-school.php?st=2bd1af6

experience, parental expectations about how starting school would affect the child, and the amount of time previously spent in preschool (Boyce, Adams, et al., 1995). Longitudinal work in our research group has examined cortisol in children transitioning to reception class at the age of 4 years, the first formal school year in the UK (Turner-Cobb et al., 2008). Controlling for previous childcare experience and life events, we followed children from 4 to 6 months before they started school, assessed them again at the end of the first week of school, then tracked any episodes of the common cold during the first 6 months of school and assessed them again at the end of those 6 months, measuring diurnal salivary cortisol, temperament and behavioural adaptation. Unexpectedly, we found an anticipatory increase in mean diurnal cortisol levels up to 6 months before starting school, as well as an expected rise in cortisol at the start of school itself, followed by an adaptive decline in cortisol levels 6 months later, shown in Figure 5.10 (Turner-Cobb et al., 2008).

In line with previous work, we found children with more extrovert or impulsive temperaments to have higher cortisol levels, and support for an interaction between the temperament of extroversion and the adaptive behaviour of internalizing social isolation (Turner-Cobb et al., 2008). In this moderation effect, children who were high on surgency/extroversion, and who had a greater increase in internalizing social isolation across the 6 months after starting school, had the highest cortisol levels at 6 months after starting school. Again, this represents

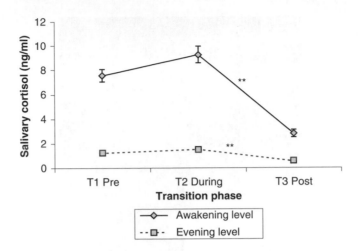

FIGURE 5.10   Salivary cortisol levels in the transition to school study: the mean (+/–s.e.m.) salivary cortisol values are given for each time point, with awakening and evening diurnal values represented separately; * p = 0.014; ** p <0.001 (using Bonferroni correction criteria p <0.016); placement of asterisks indicates significance between time points separately for a.m. and p.m. cortisol

Source: Turner-Cobb et al. (2008: fig. 1).

the congruency/incongruency between the environment and the coping resources associated with temperament, reflected in ability or inability to adapt over time.

Prenatal stress was considered at length in Chapter 4, but it is worth noting here in relation to starting school that evidence exists for prenatal stress exposure as a predictor of cortisol reactivity in 5-year-old children starting their second year of schooling (Gutteling, de Weerth and Buitelaar, 2005). This is a good example of early stress effects being observable in the response to a life event, in this case a longitudinal period of over 5 years.

So, starting school provides a point of assessment for stress reactivity which also provides an indication of accumulated life stress or early life adversity up until that point. Additionally, it also provides a useful point of assessment of health outcome as an indication of the physical impact of neuroendocrine and immune effects observed and prediction of future health. In our transition to school study described above, we also found that higher evening cortisol, and less of a decline in cortisol across the day at school transition (measured 2 weeks after starting school), were associated not with more colds but with fewer colds over the following first 6 months of school (Turner-Cobb et al., 2011). In other words, the acute stress experience of starting school appeared to enhance rather than suppress the immune response to upper respiratory tract infections. This finding is consistent with work in the adult stress literature and work in animals which supports the notion of upregulation of immune response under acute stress conditions (Selye, 1976a and b; Dhabhar and McEwen, 1997; Dhabhar et al., 2010). We also found preliminary evidence for the timing of illness since higher evening cortisol at transition was associated with poorer resistance to infection during the school holidays compared to term time.

Other work looking at the experience of starting school has examined not the first transition to formal schooling but, instead, the stress of a new school year. Similar effects have been found to those of school transition but to a lesser extent, with children (aged 6 years through to 12 years) showing an increase in cortisol on the first day of a new school year which declines by the fifth day of school (Davis et al., 1999; Bruce et al., 2002). This can be interpreted as an indication of adjustment to stress and a reduction in the challenge presented. However, in line with temperament and cortisol responses described above, cortisol reactivity was greatest not for shy or fearful children (termed high internalizers), but instead for the more extroverted children (Davis et al., 1999) and these effects have also been reported to continue through to the fifth day of school (Bruce et al., 2002).

EFFECTS OF CHILDCARE STRESS ON PHYSICAL HEALTH OUTCOME

So we know that cortisol levels can be affected by the quality of the childcare experience, and that, even in the environment of good-quality care, responses vary according to temperament. Yet what does this mean for physical health outcome? When it comes to physical health, there is relatively little research which has examined how the experience of childcare might increase or decrease the likelihood of developing physical health symptoms.

A particularly notable birth cohort study, conducted by Ball and colleagues (2002), examined the effects of childcare on upper respiratory tract infection in children attending daycare, and followed them through preschool and into formal schooling up until the age of 13 years. What they found was that, in comparison with children who were looked after at home with no unrelated children also cared for, children who attended larger group childcare with at least six other unrelated children were more likely to have a cold in their second year of life (Ball et al., 2002). However, by the age of 6 years, having attended larger-group childcare gave them some protection against upper respiratory tract illness compared to children who had been cared for at home during the first 3 years of life, and this protection continued up until the age of 11 years. Frequency of colds was the same for all children by the age of 13 years. There were also no differences between at-home and smaller-group care (defined as up to five other unrelated children). These researchers attribute the protection to increases in acquired immunity due to viral exposure in the larger daycare group, and psychosocial factors were not assessed. Nonetheless, the results show that daycare confers increased vulnerability for colds in the preschool years, but an increased protection or advantage in the childhood years preteen. It is possible that this increased protection was in part due to stress resilience developed during primary and junior school years following exposure to the social stress of daycare in the preschool years.

More recent work has reported lower cortisol levels in young adults who had a greater incidence of upper respiratory infection in the first 5 years of life (Vedhara et al., 2007). This is interpreted as evidence of postnatal programming on the HPA axis and, whilst contrary to the idea of difficulties in early life resulting in increased HPA axis activity, one explanation put forward is that increased illness in childhood leads to increased maternal caregiving behaviour which strengthens attachment processes and reduces later-life adrenocortical responses (Vedhara et al., 2007). Box 5.1 highlights a dual armed study which compares the influence of childcare stress and family stress on cardiovascular and immune reactivity and susceptibility to the common cold in a sample of 3–5-year-olds (Boyce, Chesney, et al., 1995).

BOX 5.1

Highlight on stress reactivity and the common cold

Source: W.T. Boyce, M. Chesney, A. Alkon, J.M. Tschann, S. Adams, B. Chesterman and D. Wara (1995) Psychobiologic reactivity to stress and childhood respiratory illnesses: results of two prospective studies. *Psychosomatic Medicine*, 57(5): 411–22.

Study rationale: Children experiencing greater adversity and responding to that adversity with a greater stress response are likely to have a compromised immune system which will increase their susceptibility to respiratory infection.

Hypothesis: 'Psychobiologically reactive children would have higher rates of respiratory illnesses, but only under conditions of high environmental stress.'

Research design: The researchers used two complementary study designs to explore this rationale and test this hypothesis: the first utilized a sample of 137 children aged 3–5 years attending centre-based childcare, and conducted a laboratory-based stressor paradigm plus a longitudinal assessment of childcare stressors and physical health; the second utilized 99 children aged 5 years who were transitioning to kindergarten, and conducted a field study of family stressors and illness occurrence.

In study 1, they assessed cardiovascular reactivity (heart rate and arterial pressure) in the laboratory; childcare hassle stress was measured every 2 weeks by the childcare personnel, and quality of care facility was assessed by the researchers; symptoms of respiratory infection were assessed by a paediatric nurse practitioner on site at the childcare facility.

In study 2, they assessed immune reactivity by taking a blood sample 1 week before and then within 2 weeks after starting kindergarten. During the first visit, the children also received the pneumococcal vaccine (routine school entry immunization to protect against developing pneumonia). They looked at numbers of cellular immune markers CD4+, CD8+, CD19+, lymphocyte responses to poke week mitogen, and antibody response mounted to the vaccine.

Stress was assessed through questionnaire: in study 1 measuring childcare-related hassle stress, and in study 2 measuring stressful life events in the family during the previous year and conflict in the family environment.

Upper respiratory illness was assessed over a period of 6 months in both studies: weekly by a paediatric nurse practitioner in childcare during study 1, and biweekly by parental report in study 2 recording symptoms of respiratory infection.

Age and sex were used as covariates in study 1, but were not indicated for inclusion in study 2.

Results: There was no direct association between stress and illness but, as predicted, interactions were found between physiologically reactive children and the level of stress in their environment on illness outcome:

Study 1: childcare stress and mean arterial pressure (MAP, cardiovascular reactivity; see Figure 5.11a).

Study 2: Life event stress and CD19+ (immune reactivity; see Figure 5.11b).

Overall conclusions: stress (childcare hassles or family life events) was directly associated with illness (upper respiratory infection) only for reactive (immune or cardiovascular) children such that:

(a)

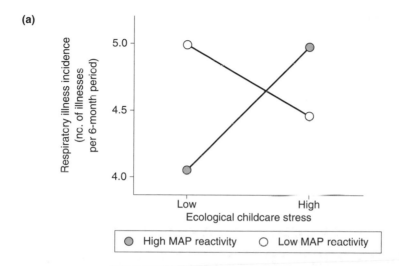

(b)

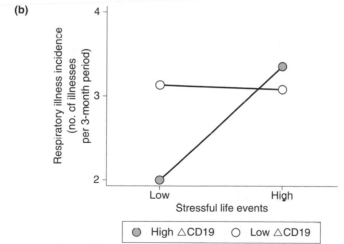

FIGURE 5.11 (a) Study 1: Interaction between ecological childcare stress and mean arterial pressure (MAP) reactivity in prediction of respiratory illness. (b) Study 2: Interaction between environmental stress and immune reactivity in prediction of respiratory illness

Source: Boyce, Chesney et al. (1995: 416, fig 1; 418, fig. 3).

(Continued)

(Continued)

1   High reactivity children showed higher rates of illness if in a high-stress environment
2   Low reactivity children did not show higher rates of illness even in a high-stress environment
3   Illness rates were lowest when high reactivity children were in a low-stress environment.

Implications of these findings: Children who are high physiological reactors represent a subset for whom high-stress environments provide particular vulnerability in terms of ill health. The authors term this a sustained 'hyperdynamic biological response' present in a subgroup of children. In essence, the data reported represent potential for psychological intervention to minimize the stressful context, whether this context is childcare or school transition, for children who have a particular vulnerability as seen by their greater physiological reactivity.

EFFECTS OF SEVERE OR TOXIC STRESS, INCLUDING POST-TRAUMATIC STRESS DISORDER

In addition to the response of healthy children to mild and moderately stressful events, we can turn to studies in which the stressor is of a much greater magnitude. Research has shown that even 'subtle' forms of child maltreatment, defined as frequent smacking or maternal emotional withdrawal, whether intentional or not, may be associated with increased basal cortisol and cortisol reactivity (for review, see Bugental et al., 2003). When it comes to more severe stress exposure, there is a wealth of literature to support the link between early childhood maltreatment and psychopathology (see Dahl and Gunnar, 2009). Our focus, however, is on the physiological effects and health outcomes that are associated with severe or extreme stress in childhood. The impact of extreme or toxic stress on physiological functioning may include cases where the stressful event or maltreatment is sufficiently severe to require psychiatric or psychological diagnosis or intervention.

The maternal environment, in particular maternal depression or distress, has been the subject of much scrutiny in understanding stress in the home environment and subsequent physiological consequences and health effects (Lupien et al., 2000; Ashman et al., 2002). For example, disruptions in circadian cortisol have been reported in a sample of 7–8-year-old children of clinically depressed mothers (Ashman et al., 2002). This study used an ingenious task in which children were asked to imagine they were flying a spaceship which was in danger of being hit by asteroids. Collision with an asteroid was, in fact, a puff of air against their throat sufficient to generate a startle response and an expected acute rise in cortisol. They report that a combination of internalizing symptoms in the child (more anxious and withdrawn) and a history of depression in the mother significantly predicted

EXPERIENCE OF STRESS DURING CHILDHOOD

elevated cortisol in the child, and maternal depression in the first 2 years of life was the best predictor of baseline cortisol at the age of 7 years (Ashman et al., 2002). Interestingly, one study has reported an increase in cortisol levels in over 503 children aged 7–8 years exposed to maternal distress (defined as clinically evaluated anxiety or depression) during the first year of life and, additionally, in those children who were exposed to maternal distress beyond one year, higher levels of cortisol were only observed in children without asthma whilst those with asthma had a decreased cortisol level (Dreger et al., 2010). This is important as it suggests chronic HPA axis activation which has led to a suppression of the glucocorticoid response mechanisms, implicated in the development and maintenance of atopic disorders such as asthma (Dreger et al., 2010).

Exposure to maternal postnatal depression during childhood has also been linked to raised or more variable morning cortisol in adolescents at 13 years (Halligan et al., 2004). As raised cortisol levels are associated with depression, this is indicated as a mechanism through which psychopathology may be transferred across the generations (Halligan et al., 2004). This longitudinal effect of stress in early childhood has been described as a 'lingering influence' on antibody profiles (Shirtcliff et al., 2009). Demonstrated in a group of 9–14-year-olds who had suffered physical abuse or who had been institutionalized shortly after birth then later adopted, latent antibodies to herpes simplex virus (HSV) type 1 were higher than in controls (Shirtcliff et al., 2009).

Childhood maltreatment or abuse, whether physical, emotional or sexual, has also been a key area of research in understanding the effects of severe stress on physiological functioning and health outcome. Whilst stress is associated with an increase in cortisol levels, a paradoxically lower level of cortisol has been frequently observed in the adult post-traumatic stress disorder (PTSD) literature (for review, see Heim et al., 2000) and can be theorized as the third type of allostatic load indicating an inadequate response (McEwen, 1998b; see Chapter 2). In children, however, the glucocorticoid landscape must also take into account the temporal aspect in order to decipher the meaning of the physiological response patterns found. For example, some research looking at maltreated children has found the most severely maltreated children to show an elevated morning (9 a.m.) cortisol level (Cicchetti and Rogosch, 2001). Similarly, Carrion et al. (2002) have reported a heightened evening cortisol response in 7–14-year-old children, particularly in girls, with a history of trauma (including one or more of separation and loss, physical abuse, witnessing violence, sexual or emotional abuse, and physical neglect) and PTSD symptoms. Also, work by Gunnar and colleagues mentioned above (Gunnar and Vazquez, 2001; Gunnar et al., 2001) has found similar patterns of cortisol elevation in 6–12-year-old adopted children who spent at least the first 8 months of life institutionalized in substandard Romanian orphanages, with a flatter decline across the day (see Figure 5.12). Interestingly, cortisol levels in children adopted at or before the age of 4 months did not show this elevated pattern. This hypercortisolaemic pattern may be a precursor to adult hypocortisolism, depending on the severity of the experience and the effectiveness of any intervention sought. Yet low cortisol responsivity or hypocortisolaemic states characteristic of adult PTSD have also been seen to emerge in childhood (e.g., in girls aged 5–7 years who had experienced recent sexual abuse; King et al., 2001). For a review of this area, see Tarullo and Gunnar (2006). Furthermore, adult

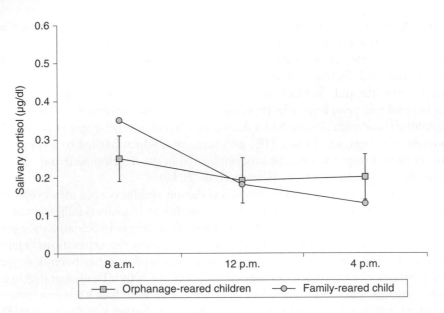

FIGURE 5.12   Effects of orphanage experience on diurnal cortisol levels in children

Source: Gunnar, M.R. (2000) Early adversity and the development of stress reactivity and regulation. In C.A. Nelson (ed.), *The Minnesota Symposium on Child Psychology: Vol. 31.The effects of early adversity on neurobehavioral development* (pp. 163–200). Mahwah, NJ: Lawrence Erlbaum. Reprinted with permission. Permission conveyed through Copyright Clearence Centre, Inc.

women (18–61 years old) who experienced physical abuse as a child have been found to display a blunted response to the TSST laboratory paradigm, even after controlling for depression and anxiety (Carpenter et al., 2011).

FAMILY ENVIRONMENT AND INTERGENERATIONAL TRANSMISSION OF STRESS

The childcare environment is, of course, not the only major environment that the child is exposed to, and should not be thought of in isolation when considering the effect of environment and experience on child health. It will come as no surprise that the home environment also plays a major role in the stress–health relationship. A major sociological study by Flinn and England (1997) longitudinally followed 264 children (aged from 2 months to 18 years) living in Bwa Mawego, an isolated rural village on the island of Dominica, across a 9-year period. They report social relationships, particularly the family unit, as one of the key influencing factors in the link between stress and health, driven by socioeconomic conditions. Interestingly, they articulate the damaging effects of 'unstable mating relationships of parents/caretakers and household composition' (Flinn and England, 1997: 33). Elevated, depressed, or unusual cortisol profiles were observed in environmental conditions such as unstable, difficult living environments, family conflict and traumatic events (parent absence or residence change).

Work in our group has examined the interaction between childcare and home environment. In a study of 56 mothers and their children (aged 3–4.5 years), we found evidence of higher cortisol in children whose mothers had lower job satisfaction or higher emotional exhaustion (a dimension of 'burnout') associated with their job (Chryssanthopoulou et al., 2005). As illustrated in Figures 5.13 and 5.14, we found that, in children whose mothers were more exhausted, spending more time in childcare was associated with lower cortisol levels. Moderate at-home levels of family expressiveness were associated with lower cortisol and lack of expressiveness or high levels of expressiveness with higher cortisol in the children. In other words, for those with high family stress at home (in the form of parental emotional exhaustion, or high or low levels of family expressiveness), the experience of childcare was beneficial in preventing hypercortisol responses (Chryssanthopoulou et al., 2005).

The chronic lower respiratory disease, asthma, is an atopic Th2 condition which is common in childhood, although can improve during adolescence and into adulthood. The balance of Th2 cytokine profile in early childhood may help to explain this age-related cytokine shift (see Chapter 2). The role of psychosocial factors in childhood asthma has been considered frequently in the literature. In a recent example, Wolf and colleagues (2008) reported higher levels of perceived stress in parents of 8–18-year-old children with asthma to predict larger increases in the production of IL-4 (Th2 cytokine) than in healthy control children over a period of 6 months. Other work supports the mechanism of Th2

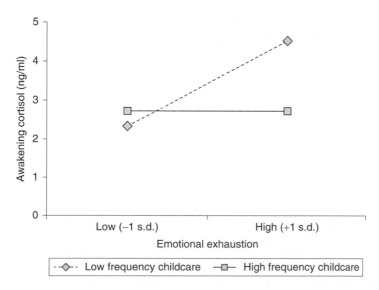

FIGURE 5.13 Interaction between frequency of childcare attendance and maternal emotional exhaustion in the prediction of awakening cortisol

Source: Chryssanthopoulou et al. (2005: 362, fig. 3).

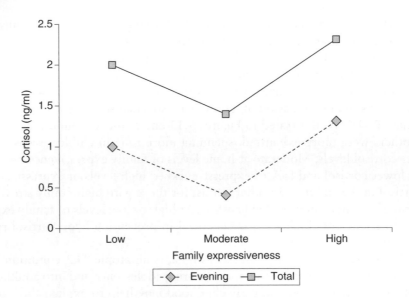

FIGURE 5.14   Mean evening and total levels of cortisol as a function of family expressiveness
Source: Chryssanthopoulou et al. (2005: 362, fig. 1).

cytokine increase in asthma under stressful conditions. For example, Marin and co-workers (2009) extended these findings to include the interactive effects of underlying chronic family stress, coupled with acute stress events, in inducing asthma symptoms and associated inflammatory Th2 profile (including IL-4 and IL-5) in children aged 9–18 years. They suggest a mechanism of HPA axis and SAM system activation over time, leading to a downregulation of the stress response in asthma, which enables and maintains the Th2 inflammatory cytokine imbalance (Marin et al., 2009). Low socioeconomic status at the age of 2–3 years has been found to be critical in influencing pro-inflammatory markers of gene expression (including glucocorticoid receptors) in adolescence (Miller et al., 2007). Citing this as evidence of the mechanism through which respiratory infection and cardiovascular disease may be influenced by stress, the authors also point out that these effects were not able to be reversed in later childhood if socioeconomic status improved (Miller et al., 2007).

The concept of intergenerational transmission of stress has been discussed in Chapter 3 on pregnancy and is relevant again here. Work by Yehuda and colleagues has found evidence of low cortisol in adult children of Holocaust survivors, indicating an intergenerational vulnerability for stress transmission particularly via mothers rather than fathers (Yehuda et al., 2000, 2001, 2008). A super-suppression of the cortisol response to dexamethasone, indicating the paradoxically low cortisol profile seen in PTSD, has been observed in a sample of young adult women in their twenties and thirties who had a history of child sexual or physical abuse in addition to an adult diagnosis of major depression. In comparison, non-abused women in the control group and abused women without a diagnosis of depression or those with depression but no childhood abuse did not show this super-suppression of cortisol (Newport et al., 2004). As with some of the other evidence we have considered, these intergenerational effects show evidence that early life adversity can create a physiological vulnerability in later life. The loss of a parent during childhood (between the ages of 3 and 15 years) has been associated with higher diurnal salivary cortisol, particularly the awakening sample, compared to a control group, who were similar on scores for anxiety and depression, in young to middle-aged adult men at age 28–55 years (Nicolson, 2004). We return to the subject of loss during childhood in more detail in Chapter 10.

HEALTH IN ADULTHOOD AND ACROSS THE LIFESPAN

From the literature reviewed so far in this chapter, there is evidence that early life experience, during the childhood years, can mould our physiological responses and possibly set our neuroendocrine and immune level of responsivity at a heightened or dampened state, at least temporarily, which, in turn, may influence our physical health status. But what about the longer-term consequences viewed from the life-course perspective that was introduced in Chapter 1? We have noted some more immediate or shorter-term effects and health outcomes during childhood and adolescence, but what about the effects of this early life stress on outcomes into adulthood? Central to this is the question of how much flexibility (or, to use the biological term, 'plasticity') exists within our physiological systems to adapt to, or compensate for, early life adversity. If you have read the preceding chapters, then these questions should be causing your own hippocampal neurons to fire excitedly and make the link with the theory of allostasis and the concept of allostatic load which fit perfectly with such questions. The effects of early adversity or maltreatment have frequently been referred to as 'casting a long shadow' (e.g., Kiecolt-Glaser et al., 2011), but exactly how far-reaching are these effects?

In a review of child abuse and its effects into adulthood, Wegman and Stetler (2009) conclude that the increased risk of child maltreatment on poorer physical health in adulthood is 'comparable' to that of maltreatment and psychological health outcomes. They point to the need for more rigorous methodologies in understanding these links and which factors may moderate the relationship with health. There is clearly a keen and growing research interest in this area, assessing the effects of early trauma experience on a range of illnesses, encouraged by recent advances in health-related biomarkers. For example, in a sample of 444 African American men and women (average age 28 years) with type 1 insulin-dependent diabetes (T1D), childhood abuse, using the Childhood Trauma Questionnaire (CTQ), was associated with an increased risk for developing cardiovascular or coronary heart disease (Roy et al., 2010). Similarly, in a cross-sectional study of men and women aged 18–50 years, self-reported emotional or sexual abuse, emotional neglect or severe abuse, measured using the CTQ, was significantly higher in patients with multiple sclerosis compared to healthy controls (Spitzer et al., 2012). The study implicates childhood abuse in adult onset of multiple sclerosis, although no evidence was found for severity of the condition as measured by level of disability (Spitzer et al., 2012). Whilst these two studies include younger adult age groups, there is variability across the ages of participants with overlaps into middle age or middle adulthood. Other studies have specifically examined patient groups in middle age. For example, in an assessment of early trauma experiences in women aged 40 years and above (mean age 53–58 years) with the chronic pain conditions of fibromyalgia or osteoarthritis, higher self-reported CTQ scores were associated with greater diurnal salivary cortisol, when sampled at 10 a.m., 4 p.m. and 8 p.m. and averaged over an impressive 30-day period (Nicolson et al., 2010). The implication from this study is that onset and severity of the condition may be linked to early childhood experience and that early abuse may be mediated by alterations in HPA axis functioning. This, in turn, has implications for intervention.

Inflammation is another important physiological marker that has been implicated as an effect of early trauma. C-reactive protein (CRP), an inflammatory marker associated with atherosclerosis and heart disease, appears key to this process. In a group of men and women, with a mean age of 42.2 years, CRP was found to be significantly higher in those who were recorded as having poorer emotional functioning (defined as inappropriate self-regulation and prone to distress) at the age of 7 years (Appleton et al., 2011). Racial differences in immune markers of inflammatory response have been reported in middle-aged adults who experienced early life adversity (Slopen et al., 2010). Higher concentrations across a range of inflammatory biomarkers, including C-reactive protein and IL-6, were observed in African Americans but not in white Americans in a sample of men and women aged 35–86 years (Slopen et al., 2010). The authors attribute this to social factors (e.g., living and working conditions) which have developed as a result of early life adversity contributing to an accelerated development of age-related disease (Slopen et al., 2010). This factor of accelerated ageing was explored in greater detail in a study by Kiecolt-Glaser et al. (2011), who directly assessed cell ageing through assessment of chromosomal telomere length, as well as assessing inflammation via IL-6 and tumour necrosis factor (TNF) alpha in a sample of Alzheimer caregivers and controls (mean age 69.7 years). After controlling for caregiving status, they found that the experience of multiple adversities during childhood (including parental death, severe marital problems or psychiatric illness in a family member) was associated with higher levels of IL-6 and shorter telomeres at this older stage of the life course compared to those who had not experienced any CTQ-defined adversity (Kiecolt-Glaser et al., 2011), as shown in Figure 5.15. What is most astounding about this study is that the reduction in adult telomere length amongst those with early trauma was projected to reduce lifespan by between 7 and 15 years. Furthermore, they also report that whilst TNF-alpha and IL-6 were higher in those who had experienced early life trauma (using the CTQ abuse scales), if this trauma was then followed by the impact of caregiving, then TNF-alpha levels were even higher (Kiecolt-Glaser et al., 2011). In other words, this study is another example of the effect of compound stress, similar to the double stressor impact or 'stress mosaic' examples referred to above.

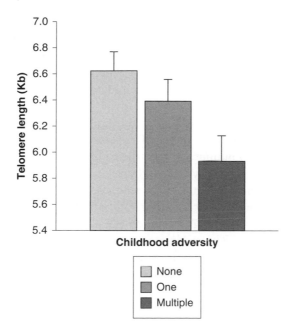

FIGURE 5.15   Childhood adversity and telomere length

Source: Kiecolt-Glaser et al. (2011: 3, fig. 1). Wolters Kluwer Health January 1, 2011. Copyright © 2011, Wolters Kluwer Health.

COMMUNICATING STRESS

Of note in many studies of stress is a disparity between the subjective level of stress reported or perceived and the physiological level of stress assessed via a biomarker such as cortisol. There may be many reasons for this, including unconscious misinterpretation or non-acceptance of emotions related to an event or, in some cases, perhaps deliberate concealment of the real impact of the effect of stress. Some events are too stressful to communicate easily, or social pressure (from parents, peers or teachers) may inhibit open communication. Being able to obtain a biological marker of stress could be considered a more definitive way of assessing the true extent of the effect of a stressful encounter or experience. Whilst this may not always be possible, what many of the studies above indicate is that children experience stress from a whole range of events and that the biological responses to them are important for both short-term and longer-term adaptation and health. Individual differences and age effects create differing responses to stressful experiences, and detecting stress in children includes sensitive interpretation of emotional and behavioural indicators.

An ongoing online survey and interview study of more than 1,000 adults and over 1,000 children aged 8–17 years, conducted by the American Psychological Association (APA) and led by Professor Norman Anderson (Anderson et al., 2010), has examined stress and health in the US (known as 'Stress in America'). In this survey, nearly one-third of the children reported having physical health symptoms of headaches, stomach aches or sleep problems associated with stress in the past month (Anderson et al., reported in Clay, 2011). One of the most telling aspects of this survey is the underestimation by parents of stress in their children. Whilst a large majority (69 per cent) of parents reported that their own stress had no impact or little impact on their children, only a small proportion of the children (14 per cent) reported that their parents' stress did not bother them (Anderson et al., reported in Clay, 2011). This is clearly a communication mismatch, possibly bidirectional, between parents and children. From the child's perspective, one of the authors states that 'it is critical that parents communicate with their children about how to identify stress triggers and manage stress in healthy ways' (Nordal, in Anderson et al., 2010).

So how do children know when their parents are stressed? According to this study, over a third of children report that a parent yelling is a sign of stress (Anderson et al., 2010). One source of stress commonly cited during childhood and adolescence is that of appearance and weight issues. This study found that children who described themselves as overweight also reported more worry in general and were more concerned about their appearance (Anderson et al., 2010). Evidence was seen for a vicious spiral of events, with overweight children responding in a less healthy way in their behavioural response to stress, managing their negative emotions through eating or inactivity (Anderson et al., reported in Clay, 2011). For more on the relationship between chronic stress and obesity during adolescence, see De Vriendt et al. (2009).

THE LONGER-TERM OUTLOOK AND OPPORTUNITIES FOR INTERVENTION

The crucial question is whether the HPA axis can be 'normalized' or at least altered to some degree through psychological intervention. Some of the work covered in this chapter demonstrates the importance of critical periods of development, such as the early years, for effective intervention (Coe and Lubach, 2003; Gunnar and Fisher, 2006) before the physiological impact becomes 'hard wired'. Early years' intervention initiatives, such as Sure Start in the UK and Head Start in the US, are aimed at prevention rather than cure, and seek to counteract the effects of disadvantage through parental support, starting in the prenatal period, coupled with childcare and an enriched learning environment for children through to school entry. A recent APA report (Novotney, 2010) highlights the impact of the economic recession on children in America and the success of a cognitive learning intervention programme developed by Leong and Bodrova, and tested and implemented by Diamond and colleagues (2007).

As seen above, there is also much potential for intervention to have an impact not only in the early years of childhood but also during the vulnerable period of adolescence (Dahl, 2004). The full extent of childhood stress on physiological functioning and the plasticity of the endocrine and immune system in adaptation to accumulated lifetime stress and its impact on physical health are still in the early stages of research. Early indications are that there is much potential for intervention if the key elements, such as those outlined in this chapter, are incorporated and outcomes accurately tested, particularly with the insight and application of new biomarkers. An increased understanding of the longitudinal impact of early life stress on adult health may result in more effective interventions to improve physical health across the life course (see Braveman and Barclay, 2009; Shonkoff et al., 2009).

CHAPTER SUMMARY

In this chapter, I have taken the life course approach referred to in previous chapters and applied it very directly to the effects of stress experienced during childhood. We considered different degrees of stress, from mild to severe, and examined both the shorter and longer physical health effects. In doing this we considered both acute laboratory stressors and naturalistic field studies examining stress in the real world environment. Implications for stress reactivity and adaptability were highlighted as central to the notion of stress having potent effects across the life course trajectory. We also considered the important role of sociodemographic, family, and individual differences. A range of stressors were considered but child care and starting school were used as key examples of naturalistic stressors. Much work, particularly in laboratory stress testing, has focused around the early years of childhood as a critical period for future health outcomes. In the current research landscape, interest in puberty and adolescence is gaining momentum as a critical period in development when stress-related illnesses may begin to emerge or when the influence of stress may shape health outcomes in later life. Stress is clearly a phenomenon that affects children but we also identified that communication about stress is often inadequate. Interventions to prevent or reduce stress offer a route to improving health across the life course, particularly if the gap between experience of stress and communication about it can be improved. This chapter concludes the first part of this book which has focused on the experience of stress and its contribution to health outcomes across the life course. In the second part we now turn to consider the experience of illness itself during childhood.

KEY CONCEPTS AND ISSUES

- Early life adversity
- Social comparison/social evaluation
- Life cycle of stress
- Stress vulnerability
- Cortisol hyporeactivity (childhood)
- Cortisol hyperreactivity (adolescence)
- Stress anticipation, responsivity and adaptation
- Childcare environment/school transition
- HPA axis normalization

FURTHER READING

Excellent review articles with a life-course perspective:

Hunter, A.L., Minnis, H. and Wilson, P. (2011) Altered stress responses in children exposed to early adversity: a systematic review of salivary cortisol studies. *Stress: The International Journal on the Biology of Stress*, 14(6): 614–26.

Lupien, S.J., McEwen, B.S., Gunnar, M.R. and Heim, C. (2009) Effects of stress throughout the lifespan on the brain, behaviour and cognition. *Nature Reviews Neuroscience*, 10(6): 434–45.

Tarullo, A.R. and Gunnar, M.R. (2006) Child maltreatment and the developing HPA axis. *Hormones and Behavior*, 50(4): 632–39.

Wegman, H.L. and Stetler, C. (2009) A meta-analytic review of the effects of childhood abuse on medical outcomes in adulthood. *Psychosomatic Medicine*, 71(8): 805–12.

A must-read, longitudinal study of respiratory infection:

Ball, T.M., Holberg, C.J., Aldous, M.B., Martinez, F.D. and Wright, A.L. (2002) Influence of attendance at day care on the common cold from birth through 13 years of age. *Archives of Pediatrics and Adolescent Medicine*, 156(2): 121–6.

For a longitudinal focus on the effects of stress including a chromosomal biomarker ('hot' research topic):

Kiecolt-Glaser, J.K., Gouin, J.P., Weng, N.P., Malarkey, W.B., Beversdorf, D.Q. and Glaser, R. (2011) Childhood adversity heightens the impact of later-life caregiving stress on telomere length and inflammation. *Psychosomatic Medicine*, 73(1): 16–22.

USEFUL WEBSITES

Stress in America (APA study): www.apa.org/news/press/releases/stress/2011/final-2011.pdf

Sure Start (UK): www.direct.gov.uk/en/Parents/Preschooldevelopmentandlearning/NurseriesPlaygroupsReceptionClasses/DG_173054

Head Start (US): http://eclkc.ohs.acf.hhs.gov/hslc

PART II

THE EXPERIENCE OF ACUTE AND CHRONIC ILLNESS DURING CHILDHOOD

THE EXPERIENCE OF ACUTE ILLNESS IN CHILDHOOD

6

Covered in this chapter

- Defining acute illness
- The relevance of illness cognitions in acute childhood illness
- Coping with acute illness in childhood
- Medical procedures and hospitalization in acute childhood illness

---

In Part II of this book, the focus turns to explore psychosocial issues of relevance to acute and chronic illness in childhood, as well as the effect of parental ill health on a child's well-being. In this chapter, I start by considering the experience of acute illness during childhood and adolescence. Being ill, whatever the condition, is a stressor in itself, at a biological, psychological and social level. From symptom onset through diagnosis, treatment and follow-up effects, key components of stress, including unpredictability, uncontrollability and fear of social evaluation, are triggered. Illness presents a threat to normal everyday functioning, and to life itself, at any age. Illness during childhood and adolescence presents its own unique set of circumstances which reflect the challenge to an individual's sense of self and intergenerational notions of the expectations of life taking a cradle-to-the-grave trajectory. Put in the context of child and adolescent sociocognitive understanding and expectations, even minor or mild acute illness can serve as a major stress-inducing threat or challenge.

DEFINING ACUTE ILLNESS

First and foremost, we need to distinguish between acute and chronic illness and to define what is meant by the term 'acute illness'. There are varying definitions of acute illness but, as highlighted in Table 6.1, it can be distinguished from chronic illness by two key criteria: (i) the speed of onset of symptoms; and (ii) the duration of time that symptoms last. Acute illness, like chronic illness, can range from mild (e.g., the common cold) to severe or life threatening (e.g., acute lymphoblastic leukaemia or meningitis). There can also be acute events associated with chronic conditions, an acute asthma attack associated with chronic asthma, for example. In addition to the illnesses, conditions and diseases listed in Table 6.1, accidents are also highly prevalent in childhood, particularly during the early years and in adolescence, and injury can result not just in an acute event but lead to acute and chronic symptoms and associated conditions (e.g., brain injury, pain and disability).

Given the dictionary definition of acute illness as 'a condition of short duration that starts quickly and has severe symptoms' (Macpherson, 1999), you may have already noted and questioned why I have included childhood leukaemias, such as acute lymphoblastic leukaemia (ALL) and acute myeloid leukaemia (AML), under the heading of acute illness and not under chronic illness. Acute leukaemia is defined as 'a rapid growth in the number of white blood cells, which is fatal if untreated' (Macpherson, 1999), ALL being associated

TABLE 6.1 Characteristics and examples of acute and chronic illnesses prevalent in children

Acute illness	Chronic illness
Characteristics:	Characteristics:
• Lasts for a relatively short duration of time • Sudden in onset • Symptoms change or worsen rapidly • May involve only one physical system or part of the body • Can be mild to severe or terminal	• Continues over an extended period of time • Onset gradual • Development gradual • Worsens over time • Can involve multiple bodily systems • Can be mild to severe or terminal
Examples include:	Examples include:
• Chickenpox • Gastroenteritis • Acute lymphoblastic leukaemia • Acute myeloid leukaemia • Measles • Meningitis • Upper respiratory tract infections, e.g. the common cold, influenza, strep. throat infection, glandular fever (mononucleosis or 'mono')	• Asthma • Cerebral palsy • Cystic fibrosis • Type 1 diabetes (T1D) • Epilepsy • Human immunodeficiency virus (HIV+/AIDS) • Juvenile chronic arthritis • Obesity • Phenylketonuria (PKU) • Spina bifida

Sources: Murrow and Oglesby (1996); Macpherson (1999); Medline Plus (2012).

with malignant lymphoblasts or lymphocyte-forming cells and AML being associated with the granulocyte precursor cells of the bone marrow (Macpherson, 1999). These severe conditions have a characteristic rapid onset of symptoms, which meets the speed of onset aspect of our criteria for acute illness above. They are more common in children than adults because of the cellular division associated with early development. Without medical intervention, symptoms will rapidly lead to death. However, medical advances have dramatically changed the prognostic landscape in childhood leukaemia. With modern treatments, an individual with AML may live with the condition for several years or, with ALL, may be 'cured' of the condition and survive into adulthood with life chances similar to those who have not had cancer. Both ALL and AML also share the chronic illness characteristic of lasting over an extended period of time. In this respect, leukaemia in children is often considered in the same way as a chronic illness with regard to psychosocial factors and quality of life.

The way I am approaching it here is to use the acute illness definition, and view ALL and AML as acute conditions, particularly as they relate to diagnosis and initial treatment. Since continuation treatment can extend over 2–3 years, this perspective is considered under chronic illness in Chapter 7. Furthermore, the threat of late effects following treatment for cancer such as leukaemia, years or even decades after 'cure', also continues into adulthood. Some more details about childhood leukaemia are given below and in the following three chapters. In Chapter 7, when we consider chronic conditions, the chronic characteristics and effects of leukaemia and its treatment are included; in Chapter 8, terminal issues and survivorship are addressed; and Chapter 9 is dedicated to the topic of pain across a range of conditions including cancer. So, in short, we follow the classification of leukaemia as an acute condition due to its rapid onset, but acknowledge that these acute illnesses in childhood are today very much associated with characteristics of chronic conditions. Whilst the physical causes and initial stages of treatment are acute, there are now long-term effects which fall under the umbrella of chronic illness.

THE RELEVANCE OF ILLNESS COGNITIONS IN ACUTE CHILDHOOD ILLNESS

In Chapter 2, amongst other things, we outlined the stages of cognitive development as applied to the understanding of illness in children. In particular, the seminal work of Bibace and Walsh (1980) was covered, based on the developmental staging models of Piaget and Inhelder (1947) and Werner (1948). In addition to age, the relevance of the child's experience with illness, the type of illness (e.g., the common cold versus measles) and socioeconomic status were all cited as contributing to a child's understanding of illness. In considering acute illness in childhood, it is vital to begin this chapter by taking another, more in-depth look at illness cognitions. Once again, we return to the useful paradigm of the common cold (acute upper respiratory tract infection) in order to do this (see Chapter 3 for a rationale about the usefulness of the common cold as a methodological paradigm).

In applying and developing work in this area to practical implications for educating children about health, Koopman and colleagues (2004) used the common cold as one example of illness that children were asked to talk about. They developed a model, referred to as the Through the Eyes of the Child (TEC) model, which provides a guide for speaking with children about illness. The responses given in their study at different age groups can be seen in Table 6.2, along with a mapping of their TEC model stages alongside those of previous key studies.

The cognitive perceptual stage of development influences how a child experiences being ill, as that experience is based in part on the causal attribution the child places on the illness (e.g., whether attributed to external causes, to contact with another person or to a combination of factors). The child's attribution is important as it may be bound up with feelings of acceptance or blame (including self-blame). The recommendation of Koopman et al. (2004: 368), when giving information to a child about their illness, is to 'build on previous knowledge of the child and moderately extend this knowledge', matching information to perceptual stage.

The study of children's understanding of illness has included a range of common acute conditions as examples, drawn mainly from healthy children but also applied to other acute or chronic illnesses. Yet aside from these studies, which are effectively retrospective or hypothetical with reference to acute illness, there is a lack of research which asks children about their acute experience at the time they are having symptoms (feasible at least for more mild or moderate acute conditions such as the common cold or common childhood viral infections). There are obvious ethical and moral constraints in doing this type of work, which might explain why the literature is not spilling over with such studies. However, that aside, a significant period of time has often elapsed between participant experience of illness symptoms and describing how it felt to have those symptoms, and often studies do not include a measure of the distal or proximal relationship (i.e., the timespan) between the two. It is important to make this distinction between a more distal perceptual understanding of illness and a direct or proximal description of the illness experience, particularly in studies which examine more mild forms of everyday acute illness which are easily forgotten once well. With serious acute illness such as ALL, the severity of the condition and its treatment make more distal studies possible. In other words, a 4-year-old child may forget how they felt when they had a common cold but the experience of chemotherapy for leukaemia is likely to remain with the child forever and shape future experiences and behaviours. Likewise, it would be unethical to ask a child to report their experience of leukaemia at diagnosis or whilst they were severely unwell, but in a longitudinal study of the common cold there is the potential to adopt a 'watch and wait' approach for symptoms, the experience of which can be reported during the cold onset. There is a much richer research literature to draw from in more severe acute illness in children, relating to their experience, coping and adjustment, than there is in milder acute illnesses. In acute illness, as in chronic, the role of the family is central, and much work has addressed parental experiences of the child's acute illness, particularly that of the mother, as well as the effect on siblings. The importance of the family, parents and siblings is integral to the issues discussed throughout this book but particularly in this

TABLE 6.2 Cognitive and perceptual development of the child

Piaget (1927), cognitive development	Werner (1948), perceptual development	Bibace and walsh (1978), illness category system	Through eyes of the child, TEC Model	Visualisation, TEC Model	Examples of Illness Interview answers
1 Senso-motorical, 0–2 years		1 Incomprehension	1 Invisible		A 'cold is during vacation'
2 Pre-operational, 2–7 years	1 Global, whole qualities are dominant	2 Phenomenism	2 Distance		'When you leave the window open, your blankets get cold which can make you a little bit sick'
		3 Contagion	3 Proximity		'Well, for example when somebody else has a cold and you get close and the next day she is better and you have a cold'
3 Concrete-operational, 7–11 years	2 Analytical, perception is selectively directed toward parts	4 Contamination	4 Contact		'Well, when you cough really hard then drops can land on your face, there are germs in there and they make you ill'

(Continued)

TABLE 6.2 (Continued)

4 Formal-operational, 11 years	3 Synthetic, parts become integrated with respect to the whole			
		5 Internalisation	5 Internalisation	"When you cough, those germs go through the air and someone else can breathe them in and then I think it gets in your blood. Then you also get a cold"
		6 Physiological	6 Body Inside	"Well the germs get into your blood and the white blood cells will fight them but if they lose you will get ill"
		7 Psychophysiological	7 Body-Mind Inside	"This can happen in different ways. Sometimes a cold is not so bad. It depends on how you feel"

Source: Koopman et al. (2004: 367–8).

chapter and throughout Part II. Here, we start by considering some of the issues relevant to parental involvement in child health as it relates to acute illness.

PARENTAL FACTORS IN ACUTE CHILDHOOD ILLNESS: CONCERN, SUPPORT AND THE USE OF MEDICATION

Before looking further at more serious acute illnesses and the experience of hospitalization, there are a number of important issues that relate to the more common childhood illnesses (e.g., common cold and flu, ear infections, headaches, and gastrointestinal viruses). Some children have a large number of such minor conditions, reported as being up to 8–10 infections per year (Ryder, 2007). For more common and relatively mild acute conditions in children, parental responses to children's symptoms can influence the child's experience of illness and help shape their long-term response to health and illness symptoms. Two important aspects are the parental perspective on the use of medication, and seeking help or advice (e.g., via consultation with a doctor or pharmacist). There has been considerable debate about antibiotic use in recent years, with the medical profession often reporting a significant and sometimes inappropriate demand from patients for antibiotics. Andre et al. (2007) conducted a prospective study over a period of one month, sampling over 800 families in Sweden with an 18-month-old child, to assess any respiratory tract symptoms, how often they visited their doctor and whether the child was prescribed antibiotics. They also measured psychosocial variables relating to parental concern about their child's health with regard to infectious illness (e.g., 'every time your child is ill, you are afraid it is something serious') and evaluated the accuracy of parental beliefs about antibiotics (Andre et al., 2007). Those parents who reported the greatest concerns about their child's health visited their child's doctor more often than parents who worried less, and the children of the high-concern parents were also more likely to have antibiotics prescribed. They also found that holding inadequate beliefs about antibiotics (i.e., believing that the infection would not go away without antibiotics) partly explained the high level of parental concern over infectious illness. Interestingly, families with only one child also reported more worry about infectious illness (Andre et al., 2007). The authors conclude that if the child's doctor can allay parental anxiety through reassurance and education during the consultation, then this would reduce antibiotic prescribing.

Other work has considered who parents turn to for advice and information about common childhood symptoms and how this translates into parental decisions about the use of over-the-counter (OTC) medication. In an Australian cross-sectional study of 325 parents with children from birth up to 2 years old, Trajanovska and colleagues (2010) report that in the previous year almost all the parents (98 per cent of their sample) had bought at least one OTC medicine to treat their child when they had common symptoms such as a cough, rash, sickness or diarrhoea, stomach ache or irritability. Parental reasons for and against buying different medicines is shown in Table 6.3. In terms of who the parents turned to for guidance about which OTC medicine to buy, 82 per cent of parents took advice from their doctor. Similarly, parents also sought advice from the doctor when their child had common symptoms such as earache, wheeziness or a rash but, interestingly, they would turn to the child nurse specialist for information and advice about sleep concerns and to friends and family for advice about issues relating to behavioural complaints ('irritability' and 'crankiness') or teething pain, as shown in Table 6.4 (Trajanovska et al., 2010).

Such studies highlight the importance of the provision of appropriate, easily accessible and up-to-date information for parents. They also highlight the opportunity for interventions to provide educational information to parents in various forms. Written information is one relatively inexpensive method of achieving this, although the effectiveness of written information in improving outcomes is frequently more assumed than it is adequately assessed. Addressing this gap, Paul and co-workers (2007) conducted a randomized controlled trial (RCT) to assess the effectiveness of a new written information leaflet for increasing parental knowledge about how to manage a febrile convulsion in their child once discharged from hospital following an initial incident. This was compared with parents receiving the standard control leaflet already given to parents on discharge. Children were aged 7–63 months, with an average age of 2 years. The majority of these parents had no previous experience of dealing with a febrile convulsion,

TABLE 6.3 Proportion (%) of parents who agreed with the following statements as reasons 'for' and 'against' the purchase of over-the-counter (OTC) medicines

Statement	Agree
Reasons for purchase of a medicine*	
'I buy medicines that my doctor has prescribed or suggested in the past because I know they work for my child' (*n* = 311)	82
'I buy medicines to have, in case of future need' (*n* = 310)	68
'The pharmacist gives me expert advice to buy a medicine' (*n* = 309)	68
'I do not want to bother my doctor for minor illness' (*n* = 308)	41
'I do not need to make an appointment to buy a medicine' (*n* = 308)	41
'I do not need to take my child with me to buy a medicine' (*n* = 305)	31
'I could choose which medicine I want' (*n* = 303)	29
Reasons against purchase of a medicine†	
'I wanted the advice of my doctor first' (*n* = 319)	58
'There was nowhere open that sold what I needed' (*n* = 314)	23
'I could not get to the pharmacy' (*n* = 312)	20
'The medicine I wanted was only available on prescription' (*n* = 313)	12
'The cost of the medicine was more than I could afford' (*n* = 312)	4
'I knew I would get it free on prescription from my doctor' (*n* = 311)	2

*Question: 'Which of the following are reasons why you have bought a medicine for your child rather than visited your doctor?'
†Question: 'Have any of the following stopped you buying medicines for your child?'
Source: Trajanovska et al. (2010: 2069, table 2).

TABLE 6.4 Proportion (%) of parents who sought advice from information sources for common childhood complaints their children had experienced

Childhood complaint	Doctor	M&CH centre	Family or friends	Pharmacist	Other*
Ear ache ($n = 132$)	95	4	4	3	3
Wheeziness ($n = 128$)	90	5	3	3	4
Sudden blotchy rash ($n = 168$)	77	11	7	7	5
Chesty cough ($n = 198$)	76	5	8	14	2
Vomiting or diarrhoea ($n = 204$)	70	10	13	3	12
High temperature ($n = 253$)	64	9	14	9	8
Dry cough ($n = 182$)	59	8	15	25	4
Abdominal pain ($n = 107$)	56	18	21	9	4
Colicky symptoms ($n = 130$)	48	38	19	8	5
Irritability or crankiness ($n = 180$)	22	37	47	1	3
Sleep difficulties ($n = 206$)	14	60	32	0	8
Teething pain ($n = 218$)	10	21	44	26	6
Other[†] ($n = 74$)	85	31	9	20	24

Row totals do not add up to 100% because some parents provided more than one source of information for each symptom.

*Other sources of information included books, community self help organisations, other healthcare professionals, hospital, Internet, mother's group, Victorian help lines and health store manager.

[†]Other childhood complaints included allergy or hay fever, cold or flu symptoms, eczema or skin irritation, constipation, infection, lack of appetite, vaccination, non-specific pain, asthma, blood nose, convulsion and dehydration.

Source: Trajanovska et al. (2010: 2072, table 5).

which emphasizes the need for information of this type. Whilst parents found the new leaflet easier to understand than the standard one, there was no difference between the experimental group and the control group with regard to the main outcome of increasing knowledge (Paul et al., 2007). In fact, the most important finding was that the new leaflet increased levels of reassurance in the parents (Paul et al., 2007). A systematic review of the support needs of parents making decisions about their child's health care, including those involved in the management of acute conditions, such as respiratory illness, and the use of OTC medication, immunization (including MMR vaccination) and prenatal screening, points to the underlying constructs which require attention in designing interventions (Jackson et al., 2008). The authors of this review report that, across 149 studies using different methodologies, three consistent underlying issues emerged with regard to decision support needs: (i) 'information'; (ii) 'talking to others'; and (iii) 'feeling a sense of control over the process' (Jackson, et al., 2008), as illustrated in Figure 6.1.

Jackson et al. (2008: 243) also highlight the need to take a biopsychosocial perspective in the provision of support, to include the psychosocial context of the information being conveyed. New sentence, insert They cite Layton et al who pointed out over two decades ago that 'solely communicating information assumes a "cognitive deficit model" which fails to take account of the fact that the way individuals use

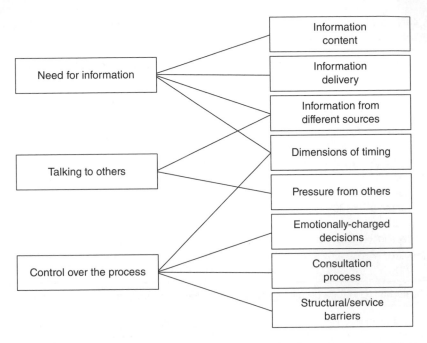

FIGURE 6.1   Emerging themes of the decision support needs of parents making child health decisions

Source: Jackson et al. (2008: 239, fig. 3).

information is contingent on multiple factors including their social environment'. The last theme of 'control over the process' relates back to one of the underlying constructs in the experience of stress as discussed in Part I of this book, particularly Chapters 2 and 5. Such findings emphasize that the experience of illness in the child is also experienced directly as well as indirectly by the parent, whether it is treatment for the illness itself that is being sought (medication) or the avoidance of ill health through preventive measures which the parent has to make decisions about (e.g., vaccination or prenatal screening). Cultural and religious factors also contribute to health outcomes via parental influence. An extreme example of religious beliefs affecting medical treatment is given in Box 6.1.

MEDICALLY UNEXPLAINED SYMPTOMS AND SOMATOFORM DISORDERS

It is also worth being aware of some related terms and concepts with regard to acute illness in children. These relate to symptoms without any definable or detectable underlying cause and are referred to as 'functional somatic symptoms', 'medically unexplained symptoms' or 'somatoform disorders'. Whilst they are receiving a mention under the heading of acute illness, such symptoms may in some cases lead to

---

BOX 6.1

Parental influences on child health

The influence of parental religious beliefs on a child's health could be very positive, associated with a healthy lifestyle and supportive, nurturing family values conducive to good health outcomes. However, where these beliefs are so extreme that they override and operate independently of mainstream medical care, the outcome can become critical. Some extreme examples have made the media headlines in recent years, drawing attention to the ethical dilemma faced when parent or child refuses life-saving treatment due to religious convictions. In 2009, the *New York Times* (www.nytimes.com) reported that in the US approximately 300 children had died in the previous 25 years after parents had refused medical treatment on religious grounds (Swan, in report by Johnson). Cases reported include a 15-month-old girl who died from pneumonia, a 16-year-old boy who died after not receiving treatment for a urinary tract infection, and a 16-month-old boy who died from meningitis after his mother delayed hospital treatment. Perhaps most well-known cases are those in which Jehova's Witnesses have refused a blood transfusion for their child. A recent case in the UK documented a 15-year-old boy who, following a car accident as a pedestrian, died after he himself refused a blood transfusion and his decision was not overruled by his family (www.telegraph.co.uk/health/healthnews). There are obvious ethical, moral and legal issues involved with these and other high-profile cases which are hotly debated. For example, whose right is it to determine treatment? Are parents not simply doing what they think is best? What do you think? Here these cases serve to highlight one extreme end of the spectrum with regard to the influence of parental beliefs on medical treatment and health outcome in children.

---

chronic disorders. Symptoms can include, amongst others, headache, abdominal pain or a range of neurological symptoms, all of which can impact severely on the quality of life of the child and those around them (see Rask et al., 2009; Wallace et al., 2012). Interestingly, a recent review of the appropriateness of the clinical classification of somatoform disorders as applied to children and adolescents emphasizes the role of child environment, in particular parental influence, in these disorders (Schulte and Petermann, 2011). The authors of the review call for the addition of two further criteria in the diagnosis of complex somatoform disorders in children and adolescents: (i) 'parental excessive concern and preoccupation with the child's symptoms'; and (ii) 'high parental health anxieties' (Schulte and Petermann, 2011: 223, 224). This highlights the potential parental involvement in such disorders, although there is much debate surrounding this issue. The symptomatology in these types of condition is frequently pain related and we touch on medically unexplained symptoms again in Chapter 9 when we focus on pain. In consideration of acute conditions in this chapter and throughout the book, we are considering medically *explained* symptoms which have an underlying physical basis, but it is worth bearing in mind this subset of the literature which deals with symptoms which are medically *unexplained*. As is documented in Chapter 8, 'medically unexplained' can in some cases mean medical conditions which are slow to be diagnosed but eventually become medically explained.

COPING WITH ACUTE ILLNESS IN CHILDHOOD

Having eased you into the experience of acute childhood illness and, I hope, steered your thinking towards considering it as an experience shared by the parents and family, we now consider the role of coping. So how do children cope with acute illness? The concept of coping has already been referred to on many occasions throughout this book, particularly in Chapters 2 and 5. We now need to look at coping in children and adolescents in more depth, since coping is central to the experience of illness, whether we are referring to the experience of acute illness or chronic illness, a condition that is mild or severe, or one that is life-threatening. Different characteristics of the illness, and stages in the journey of the experience of that illness, will elicit different coping responses, and the responses chosen may influence the physical as well as the psychological health outcome.

Coping has attracted many definitions by different researchers seeking to capture the meaning of the term, to wrestle with it and tie it down, in order really to understand this seemingly amorphous, often rather slippery, concept. But herein lies the problem. Trying to constrain the concept, and reduce the 'noise' associated with defining different types of coping, can lead to an oversimplification. For example, coping research in the 1990s attempted to pigeon-hole coping into square-shaped boxes wherein it was conceptualized as 'emotion-focused' versus 'problem-focused' coping, or 'adaptive' versus 'maladaptive' coping. Whilst these are all useful and relevant terms in understanding coping, they somewhat constrain the concept, our understanding of it and the development of the theory and application of coping to different types of stressful situations. These terms are still very much in use within the coping research literature, but the field has also moved beyond this to categorize coping into more sophisticated groupings dependent on the situation being faced.

One of the key researchers in the field of coping responses in children provides an excellent workable definition of coping as 'conscious volitional efforts to regulate emotion, cognition, behavior, physiology, and the environment in response to stressful events or circumstances' (Compas et al., 2001: 89). These 'conscious volitional' responses are secondary to the automatic responses to stress, which include sympathetic adrenomedullary (SAM) system and hypothalamic-pituitary-adrenal (HPA) axis activation and their associated emotional and behavioural effects (see Chapter 2). Coping responses are self-regulatory responses but compose a subset of this broader umbrella term and specifically deal with stressful events (Compas et al., 1997, 2001, 2012). Developmental aspects heavily influence the resources available, whether biological, psychological, or social, for coping with the stressor and the repertoire of behaviours that the child or adolescent is able to utilize in the expression of the coping response (Compas et al., 2001).

TABLE 6.5 Three coping subgroups proposed by Compas and colleagues

Coping subtype	Definition	Coping responses
Primary control coping	Efforts to directly *act* on the source of stress or one's emotions	Problem solving Emotional expression Emotional modulation
Secondary control coping	Effort to *adapt* to the source of stress	Acceptance Distraction Cognitive restructuring Positive thinking
Disengagement coping	Efforts to *withdraw* from the source of stress and one's emotions	Avoidance Denial Wishful thinking

Source: Compas et al. (1997, 2001); Connor-Smith et al. (2000).

One popular and well-used questionnaire measure of coping in children and adolescents is the Responses to Stress Questionnaire (RSQ; Connor-Smith et al., 2000) based on earlier theoretical work by Compas and colleagues. Originally designed for use in adolescent populations, this measure has since been developed for use in children as young as 9 years old and deals with specific stressors identified at the start of the questionnaire. Versions of the RSQ have been developed for use across a range of stressful situations (including those relating to family or peer stress), in response to specific acute and chronic paediatric illnesses (including headaches, paediatric cancer), and in response to parental depression or cancer, as well as parental versions. Compas and colleagues have defined three major subtypes of coping in children and adolescents, based on factor analysis of their RSQ measure: 'primary control coping', 'secondary control coping' and 'disengagement coping' (Connor-Smith et al., 2000). These three subgroups, when set against the complex backdrop of other coping research in children, using various questionnaire assessments as well as interview and observational methods, show good consistency (see Compas et al., 2001 for review) and are a development from the earlier emotion-focused versus problem-focused coping dichotomy which was based on the adult literature and is set out in Chapter 2. Table 6.5 illustrates the three coping subgroups proposed in the model of coping of Compas and colleagues (Compas et al., 1997, 2001; Connor-Smith et al., 2000). As can be seen from the definitions of the subgroups, these refer to whether a child employs 'action', 'adaptation' or 'withdrawal' to deal with the problem.

This multidimensional aspect of coping is also a key feature of a study by Holen et al. (2012) in a non-clinical sample of 1,324 Norwegian children aged 6–8 years. They used the Kidcope, another popular questionnaire measure of coping designed specifically for use in children aged 7–12 years (Spirito et al., 1988). These researchers emphasize that coping with a stressor may require navigating through a repertoire of responses, and that it makes more sense to talk about coping patterns than individual responses. They suggest that children would benefit from learning a range of different coping strategies, including emotional coping responses and those termed 'secondary coping', such as distraction, rather than a focus solely on active coping as is often the case in school health promotion. Interestingly, they single out the coping strategy of 'wishful thinking' as one of the most common strategies used by young children and worthy of further study (Spirito et al., 1998). This study and the review by Compas et al. (2001) are more than 10 years apart, but many of the same issues raised in these studies remain, predominantly that, in coping research with children: (i) we know more about coping in older children and adolescents and relatively little about coping in younger children; (ii) we need to develop better assessment measures of coping (e.g., via questionnaire, interview and observational methods) and to include multi-informant input from parents and peers, as well as the child; (iii) we need to look at the pattern in which coping responses occur and the temporal effects which delineate the order in which responses or patterns of responses occur; and (iv) research findings need to be applied more directly and specifically to interventions delivered to children.

In some of the early work on coping conducted in the 1990s referred to above, we used the Kidcope questionnaire (Spirito et al., 1988) to assess children's coping styles in response to a recent problem at home or at school (Turner-Cobb and Steptoe, 1998). Rather than looking at how children coped with the common cold, we explored whether different styles of coping in children were associated with the likelihood of getting a cold (onset) and the severity of the symptoms following onset. In children who used a more avoidant style of coping, the likelihood of having a cold significantly increased as hassle stress increased. Children were more likely to remain healthy under stress if they did not use avoidance as a coping style. Similarly, the use of problem-focused coping strategies was associated with having a cold which lasted for a shorter amount of time, and children who used avoidant coping were ill for a longer period of time. In other words, problem-focused coping was associated with better health outcomes, and avoidant coping with poorer health outcomes, in this sample of otherwise healthy children (Turner-Cobb and Steptoe, 1998). Interpreted in light of the model proposed by Compas and colleagues, which promotes secondary control coping as the most effective type of coping response, the primary control coping subtype of problem-solving was unusually effective in these minor everyday situations in terms of being protective in acute health. Avoidant coping, on the other hand, in line with the Compas et al. (1997, 2001) and Connor-Smith et al. (2000) model, was not a useful coping strategy in staying healthy. Consideration of stressor type and severity, and the outcome measure under consideration, are therefore important factors, and in some cases primary control coping may have advantages.

Central to research on how children cope with acute or chronic illness is the rationale that illness is itself a stressor. The diagnosis of illness can be an acute stressor, generating a range of coping responses, as can dealing with treatment or medication and ongoing symptoms. There is relatively little research investigating how healthy children cope with minor common illnesses such as the common cold. Forsner and co-workers (2005b) point out that, whilst research has addressed how children cope with hospitalization and the experience of illness over a longer period of time, 'being ill for a short time has not been studied from a child's perspective' (p. 154). In their qualitative study of seven, previously well, Swedish children (aged 7–10 at time of illness), admitted to hospital with sinusitis, a fractured arm or leg, encephalitis, appendicitis or femoral osteotomy, an open interview technique was used to encourage the children to talk informally about their experience of being acutely ill or injured. They found an interesting series of 'contrasts' (pp. 157, 162) between children and within the same child in describing their experiences, all of which drew from a combination of 'reality and imagination' (p. 157) (Forsner et al., 2005b). These composed of: 'being scared' yet 'confident' (p. 157); feeling 'sad' yet 'cosy' (p. 158); 'being hurt' yet 'having fun' (p. 159); and 'being caught' yet 'trying to escape' (p. 160) (Forsner et al., 2005b).

So far in this chapter, we have really been dancing around the periphery of acute illness experience in children. What about coping in response to more serious or severe physical symptoms and conditions, and the experience of medical procedures and hospitalization? The case of acute leukaemia in children highlights some of the characteristics and issues associated with more severe illness. Acute lymphoblastic leukaemia (ALL) is one example which will be considered here and was introduced earlier in the chapter. ALL is the most common cancer in children, reported to account for about a quarter of all childhood cancers and three-quarters of childhood leukaemias (Stanulla and Schrauder, 2009). It can occur in children of any age but peaks in incidence between the ages of 3 and 6 years (Tucci and Arico, 2008). With the development of more effective chemotherapy drugs and regimens, the treatment of ALL, a disease once considered largely incurable, has become one of the success stories of modern medicine (Tucci and Arico, 2008). Five-year survival rates are reported to have increased from less than 10 per cent in the 1960s to a current figure of just over 90 per cent based on statistics gathered between 2000 and 2005 (Hunger et al., 2012). ALL contrasts with the less prevalent acute myeloid leukaemia (AML) which has an earlier age of onset (during the first couple of years of life), a lower incidence and a much lower survival rate of 40–50 per cent (McGrath et al., 2005). Treatment for ALL involves a series of stages, including remission induction therapy, induction (consolidation) therapy, and continuation treatment, using a combination of chemotherapeutic medications including glucocorticoids (Pui and Evans, 2006). The initial intensive stages of treatment involve hospital admission; the later stage of continuation therapy occurs at home and can continue for at least 2 years (McGrath and Rawson-Huff, 2010). Whilst new advances in medical treatment have led to this very optimistic outlook for survival, children diagnosed with ALL face a whole range of potentially stressful situations related to these treatments, the associated hospital and medical procedures that are necessary, and the side-effects of treatment. Of particular interest in this chapter are the acute illness effects associated with ALL diagnosis and treatment, as explained above. Late effects of cancer treatment are considered in Chapter 8 under survivorship issues.

Of course, it is not just the child who may experience distress because of the diagnosis of ALL, but also their family for whom the diagnosis might be associated with a fuller understanding of the possible implications or outcomes. There has been extensive work in this area, which has led to significant interventions for children and their families. A key researcher who has explored the experience of the child with ALL, and the family impact, is Christine Eiser with her team in the UK (for a full review of the area, see Eiser, 2004). Recent aspects of this work have considered the importance of the style and content of communication between parents and their child following diagnosis. For example, Clarke and colleagues (2005) highlight a turnaround regarding how parents should talk to their children, which appears almost as dramatic as the improvements in medical treatment. There has been something of a social and cultural revolution in the past half-century which has moved professional practice and government policy away from one of protectionist avoidance in communicating with children about their cancer diagnosis (e.g., unpleasant effects of treatment and life-threatening potential) towards an enhanced, more open and honest communication (for recent review, see Ranmal et al., 2012). This is based on research which provides evidence that children adapt better if they are told more about their diagnosis and its consequences early on. Yet parents, who are frequently the go-betweens or 'gate-keepers' in communicating from health professional to child, may understandably find this a daunting task and feel that they lack the skills to do it effectively. Using a qualitative thematic analysis, Clarke et al. (2005) directly explored the content and style of parental communication in a sample of 55 mothers of children diagnosed with ALL. They categorized factual information provided by the mother to the

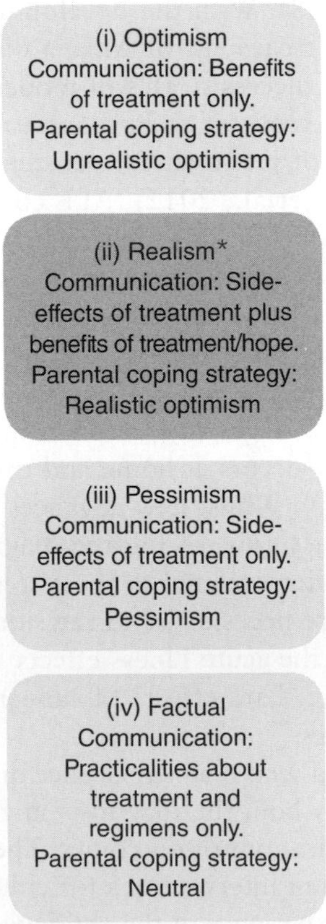

(i) Optimism
Communication: Benefits
of treatment only.
Parental coping strategy:
Unrealistic optimism

(ii) Realism*
Communication: Side-
effects of treatment plus
benefits of treatment/hope.
Parental coping strategy:
Realistic optimism

(iii) Pessimism
Communication: Side-
effects of treatment only.
Parental coping strategy:
Pessimism

(iv) Factual
Communication:
Practicalities about
treatment and
regimens only.
Parental coping strategy:
Neutral

FIGURE 6.2   The ways parents communicate factual information about cancer and its treatment to their child. *Realism is the most effective strategy based on coping and intervention literature across many illness domains

Source: Based on Clarke et al. (2005).

TABLE 6.6 Parental communication style by mean age of child in a sample of children diagnosed with acute lymphoblastic leukaemia (ALL)

Parental communication style defined by degree of openness, sophistication and detail of the information given	Mean age of child (s.d.)	No.
Minimal information, without severity, e.g., 'poorly blood'	4.24 (1.71)	17
Ambiguous information, e.g., used term 'leukaemia' but avoided using word 'cancer'	5.63 (2.67)	8
Factual information, e.g., used the word 'cancer' but did not include life-threatening aspect (death)	8.73 (3.71)	15
Full information including life-threatening aspect (death)	12.0 (2.65)	3

Source: Adapted from Clarke et al. (2005: 278, table 1).

child as: (i) 'optimism' (e.g., encouraging the child to take medication as it will help them get better but not detailing side-effects); (ii) 'realism' (e.g., explaining that the medication will have side-effects but should then help them feel better); (iii) 'pessimism' (e.g., communicating the side-effects without focusing on the benefits); and (iv) 'factual' (e.g., providing medication and regimen details without benefits or side-effects (Clarke et al., 2005: 277). These categories could be interpreted along the coping strategy dimensions of unrealistic optimism, realistic optimism, pessimism and neutral realism as shown in Figure 6.2. Realistic optimism is highlighted as the most effective strategy based on coping and intervention literature across many illness domains (see Chapter 2).

However, the majority of parents in the Clarke et al. (2005) study used a communication style which was minimal in openness of information, but this increased with age, although only three of the sample gave full information including potential death, as shown in Table 6.6. It is interesting that these researchers also found evidence for parental beliefs influencing the amount of information provided to their child. Parents who believed that a diagnosis of leukaemia was terminal tended to provide less information to their child, but those who expressed shock were found to be more open with their child about what they knew of the disease (Clarke et al., 2005). Such issues relate not just to coping in the child but also to parental coping, creating a dual interactive stress process, as parent(s) and child attempt to cope with the experience of illness.

These findings of Clarke et al. (2005) are consistent with other evidence that a greater degree of openness about the diagnosis and treatment, in conjunction with an age-appropriate style of communication, is associated with better adaptation in terms of mood and behavioural outcomes. Those children given the middle two categories of information (i.e., being told they had 'leukaemia' or 'cancer') demonstrated better behavioural adaptation (Clarke et al., 2005). The majority of research in childhood leukaemias has considered ALL rather than AML, but many of the issues raised are also relevant in AML, with particular relevance for issues relating to the life-threatening nature of the condition (for more detail, see McGrath et al., 2004, 2005).

Parents may struggle to put into practice the advice by health-care providers to maintain a normal life following their child's diagnosis of ALL, particularly in the continuation phase of treatment (Earle et al., 2006). Whilst much of the research looking at the effects of ALL on the child and family has focused on the mother, there is a small body of work that has considered the father's view in coming to terms with their child's diagnosis and treatment. McGrath and Chesler (2004) talk about the 'emotional shock and pain' felt by fathers during the initial induction-remission treatment phase for their child's ALL. In particular, this work emphasizes the importance of considering the role of fathers in family adjustment since they may feel shut out of the process despite shouldering responsibility for coping with the illness at both the level of the child and the family (Hill et al., 2009). In this qualitative study by Hill et al. (2009), fathers reported a preference for problem-focused coping in contrast to emotion-focused types of coping, which links to a need to retain control over the situation. Furthermore, the fathers mentioned a feeling of being on the 'periphery' of their child's care as the mother took the primary role, sometimes termed maternal 'gate-keeping'. In particular, the idea of returning to normal life during the post-hospitalization phase of treatment was a high priority for the fathers and a role they were keen to adopt (Hill et al., 2009). This notion of bringing back some normality to the situation, for both themselves and their family, is a theme that is repeated across studies (e.g., see also McGrath and Chesler, 2004). In contrast, whilst nearly two-thirds of the mothers in the Clarke et al. (2005) study assumed responsibility for medication, of these almost half reported that their partner did not give enough support with medication at home. The issue of single parenting deserves at least to be flagged here and noted, given the dual role expectations and increased responsibility that single parents face when caring for an ill child, although there is scant coverage of the experience of lone parenting in acute illness in the literature. Lone parenting of an ill child is discussed further in Chapter 7 under chronic illness.

Other work has incorporated the characteristic of temperament in coping with childhood cancers (including leukaemias, lymphomas, brain and other solid tumours; Miller et al., 2009). Primary control coping has been found to moderate the relationship between negative affect and depression, since depressive symptoms were less likely to be associated with negative affectivity when primary control coping was used, but this effect did not hold for anxiety (Miller et al., 2009). Primary and secondary control coping each individually mediated this link between negative affectivity and depression (Miller et al., 2009). Both effects indicate that it is not the negative affectivity characteristic *per se* that is important, but the relationship with the pattern of coping responses.

Much of the work in this area looks at the experience of hospitalization since the hospital is the acute care setting. In this next part of the chapter, we go on to consider the various experiences and challenges faced by a child in this acute care setting.

MEDICAL PROCEDURES AND HOSPITALIZATION IN ACUTE CHILDHOOD ILLNESS

The hospital experience, whether as an inpatient or an outpatient, presents many challenges at a biological, psychological and social level, and as such there is a vast and growing literature which has examined medical procedures and hospitalization.

Receiving treatment in an acute care setting can be a highly stressful experience for both adults and children. Based on the definitions of stress given in Chapter 2, receiving medical treatment, which is likely to be unpleasant, intrusive and frequently painful, in the context of an alien social environment, has the potential to score very highly in terms of stress appraisal and allostatic impact. We have already discussed the developing cognitive understanding, social and behavioural skills of children, based on age and experience. Children are less able to make sense of the hospital experience and less likely to be able to rationalize what is happening to them, creating greater potential for misattribution (e.g., being physically confined in a hospital bed or receiving a blood test may be perceived as punishment, or surgery and pain as mutilation; Rokach and Parvini, 2011). In an excellent review of adult and child experience of hospitalization, Rokach and Parvini (2011) describe hospitalization stress as stemming from a number of sources including the:

- Practical lack of home comforts; for example, sleeping in a different bed away from home, eating the hospital food, lack of sunlight.
- Uncontrollable, excessive noise and sensory overload; for example, from medical equipment, day-to-day activities of the nursing staff, noise from other patients and visitors.
- Personable nature of care; for example, perceived lack of emotional involvement from hospital staff or feeling that concerns are disregarded.

They highlight the importance of these factors not only for addressing the quality of life of the hospitalized patient, but from a psychoneuroimmune (PNI) perspective, since these factors may influence recovery rate, whether indirectly via their effects on heath behaviours (e.g., sleep) or directly (e.g., rate of wound healing; Rokach and Parvini, 2011). Children are particularly vulnerable to these influences given their limited ability to comprehend the hospital environment, and their need for parental attachment and support. For children, then, the hospital experience, in addition to the illness itself, puts them in a vulnerable, high-stress situation which may have psychosocial effects not only on the child but also on their family (Rokach and Parvini, 2011). Citing 'fear', 'loneliness' and 'frustration' as key emotions that are evoked in children in response to the experience of hospitalization, Rokach and Parvini (2011: 711) go as far as saying that 'hospitalisation can be considered as a "life crisis" for children', which might harm their sense of identity or self-esteem. A number of studies have categorized children's fears and anxieties around hospitalization, based upon these recurring themes of separation and attachment, symptoms and medical procedures, restrictive features of the environment, and threat to self-identity. A particularly useful classification has been put forward by Coyne (2006) based on interviews with 11 UK children between the ages of 7 and 14 years of age, admitted to hospital with a range of acute (cellulitis, constipation) and chronic (asthma, skin conditions) illness. As shown in Table 6.7, these fears and concerns fell into four categories, including separation from family and friends, the unfamiliarity of the hospital environment, treatments received, and what Coyne (2006) refers to as 'loss of self-determination'.

TABLE 6.7   Children's fears and concerns about hospitalization

Separation from family and friends	Disruption to:
	  Family routines
	  Normal activities
	  Peer relationships
	  School achievement

Being in an unfamiliar environment	Fears of:
	  The unknown
	  Strange environment
	  Professionals

	Dislikes:
	  Noisy ward
	  Bright lights at night
	  Hot environment
	  Inadequate play facilities
	  Food

Receiving investigations and treatments	Fear of:
	  Operations
	  Needles
	  Mistakes in treatment
	  Harm to body
	  Mutilation
	  Pain
	  Altered body image
	  Dying

Loss of self-determination	Loss of independence
	Restricted activities

	Lacking control over:
	  Personal needs
	  Sleeping/waking time
	  Food/meal times
	  Timing of procedures

Source: Coyne (2006).

PARENTAL INVOLVEMENT IN HOSPITAL CARE

Back in the 1950s (before what is often termed the 1960s' revolution in treatment and health care), James Robertson, a London-based psychiatric social worker and psychoanalyst, conducted pioneering work which raised awareness within the medical profession. In 1952, he produced a film which follows the experience of a 2-year-old girl who is hospitalized in order to undergo minor surgery. In the black and white footage of its time, this rather disturbing film shows the distress experienced by the toddler. Despite good practical care, restricted visiting hours for parents resulted in separation anxiety and depressed mood, and lack of a child-centred environment in the hospital further increased the apparent fear, loneliness and frustration felt by the child. By contrast, a second film was made by Robertson 6 years later in 1958, entitled *Going to Hospital with Mother*, in which a young child admitted to hospital for a minor operation (repair of an umbilical hernia) has her mother remain with her for the 5-day hospital stay. These emotive films worked wonders on the medical profession and, by the majority of accounts, moved the field of paediatric care forward by leaps and bounds. The toddler who featured in the first film is pictured in Figure 6.3; contrast this with the mother and toddler from the second film in Figure 6.4.

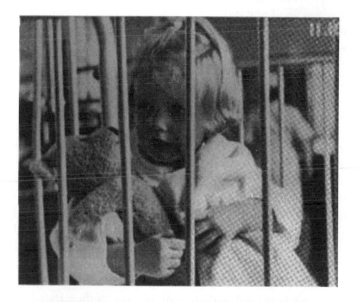

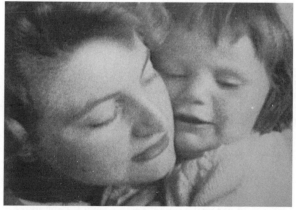

FIGURES 6.3 and 6.4   Contrasting pictures of toddlers from James Robertson's two films

These films were clearly instrumental in creating change in hospital care, encouraging the inclusion of parents, with increased visiting hours, the provision of facilities for parents to stay with their children, and in general creating a more child-friendly hospital environment. However, a paper published to mark the 50-year anniversary of the first film gives a refreshing perspective, not on the importance of Robertson's work, but on the degree to which hospital care had already begun to change prior to these films (Lindsay, 2003). As Lindsay (2003) points out, in considering the current state of the hospital environment, it is worth considering this historical perspective. Before the advent of children's hospitals in the 1850s, it was unusual for children to be admitted for hospitalization, but when they were, their mothers usually accompanied them and helped out with their care (West, in Lindsay, 2003). Once children's hospitals existed, visits by parents and other children were encouraged and restricted visiting access was lifted if the child was seriously ill or dying (Lindsay, in Lindsay, 2003). Furthermore, there is evidence that toys and books were also encouraged to provide a stimulating and reassuring environment. According to Lindsay, it was not until the late nineteenth century that parents began to be excluded from some children's hospitals, at a time when children would routinely stay in hospital for several weeks for what we would now consider routine operations. Exclusion or restriction was for many reasons, including the risk of infection, concerns over parental emotions interfering with care, and the professionalization of nursing, which continued into the 1930s. With the development of theories on attachment and an increased interest in the care of children, a disparity occurred between hospital practice and emerging theory, and change began to gain momentum in the 1940s (Lindsay, 2003), creating a suitable climate for the Robertson films to have maximum effect.

Following this mid-twentieth century resurgence of interest in the provision of a more child-centred hospital environment, the landscape of acute care for children and adolescents now looks very different. Modern-day hospitals in the Western world comprise much more positive environments, with effort made to accommodate not only their physical needs, but also the psychosocial comfort of the child and of the family, including parents and siblings. The notion of the 'healing environment' has received significant attention in hospital design in recent years, particularly with respect to the care of children. Contrast

Central considerations in child-centred hospitals

- Alleviating fear and anxiety
- Maximizing security and safety
- Reducing boredom
- Creating a healing environment

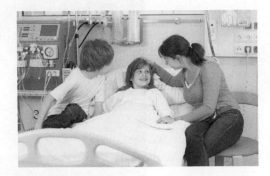

FIGURE 6.5　Modern-day child-centred hospital environment for children and young people

Source: NHS Estates (2004); iStock picture: stock-photo-19023099-visit-in-hospital.

the stark and frightening hospital environment highlighted by Robertson in his book *Young Children in Hospital* published in 1958, with present-day Department of Health (UK) guidance for best practice in building or upgrading children's hospitals. As illustrated in Figure 6.5, current recommendations for the design of children's hospitals are based on the aim of 'creating a child-centred built environment' (NHS Estates, 2004).

Parental involvement in hospital care has enormous benefits for the reduction of hospitalization stress in the child, through a reduction in separation anxiety and fear associated with medical treatments and hospital routines. It is, of course, also highly cost-effective for the health-care services or provider since parents constitute an extra pair of hands both physically to help with daily care and play, but also to assist in the social and emotional care of their child. A cynical stance on this might indeed argue that parental involvement or 'active parent participation' is tolerated primarily to enable administrative efficiency, and nurses do not receive sufficient training in the support of parents on the ward (Coyne, 2007). Indeed, there is evidence that, in some cases, parents are not adequately supported in this role, with nurses employing complex strategies of reward and punishment towards the parents in order to socialize them into compliance (Coyne, 2007).

As well as the advent of parental involvement in the hospital setting, health and social policy has seen a recent move away from inpatient hospital care towards out-of-hospital care, in the community, wherever possible. In the case of children, out-of-hospital care frequently means the parents taking over as care providers at home. As well as day-to-day physical care, this may include responsibility for administering medication, as directed by medical professionals, and for remembering appointments, in addition to their role as parent. Similarly, when hospitalization is required, unlike the lengthy stay of several weeks for minor surgery in decades gone by (e.g., see reports of the Sheffield Children's Hospital in Lindsay, 2003), length of stay is now kept to a minimum, with discharging back home for rest and recuperation or continued care away from the hospital. Similarly, since the middle of the 1980s, there has been a move towards greater use of 'ambulatory care', including a range of outpatient appointments, such as day-case surgery for children (Hughes and Callery, 2004). Box 6.2 describes a study which explored the impact of child day-case surgery for both the child and their family, using a diary methodology (Hughes and Callery, 2004).

ACCIDENT AND EMERGENCY CARE

One area of note concerning child admissions to hospital is that of accident and emergency care (A&E). An increase in the admission rates of children following A&E visits, albeit frequently for less than 24 hours, has been reported, particularly in the under-fives age group (for review see Small et al., 2005). Children may present at A&E with a range of acute symptoms, from mild to life-threatening. The condition of gastroenteritis represents one of the most common acute illnesses in children and, whilst often self-limiting, runs the risk of causing premature death (Stewart, in Small et al., 2005). To address the question of whether children have a better outcome in terms of clinical status and psychological state depending on whether they are admitted to hospital or discharged and

BOX 6.2

The impact of child day-case surgery for both the child and their family

Source: J.M. Hughes and P. Callery (2004) Parents' experiences of caring for their child following day-case surgery: a diary study. *Journal of Child Health Care*, 8(1): 47–58.

Rationale: Despite a move towards increases in day-case surgery for children, relatively little is known about the wider impact of this style of treatment on the patient and their family.

Methods: Eleven families of children undergoing day-case surgery for minor procedures, including circumcision, squint correction, metatarsal tenotomy, and hernia repair, were provided with a diary in which to record their experiences and feelings about the surgery and following surgery (via writing or drawing). Participants used their diaries for an average of 7.6 days (range = 1–10 days) post-surgery. As well as one parent per family, four children used the family diary and, in two cases, both parents contributed. Qualitative analysis employed an inductive and thematic approach.

Results: Six themes were identified from analysis of the diary information (see Figure 6.6).

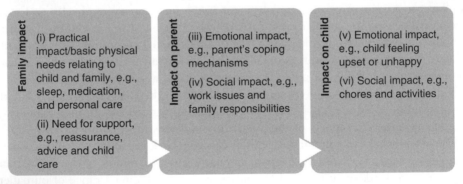

FIGURE 6.6   Six themes identified from analysis of diary entries following day-case surgery in children

Source: Hughes and Callery (2004).

Conclusions: Managing care following day-case surgery raises a range of practical, social and emotional issues for parents and children. Adequate preparation of families prior to day-case surgery is needed beyond that which is currently provided.

cared for at home, Small et al. (2005) focused on children presenting at A&E with gastroenteritis. In their sample of 112 children, they found no differences between hospital admissions or discharge home in terms of clinical outcomes and no difference in psychological outcomes a month after discharge. However, at one week post-discharge, those children admitted to hospital exhibited greater separation anxiety. Parental concerns and need for reassurance from the medical profession was similarly high in both groups (admitted and discharged). This study shows that the effects of short-term hospitalization were not damaging to children in the longer term (one month), yet it also shows that discharge home does not necessarily produce a better outcome. It emphasizes the need for allaying parental anxieties whether due to concern over the hospital admission of their child or the responsibility of taking care of them at home. This study also highlights the lack of research on children with acute conditions when not admitted to hospital, whether a visit to A&E is warranted or not.

INTERVENTIONS IN HOSPITAL CARE

Despite such significant improvements in the delivery of care to children in the past half-century, there is no escaping the fact that being ill is an unpleasant and highly stressful experience. Within this child-centred built environment, the context of care and interventions to enable adjustment are extremely important in facilitating psychological adjustment and they improve health outcomes. In order to minimize the negative effect of illness and hospitalization on social and emotional development in children (e.g., to avoid a decline in positive self-concept), adequate information provided to both children and parents in an appropriate form is essential, taking into account age and culture (Gultekin and Baran, 2007). A style of open communication is emphasized by Forsner and colleagues (2005a) in order to empower children to cope most effectively with being ill. Indeed, there is unanimous support by researchers in this field for greater age-appropriate communication and psychosocial intervention to continue to address the fear of hospitalization and medical procedures and reduce the damaging state of high alert that hospital stress can induce (Rokach and Matalon, 2007). There is also a growing interest in the use of the performing arts, such as theatre, in the context of health education in hospitalized children, which focuses on building children's self-concept and self-esteem, leading to empowerment in the face of illness and medical treatment (Rokach and Matalon, 2007).

PROMOTING HEALTH AND UNDERSTANDING OF ILLNESS IN WELL CHILDREN

Facilitating a greater understanding of illness and medical treatment in children who are well is perhaps the ultimate goal. Promoting a culture of understanding about illness and treatment under conditions of health may be the best route to health empowerment and optimum coping when ill health occurs. Support for this is provided in a study conducted by McGrath and Huff (2001) in a sample of 27 healthy preschool children (aged 3–5 years) who, as well as standard age-appropriate toys (e.g., crayons, farm animals), were given medical equipment to play with (e.g., swabs, bandages, chemo glasses, syringes, and an intravenous bag and tubing), and their responses were recorded. Interestingly, children who had no previous experience of hospital treatment approached the equipment with a 'naïve, joyous curiosity' (McGrath and Huff, 2001: 460), incorporating it into their play, asking questions and coming up with explanations about how the equipment worked. Yet those children who had previous treatment experience did not play with the medical equipment and instead chose the non-medical toys, and even the children who had indirect experience of hospitals via a close relative were fearful towards the medical equipment and less keen to play with it. Whilst this study shows the effect of hospital treatment on the child, it also highlights a need to promote understanding of medical treatment in healthy children in order to minimize the negative psychological impact that their naïvety may otherwise foster if subsequently faced with illness.

INTENSIVE CARE TREATMENT

A further area that it is essential to mention in this chapter is that of intensive care units (ICU). Paediatric intensive care units (PICUs) provide intensive care treatment for child and adolescent patients up to 16 years of age, and neonatal intensive care units (NICUs) specialize in treatment for newborns, during the first month of life, frequently when born prematurely. As for adult intensive care, patients are admitted to PICU for acute emergencies (including road traffic accident, burns, fractures and secondary bacterial infections or complications of common illnesses) as well as following planned surgery. The effects of the intensive care experience on patients and close family members are increasingly being documented in adults (Turner-Cobb et al., 2013). In an excellent review of intensive care for children, Colville (2012) points out the impact of the intensive care experience on the child and the parents. In particular, Colville points to recent work which has discovered that, although frequently sedated during their time on the PICU, children frequently experience traumatic memories and hallucinations relating to their hospital experience. Coupled with recurring memories of events leading to PICU admission, this can leave children feeling troubled and affect their long-term psychological recovery (Colville, 2012). Similarly, parents frequently find the experience of their child receiving intensive care highly distressing, as well as the experience of leaving the safety of the intensive care ward and returning home, to the point that some may develop clinical levels of anxiety and post-traumatic stress (Colville, 2012). Provision of adequate care in dealing with psychological distress in the child and providing psychological support to the parents is vital not only for reducing psychological distress but also as a route to prevent relapse and readmission in survivors of intensive care. I return to this topic in Chapter 8 when we consider survivorship and terminal issues.

CHAPTER SUMMARY

In this chapter, I have considered the experience of acute illness in children, with examples from mild to severe conditions of ill health. Key themes discussed have been the experience of illness as a stressor, the role of and impact on the family, developmental stage, cognitive understanding, coping responses and social effects. Much of the research in this area has been on the experience of hospitalization, and pioneering work has led to significant developments in the care of children over the past half-century. Given parallel advances in medical treatment and care, many diseases once considered terminal are now fortunately curable and/or chronic. This raises different issues about the experience of chronic illness and also about the quality of survival. These are the issues covered in Chapters 7 and 8.

KEY CONCEPTS AND ISSUES

- Definition of acute illness
- Parental support, parental influence and parental involvement
- Over-the-counter medication (OTCs)
- Illness as a stressor
- Definition of coping: automatic and conscious volitional responses
- Coping as a multidimensional construct
- Realistic optimism
- Day-case surgery
- Outpatient/ambulatory care
- Hospitalization stress
- Medically explained/unexplained symptoms
- Neonatal intensive care unit (NICU) and paediatric intensive care unit (PICU)
- Child-centred built environment

FURTHER READING

For an excellent review of the theory and measurement of coping in children and adolescence:

Compas, B.E., Jaser, S.S., Dunn, M.J. and Rodriguez, E.M. (2012) Coping with chronic illness in childhood and adolescence. *Annual Review of Clinical Psychology*, 8: 455–80.

For the original writings of Robertson about children's experience of hospital and recommendations for change:

Robertson, J. (1958) *Young Children in Hospital*. London: Tavistock.
Robertson, J. (1970) *Young Children in Hospital*, 2nd edn with postscript. London: Tavistock.

Robertson, J. and Robertson, J. (1989) *Separation and the Very Young*. London: Free Association Books.
DHSS (Central Health Services Council) (1959) *The Welfare of Children in Hospital*. Report of the Committee (Platt Report). London: HMSO.

For official guidance on modern-day child-centred hospital environments:

NHS Estates (2004) *Hospital Accommodation for Children and Young People*. London: The Stationery Office/Department of Health, UK.

For an informative and very readable review of paediatric intensive care:

Colville, G. (2012) Paediatric intensive care. *The Psychologist*, 25(3): 206–9.

USEFUL WEBSITES

For further information on the various forms of the Responses to Stress Questionnaire, see the Stress and Coping Research Laboratory (Director: Dr Bruce Compas): http://kc. vanderbilt.edu/stressandcopinglab/products_rsq.html

Link to James Robertson's films, including *A Two-year-old Goes to Hospital*: www. robertsonfilms.info

THE EXPERIENCE
OF CHRONIC ILLNESS
IN CHILDHOOD

7

DEFINING CHRONIC ILLNESS

The definition of chronic illness is not as simple as it may at first appear. In Chapter 6, we considered the characteristics of acute illness, and in this chapter, I contrast these characteristics with those of chronic illness, as highlighted in Table 7.1.

The overriding characteristic that distinguishes acute from chronic illness is the time course of symptoms. Chronic illness is usually characterized by a gradual onset and development of symptoms in comparison with the rapidity of symptoms in acute illness. A number of additional characteristics relating to duration of symptoms contribute to the definition of chronic illness in childhood and adolescence, and some ambiguity exists. Eiser's (1990: 3) description of chronic diseases as 'conditions that affect children for

TABLE 7.1 Characteristics and examples of acute and chronic illnesses prevalent in children

Acute illness	Chronic illness
Characteristics:	Characteristics:
• Lasts for a relatively short duration of time • Sudden in onset • Symptoms change or worsen rapidly • May involve only one physical system or part of the body • Can be mild to severe or terminal	• Continues over an extended period of time • Onset gradual • Development gradual • Worsens over time • Can involve multiple bodily systems • Can be mild to severe or terminal
Examples include:	Examples include:
• Chickenpox • Gastroenteritis • Acute lymphoblastic leukaemia • Acute myeloid leukaemia • Measles • Meningitis • Upper respiratory tract infections, e.g., the common cold, influenza, strep. throat infection, glandular fever (mononucleosis or 'mono')	• Asthma • Cerebral palsy • Cystic fibrosis • Type 1 diabetes (T1D) • Epilepsy • Human immunodeficiency virus (HIV+/AIDS) • Juvenile chronic arthritis • Obesity • Phenylketonuria (PKU) • Spina bifida

Sources: Murrow and Oglesby (1996); Macpherson (1999); Medline Plus (2012).

extended periods of time, often for life', which are 'managed' rather than 'cured', is still a useful working definition, although it lacks both disease duration and specificity. Eiser also cites leukaemia as an exception to the rule since it can be 'cured', thus contradicting the definition. In a thorough systematic review of the way chronic illness in children (0–18 years) has been defined and measured, van der Lee and colleagues (2007) point to four different definitions of chronic health conditions which have been used across US and UK studies. These include a time specification: for the illness to have lasted from 3 months, in two of the definitions, to a year, in another definition, while the time course is not specified in the fourth definition. Van der Lee et al. (2007) point out that the wide range in prevalence rates for chronic illness in children (estimated anywhere between 0.22 and 44 per cent of the population) is explained by the different definitions and measures used. Later work by this research group devised a specific definition of chronic illness in childhood (0–18 years), based on a Dutch national consensus, to include a disease or condition which has lasted longer than 3 months or is likely to last longer than 3 months, or has occurred at least three times in the previous year and is likely to occur again (Mokkink et al., 2008). They further differentiate chronic illness as a long-term condition which is not curable (as opposed to a short-term condition or a long-term condition which is curable). A chronic illness defined in this way is likely to incur frequent hospital visits and medical treatment, and would normally have an impact on the child's

social life, normal activities and school attendance, and these are taken into consideration in some of the definitions (van der Lee et al., 2007). Yet, even with these caveats, a
straightforward description of chronic illness in children is not possible. The fact that
there have been several high-quality systematic reviews and empirical studies in this area
in the past few years, published in high impact journals, shows the importance and interest in this issue.

In this chapter, we consider chronic illness as distinct from acute illness, defined, as
before, not by severity but by its speed of onset and the length of time that the illness
lasts. Many of the characteristics of chronic illness are now shared by some cancers,
which previously had a much poorer prognosis and for which early death was frequent
(e.g., acute lymphoblastic leukaemia [ALL]). Despite rapid onset of symptoms, conditions such as ALL now have a much higher survival rate (see Chapter 6) and, in many
respects, have taken on the same psychosocial features of chronic illness. For the sake of
clarity, issues surrounding the acute onset, diagnosis and initial hospital treatment in
leukaemia are considered under acute illness (Chapter 6) given the rapid onset and
intensive treatment needs in the initial stages. Yet as ALL involves treatment extending
substantially longer (i.e., 2–3 years) than those normally attributed to acute illness (i.e.,
up to approximately 3 months), we also consider the chronic illness characteristics of
this acute condition in this chapter. This reflects the changing nature of some childhood
diseases, as described above, but also the multifaceted trajectory of psychosocial needs
in patients and their families facing cancer diagnosis in their child. It also fits with our
focus on illness as being both an acute and a chronic stressor, depending on the characteristics of the illness. Post-treatment effects for the child and family, including life-long
implications and threat to survival, are covered in Chapter 8 under terminal issues and
survivorship. The reason for this division will, I hope, become clear as the psychosocial
characteristics of different types of conditions are described. It is worth being aware
that, for these reasons of definition and treatment course, cancers such as ALL are frequently considered as chronic illness in the literature. Suffice it to say, such conditions
are ambiguous in definition but, whatever the categorization, the psychosocial aspects
and impact remain the same.

So, in this chapter, I consider chronic illness defined as 'a persistent or recurring condition which may or may not be severe, often starts gradually and changes will be slow'
(Macpherson, 1999). Whilst some chronic conditions may be congenital (i.e., genetically
inherited) and emerge at birth (e.g., phenylketonuria [PKU], spina bifida), others emerge
in the first year of life during infancy (e.g., cystic fibrosis and sickle cell anaemia), or during early childhood (e.g., muscular dystrophy, which emerges after 3 years of age; see
Gortmaker, in Eiser, 1990). Other non-congenital chronic conditions develop during
childhood: for example, the autoimmune condition of type 1 diabetes (T1D; also referred
to in the past as insulin-dependent or early onset diabetes) which has a peak developmental age of 12 years; or the allergic atopic condition of asthma, which, although variable,
frequently develops during the first couple of years of life (see Gortmaker, in Eiser, 1990).
Table 7.2 gives a description of some of the most prevalent chronic childhood illnesses
and conditions based on age of onset, incidence and survival rate.

TABLE 7.2 Incidence rates for prevalent chronic illnesses in children (0–18 years)

Disease/illness	Age of onset	Incidence	Survival estimates
Asthma	Variable: first 1–2 years	2005: 8.9% children (6.5 million) (US) 2007: 9.1% of children (6.7 million) (US)	Similar to typically developing children
Cystic fibrosis (congenital)	Variable: usually during first year, most by age 2	1 out of 3,200 children (worldwide)	Median life expectancy is 40 years
Type 1 diabetes (T1D)	Variable: childhood	1 in every 400 individuals (under 20) (worldwide)	With treatment, few children die
Obesity	Variable: childhood	2010–2011: 22.6% obese ages 4–5 (33.4% ages 10–11) (UK)	With treatment, few children die
Developmental disabilities (learning disability and ADHD)	Variable: anytime during development	1997–2008: 13.87% ages 3–17 (US); 1.4% (worldwide)	Similar to typically developing children
Cerebral palsy	Neonatal up to age 3	2007: 2.12–2.45 per 1,000 live births (US)	Usually a normal life expectancy
Congenital heart disease	Birth	Between 4 and 9 per 1,000 live born infants (UK)	78% of babies will survive until adulthood
Acute lymphocytic leukaemia (ALL)	Peak incidence aged 2–5 years	2009: 3.7–4.9 cases per 100,000 children age 0–14 years (US)	2010: 5-year survival rate for ALL is 89%
Spina bifida	Birth	1–2 cases per 1,000 live births (worldwide)	Majority live until early adulthood
HIV/AIDS	Most commonly transmitted during pregnancy, delivery and after delivery	2010: estimate 3.4 million (worldwide); 68% of all HIV cases are in Sub-Saharan Africa	With treatment, (AIDS) life expectancy is ~10 years
Juvenile arthritis	Most common in ages 7–12 (may also occur in adolescents)	2007: 1 in 250 children (US)	In most cases, similar to typically developing children
Muscular dystrophy	Birth	Approximately 1 in 544,000 (US)	Varies according to the type of MD and the progression of the disorder

Source: Based on Gortmaker, in Eiser (1990), with additional sources: Elborn et al. (1991); Klinnert et al. (2001); Knoll et al. (2007); Akinbami et al. (2009); Ribera and Oriol (2009); Hunger et al. (2010); Jemal et al. (2010); Torpy et al. (2010); Boyle et al. (2011); Compas et al. (2012).

BOX 7.1

What is the difference between incidence and prevalence of a disease?

Both incidence and prevalence are measures of the 'frequency' of a disease or illness within the population:

Incidence is the number of 'new' cases of a disease over a certain period of time.

Prevalence is the 'total' number of cases (new and previously existing) at a certain point in time.

(Macpherson, 1999)

THE PREVALENCE OF CHRONIC ILLNESS

One factor that makes the definition of chronic illness another of our slippery, amorphous terms (albeit, in a good way) is the development of new treatments. New procedures and medications can reframe once-acute terminal illnesses into chronic conditions and provide curative treatment for once-chronic illnesses (see Chapter 8 for a discussion of the term 'cure'). Furthermore, a change in prevalence rates across different illnesses in children and adolescents can dramatically change the profile of chronic disease. A case in point is an epidemiological study by Van Cleave and colleagues (2010) described in Box 7.2.

BOX 7.2

The changing profile of chronic disease in children

Source: J. Van Cleave, S.L. Gortmaker and J.M. Perrin (2010) Dynamics of obesity and chronic health conditions among children and youth. *Journal of the American Medical Association*, 303(7): 623–30.

    Background: Prevalence rates for chronic conditions, such as obesity, asthma, behavioural and learning problems, in children and adolescents have increased considerably over the past quarter of a century or so. Some conditions which were once rare have now increased in prevalence due to advances in neonatal care, and other conditions have seen advances in treatment, increasing life-expectancy and survival time.

    Aim of the study: To examine changes in prevalence rates and patterns in chronic childhood illness.

    Populations and methods: Chronic illness was examined in over 5,000 children across three cohorts in the US, using data from a national longitudinal survey. Participants were mothers with children aged 2–8 years at baseline, followed up once every 2 years over a 6-year period until the ages of 8–14 years. Three cohorts were studied, assessed across the years 1988–2006 as illustrated in Figure 7.1.

(Continued)

(Continued)

In an interview, mothers reported whether their child had 'any physical, emotional or mental condition' which affected their school work, attendance at school, or doing usual childhood

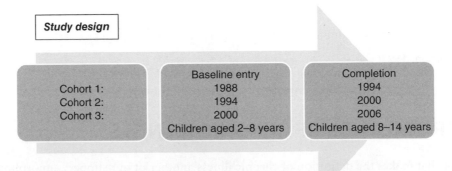

FIGURE 7.1   Study design showing the three cohorts assessed from 1988 to 2006
Source: Van Cleave et al. (2010).

activities, and whether the condition required frequent medical appointments or medication. The type of condition and length of time the child had reported it were recorded, and chronic illness was defined as a condition lasting at least a year. Chronic conditions were divided into four categories: (i) asthma; (ii) obesity; (iii) other physical conditions (including sinus infections, sight or hearing problems, allergies, and epilepsy); and (iv) behavioural or learning difficulties.

Results: The authors found a high prevalence rate of having a chronic condition across the 6 years that each cohort was followed. They observed an increase in chronic illness prevalence across the subsequent cohort waves (for children aged 8–14 years, prevalence was 27.8 per cent in the earliest cohort examined between years 1988 and 1994, compared to 51.5 per cent in the later cohort examined between the years 2000 and 2006) with the same cohort pattern for each illness. The increase in prevalence was greatest for obesity, followed by the range of conditions classified as other, then lastly for asthma and behavioural or learning problems. Interestingly, as well as this pattern of increase across cohorts, they also reported a 'dynamic' pattern to the prevalence. In other words, chronic illness in children did not always remain or get worse but in many cases improved or 'remitted' throughout the course of childhood (9.3 per cent of sample), although some then developed new conditions. Prevalence rates were associated with sociodemographic factors such that illness incidence was greater in males, children from a racial minority, and those whose mothers were recorded as obese.

Conclusion: Chronic illness in children and adolescents is described as both 'common' and 'dynamic'. This dynamic nature, including remission in some cases, was a surprise finding for the authors who conclude by recommending the need for health care to 'adapt' to the dynamic nature of chronic conditions, to 'promote' remission, as well as to 'prevent' the onset of new conditions.

It is important to document changes in chronic illness prevalence rates as they serve as a barometer for changes, not just in medical treatment, but also in psychosocial factors which contribute to changes in illness rates. Knowledge of changes in prevalence also helps inform treatment and prevention practices since psychosocial factors interplay with prevalence in chronic conditions. A good example of this caught the attention of the international media (see www.bbc.co.uk/news/health-17942181) when a massive increase in prevalence levels of myopia (short-sightedness or near-sightedness) in children growing up in East Asia was identified in a review of reported myopia prevalence rates (Morgan et al., 2012). Myopia is considered a major visual impairment by the World Health Organization (WHO) and, if not treated, can lead to severe impairment in sight or even blindness in 10–20 per cent of those affected (Morgan et al., 2012). In East Asian countries, such as Singapore, prevalence rates for myopia in children of Chinese, Indian and Malay ethnicities graduating from high school have increased from 20 to 30 per cent to rates of between 80 and 90 per cent in the past 25 years (Morgan et al., 2012), as shown in Figure 7.2.

This increase in prevalence rates is attributed to a combination of cultural academic pressure to obtain high grades, coupled with a lack of exposure to natural outdoor light (not necessarily to sun but light exposure), as a result of staying indoors for long periods of each day engaged in intensive reading and study. Morgan et al. (2012) also report early evidence of increases in myopia in children in North America and Europe, although to a lesser extent. Such changes are perhaps an ominous indication of the future picture of health in developed

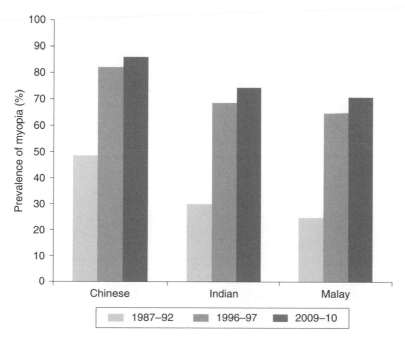

FIGURE 7.2 Changes in the prevalence of myopia in the three major ethnic groups in Singapore: Chinese, Indian and Malay

Source: Morgan et al. (2012: 1741, fig. 2).

BOX 7.3

Nature deficit disorder: spotlight on lifestyle factors contributing to chronic illness

In March 2012, the National Trust (an independent registered UK charity) caused a media storm by adopting the term nature deficit disorder (NDD) in their report on the plight of UK children suffering from a 'sedentary, indoor childhood' (www.nationaltrust.org.uk). They were responding to an increased pattern of children staying indoors – staying in becoming the new going out, to use a common phrase. They identified a number of factors responsi-

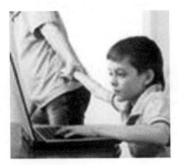

FIGURE 7.3 'Virtual play': implicated in nature deficit disorder

Source: shutterstock-98100608?

ble for this trend, including health and safety restrictions, parental fear of strangers and traffic dangers, children's use of technology, electronic devices and the Internet, and a focus on 'virtual play' rather than 'real play' (Figure 7.3). Coined by Louv (2010), NDD is a descriptive phrase, not a recognized medical condition (see the British Psychological Society's coverage of this report at www.bps.org.uk/news/uk-kids-are-not-experiencing-great-outdoors). The NT report (Moss, 2012) makes use of this term to illustrate the 'human costs of alienation from nature'. In addition to a 'diminished use of the senses' and 'attention difficulties', these costs include 'higher rates of physical and emotional difficulties' (Louv in Moss, 2012: 2). It is this last characteristic which is important with respect to chronic illness, and links to illness prevalence as described above, particularly the examples given of obesity and myopia. The report also cites increases in asthma, vitamin D deficiency leading to rickets, and overall decline in muscle strength and cardiovascular fitness. This not only has implications for childhood, but for long-term health complications into adulthood. Health is one of the four categories outlined by the NT report as having the potential to benefit children if the generational trend towards NDD can be 'reversed'.

Points to consider

- Does NDD exist or is the use of the term a resistance to adaptation to new technology and modern ways of living in childhood?
- How do psychosocial factors contribute to NDD and which further types of chronic illness might increase as a result of a sedentary, indoor lifestyle in the future?
- How might psychosocial intervention programmes encouraging children to play outdoors be able to alter the prevalence of chronic illness in children?
- How is stress implicated in the relationship between NDD and illness?

countries. This is a good example of a chronic condition for which prevalence rates are being increased through changes in lifestyle and health behaviours, and which presents both a challenge and an opportunity for intervention to change behaviour to prevent and reduce the severity of the chronic condition. Morgan et al. (2012) report early trials currently underway in China and Singapore to increase the amount of time children and their families spend out of doors in order to increase exposure to natural light. Such interventions are not in opposition to medical treatment and ophthalmic correction, but work alongside and help to prevent the need for them. Similarly, genetic factors are implicated in myopia, but it is the important gene–environment interaction that is at play here.

THE IMPACT OF CHRONIC ILLNESS: THE STRESS CONTEXT

Chronic illness is a major ongoing stressor and, as such, fits with the second type of allostatic load as described by McEwen (1998b; see Chapter 2). Yet the stress trajectory of chronic illness also involves phases of acute illness events or characteristics (e.g., diagnosis and initial treatment, periods of heightened symptom severity or surgical procedures) which constitute acute stressors. These acute stressors reflect the first type of allostatic load as referred to by McEwen (1998b; see Chapter 2). Together, this mix of underlying chronic stress coupled with periodic acute stress make up a complex 'stress mosaic' (Miller et al., 2007) and the 'double exposure' of the stress pattern referred to by Marin and colleagues (2009).

So chronic illness is a major stressor at any age but, starting in childhood, it presents additional hurdles associated with every stage of development. In the earliest stages of life, parental attachment and bonding may be affected, the ability of the preschool child to learn through play and socialization may be hampered, and once of school age, doing regular activities, such as sports, games and music, perhaps taken for granted by other children, may present a range of challenges and difficulties. Once the storm of adolescence begins, the challenges and difficulties take on a new dimension, with additional social pressures and self-consciousness which may compound the usual turbulence of the teenage years. Across childhood and adolescence, chronic illness presents a potential disruption to schooling, social life (friends and friendship groups), relationships, identity, and self-concept. The impact and influence on family life may also be considerable, and for parents and siblings there is enormous potential for stress in facing the challenges of having a child or sibling with a chronic illness. It may involve regular hospital appointments, compliance with medication, general disruption to lifestyle, and concern for future well-being, as well as possible financial implications of parental caregiving for the chronically ill child. Chronic illness in childhood is not static but presents an ever-changing landscape as new developmental milestones and expectations require adaptation within the restrictions of the condition.

In the light of these recognized substantial potential needs for support and appropriate information, children with chronic illness and their families are often reported to cope well. Both the difficulties in coping and the resilience observed provide a rich source of evidence for understanding the process of coping in the face of the stress mosaic confronted by children with chronic illness, their parents and siblings. This notion of resilience and positive coping should not be underestimated. For example, in a review of quality of life following bone-marrow transplant in children up to the age of 18 years as part of the treatment for cancer, Clarke, Eiser, and Skinner (2008) report a good quality of life (as good as or better than population norms) at 6–8 months after transplant surgery. This study highlights the psychosocial variables of family functioning and individual resources, including social skills as predictors of quality of life outcome.

As with adult chronic illness, the visibility of the condition is an important characteristic. A child in a wheelchair obviously has a disability, and a child who has lost their hair and is wearing a headscarf has become a symbol of cancer chemotherapy treatment. Such obvious signs of illness may generate a range of reactions from peers and strangers who make their own interpretations of the condition. For the child with an unseen condition – for example, diabetes, phenylketonuria (PKU) or human immunodeficiency virus (HIV+) – the illness is masked from public view, but the psychosocial effects may still be significant. Whether the condition is visible or not, the effects act as a double-edged sword in their impact on the child or adolescent. The genetically recessive inherited condition of PKU is a metabolic illness, characterized by a deficiency of the enzyme phenylalanine hydroxylase, and can result in severe mental retardation if left untreated, due to high levels of phenylalanine in the blood. The presence of PKU is now routinely assessed from blood tests a few days after birth and, as such, is generally detected early and managed well, avoiding the effects seen in previous decades. Treatment is through a strict dietary regimen, involving intake of only very limited levels of phenylalanine-containing food found in protein substances, which needs to begin during the first month of life. Such dietary restraints are similar to those in diabetes, but there is relatively little research on this condition in the psychosocial domain. In a qualitative study by Vegni and colleagues (2010), of 47 participants with PKU aged 8 years up to 31 years, characteristic themes were evident across different age groups. A common theme across all age groups was that having PKU was invisible ('transparent') until it came to eating in a social context, which meant that PKU patients often felt they had to choose between being isolated socially from events involving food in order to retain a feeling of normality or to let their condition become visible in order to take part socially. Specifically for the youngest group, of 8–12 years, the sense of feeling 'different' was evident, and dealing with disclosing their condition to others both their choice and that of their parents. They had to (i) 'make the disease a part of the self' and (ii) 'affront the irony of their peers' (Vegni et al., 2010: 544). In comparison, in the adolescent group aged 13–17 years, PKU patients were progressively taking responsibility for their diet and sometimes deliberately 'violated the rules'. Disclosure of PKU status to friends during adolescence was their decision, and the authors note that friendships were often based on whether or not they felt they could disclose. Parental involvement in diet during this age is described as complex, as some felt supported by their parents' attempts to assist with their diet, whilst other battled against feelings of control (Vegni et al., 2010). Similar themes arise in research with adolescent diabetic patients described below.

Another example of a condition with unseen or non-visible effects is that of children with the human immunodeficiency virus (HIV+). Yet they may experience a number of stressors which could be classified as medical, psychological or social in nature and their effect 'accumulative' as listed in Figure 7.4 (Moss et al., 1998). Moss and co-workers (1998) prospectively studied a group of 24 children aged 8–15 years who were HIV+ (over 80 per cent of whom had contracted the virus through blood transfusion) and receiving anti-retroviral treatment, over a 2-year period. They report a decrease in positive social self-concept over time, but, interestingly, they note that psychosocial adjustment scores (e.g., on depression, anxiety, social competence and resiliency) were within the normal range and hence comparable with non-infected children. In this study, the child's life event score was significantly correlated with psychosocial adjustment and also with survival. Five out of the 24 children died before the 2-year follow-up, and these children were found to have a greater life event score (more adversity), a lower resiliency score and poorer immune profile (lower CD4 percentage). It is important to note that just over a third of the sample also had haemophilia and, as such, would have had the additional impact of this condition to cope with. Of course, these stressors are not exhaustive and, characteristic of the biopsychosocial model, there is considerable overlap and interplay between them. The stressor of pain, for example, may be a medical source, but psychosocial factors influence the experience of pain, and similarly the threat of a shortened life may trigger psychosocial stressors (see Chapter 9 for more on

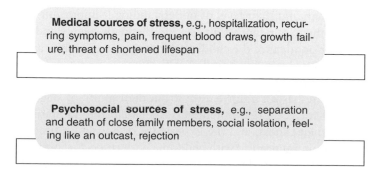

FIGURE 7.4 Examples of accumulative stressors from medical, psychological, or social sources in children with HIV+

Source: Based on information in Moss et al. (1998).

these specific topics). Although this study is of children with HIV+, it could be seen as a model for other diseases as well.

In HIV+, a central issue is that of disclosure; in other words, if and when individuals tell others about their disease status. Having to keep something a secret is associated with negative health outcomes and, conversely, being able to disclose information, with positive outcomes. A study by Sherman et al. (2000) found evidence for disclosure of HIV+ status in a sample of children aged 8–18 years to be associated with a better immune profile (greater CD4 percentage) relevant to HIV+ progression. Disclosure therefore had a positive effect on their immune profile, although it had no effect on their behaviour or self-concept (Sherman et al., 2000). It is noteworthy that studies frequently report changes in physiological impacts, such as alterations in immune functioning, whilst psychosocial factors may remain comparable with HIV-children. This emphasizes the need to explore the physiological impact of psychosocial stressors in order to understand changes at an objective hormonal or immune level rather than relying solely on more overt behavioural or self-report indices. Changes at a physiological level may occur in a different temporal mode from (e.g., in advance of) reported or observable psychosocial effects and provide an early warning signal or biomarker.

THE RELEVANCE OF ILLNESS COGNITIONS IN CHRONIC CHILDHOOD ILLNESS

There are specific features of chronic illness that may influence psychosocial cognitions in a child. By its nature and definition, chronic illness starts relatively slowly (an acute event precipitating the illness notwithstanding) and is likely to be with the child for the entirety of his or her life, even if in varying degrees of severity. Given that we are considering conditions that start early in life, in some respects the illness becomes a way of life that is normal, at least for the child. Whilst children's cognitive capacities become more complex throughout development, and their level of understanding is important in chronic illness, there is evidence that the experience of illness, and the many events and procedures associated with it, can alter or advance the child's stage of cognitive understanding. How these medical events and procedures are handled is therefore important as they present an opportunity for developing cognitions.

Rushforth (1999) emphasizes a move away from the rigidity of staged models of children's cognitions to a focus on the 'potential' rather than the 'limitations' of children's understanding about their illness, and the experience of hospitalization and the implications that this has for communicating with children. With respect to preparation for hospital procedures, Rushforth (1999) describes the child as having 'considerable' potential for understanding. She points out the vital role of hospital practitioners in gathering information about the specific level of knowledge and understanding of each individual child, in connection with their illness and its treatment, prior to providing appropriate information in accordance with this level. Checking and confirming that the information given has been understood correctly is also vital. Rushforth highlights the importance of explaining medical terminology to children, who may hear words that are unfamiliar to them and, in trying to make sense, may wrongly misinterpret (giving the example of a child mistakenly believing they had 'ivy' growing inside them on hearing the term 'IV'). The importance of the careful use of metaphors in explanation, often used to aid understanding, is also highlighted, since they may give particular scope for misunderstanding; for example, whilst a balloon may be the obvious metaphorical aid to an explanation of the lungs or bladder, a child's most frequent experience with balloons is that they may 'burst' (Rushforth, 1999). Such explanations may be counterproductive to a well-meaning explanation if understanding is not checked. Similarly, parental understanding cannot be assumed, and a thorough knowledge of this is important before a parent is charged with explaining a procedure to their child (Rushforth, 1999).

COPING AND ADAPTATION IN CHRONIC CHILDHOOD ILLNESS

Given the characteristics of chronic illness described above, unlike the sudden onset of acute illness, in some cases a chronic illness condition and the many demands it makes may be viewed as the norm for a child who has lived with a condition since birth. Under these circumstances, adaptation to the condition may take a different form to that of acute illness since life without the illness or condition may be difficult to imagine. For the parents and family, however, the need for adaptation may be greater from the start, since their point of reference for normality, their hopes and expectations of life without illness, may be somewhat different. For the child, increasing realization of the impact of the condition on their lifestyle may come with age and comparison with the external world, and peer rejection is perhaps no more apparent than in the teenage or adolescent years.

Coping responses to stress were introduced in Chapter 2, and further detailed in Chapter 6, under acute stress. I considered the development of the taxonomy of coping in children and adolescents and introduced coping as a mediator of stress. Specifically, we focused on the dominant stress-control model of coping in children and adolescents, based on the work of Weisz, McCabe, and Dennig (1994), and applied to children with cancer undergoing medical procedures by Rudolph, Dennig, and Weisz (1995). Built upon by Connor-Smith and colleagues (2000), a further distinction was made between automatic components of the coping process and volitional or controlled components. The former are those responses, whether emotion or physiological, which are not under conscious control and are linked to temperament or influenced by past conditioning, whereas the latter are the coping responses themselves over which individuals have freedom of choice (Connor-Smith et al., 2000). It is these coping responses that are most open to change via psychosocial intervention and can be divided into primary control, secondary control and disengagement coping (Connor-Smith et al., 2000). These theories of stress and coping are just as relevant, if not more so, when considering adaptation in chronic illness.

Seminal work in the 1980s and 1990s by researchers such as Christine Eiser and her team drew attention to the experience of the child with chronic illness and their family in the context of stress and coping, both in a generic sense and with factors specific to each type of illness. Emphasizing the dynamic nature of coping, Eiser (1989) highlights the daily, ongoing stresses and coping needs of children with chronic illness as falling into three inter-related areas: (i) those associated with management of the illness itself (medication, diet, exercise, changes in appearance); (ii) indirect issues associated with treatment, such as negotiating school in conjunction with continuing treatment; and (iii) everyday stressors not associated with the illness but which all children have to deal with whether these are exams or peer relationships. Viewing coping as a dynamic process allows for different styles of coping to be seen as effective in different situations for the same person, allowing for changes over time in what may be effective. Rudolph et al. (1995) also describe the notion of a temporal pattern to coping responses in children, using terms such as 'coping repertoires', 'profiles' and 'temporal sequences' to describe the complexity of coping, and they refer to the concept of 'layered coping' or a 'hierarchy of ordered strategies' (Weisz and Dennig, in Rudolph et al., 1995). In other words, it is necessary to have a range of coping responses available to operationalize, depending on the characteristics of the challenge. Combinations of coping responses are also referred to by Rudolph et al. (1995) which may utilize 'concurrent' or 'reciprocal' ways of coping (i.e., several responses used at once in order to deal with the different aspects of the stressor). This is particularly relevant to the mosaic stressor patterns seen in chronic illness, in which variable ongoing chronic stress is coupled with acutely stressful events over a prolonged period of time.

This early work also emphasized the need for family support, parental involvement and awareness of the effect of chronic illness on siblings. As well as coping with the stress of having a brother or sister who is chronically ill and the distress that may generate, it may also create a dynamic of competition or feelings of isolation in the well sibling because of the demands placed upon the parents' attention towards the ill child. Person-specific moderating variables (e.g., gender, developmental level, prior experience, temperament) and situation-specific moderating variables (e.g., stressor type, stage and controllability, parental influence) are also important, as outlined by Rudolph et al. (1995). As work by Houtzager and colleagues (2004) points out, the acute stress response to having a sibling diagnosed with cancer usually 'normalizes' in most children by the time the condition is seen as long term or chronic (in this study measured at 2 years after diagnosis) but, for some, the feeling of emotional distress may continue. For younger siblings (7–11 years at follow-up), this was observed in reduced quality of life, whereas for adolescents (12–18 years at follow-up), the effects showed themselves in symptoms of depression, anxiety and social withdrawal (Houtzager et al., 2004). Houtzager et al. also point to the lack of longitudinal research on the emotional impact on siblings of cancer patients during the chronic phase of the illness.

As Eiser (1989) points out, work in this era was heavily concentrated on children with diabetes or cancer, and focused more on the family response and coping rather than how the child coped with the actual illness or treatment. So has this changed in recent years? Has this gap in the literature been addressed and do we now know more about how children cope with illness and treatment in chronic conditions? Cancer and type 1 diabetes (T1D) are still amongst the most prevalent chronic illnesses in children, and interest in the characteristic stresses they present has been sustained across several decades of psychology research into chronic illness in children despite advances in treatment. As demonstrated in a much-needed, thorough review of child and adolescent coping in chronic illness (Compas et al., 2012), the literature has moved forward significantly with regard to understanding the psychosocial aspects of coping responses in children and adolescents with chronic illness (e.g., see Weisz et al., 1994; Connor-Smith et al., 2000). The dominant theories and models view stress and coping as a transaction between the individual and the environment, in which the individual tries to achieve a 'goodness of fit' (Weisz et al., 1994) between the demands of the stressor and the way in which they respond to it. Yet, even in the review by Compas et al. (2012), over 20 years after Eiser (1989), the authors still point out a lack of research directly examining illness-specific stressors in children themselves, particularly those at the time of treatment and post-treatment.

For children receiving treatment for cancer (leukaemia, lymphoma, brain and other solid tumours) and their parents, stressor characteristics have been categorized as falling into three domains: (i) 'daily role functioning'; (ii) the 'physical effects of treatment' (child) or 'cancer communication', i.e., communication about the treatment (parents); (iii) 'uncertainty about cancer' and the future (child) or 'cancer caregiving' (parent) including future concerns (Rodriguez et al., 2012). In this range of cancers, parents and children have been reported to be moderately to highly stressed on all three domains, but the domain of daily role functioning has been reported by both parents and children as being more stressful than uncertainty about the future (Rodriguez et al., 2012). For parents, this domain of 'daily role functioning' refers to 'paying bills and family expenses', concerns about their job or that of their partner, or 'having less time and energy for other children and/or spouse'; and, for children, this refers to 'missing school', 'falling behind in school work', not being able to do the things they used to, frequent visits to hospital, or being concerned about family or friends. These cancer-specific daily role stressors are similar to the indirect cancer stresses described by Eiser (1989), as cited above, and are relevant to chronic illness and chronic phases of cancer with ongoing treatment.

Compas et al. (2012) specifically consider type 1 diabetes (T1D), chronic pain and cancer as three prevalent health conditions affecting children and adolescents. Pain is covered here separately in Chapter 9. The illnesses of T1D and cancer are interesting as they represent contrasting conditions in terms of symptoms and treatments, and each has its own characteristic profile of stressors which require a range of coping responses. In contrast to the cancer stressors described above, diabetes requires repeated daily monitoring of blood glucose levels (at least four per day), 3–4 daily insulin injections or use of a pump, attention to carbohydrate intake and careful matching of insulin with diet and exercise, and checking of urine for ketones (Compas et al., 2012). As peak onset for T1D is around puberty, the medication regimen, which may require parental input and monitoring at least in the initial stages following diagnosis, is in 'direct conflict' with the natural adolescent striving for autonomy (Compas et al., 2012). During adolescence, monitoring and medication in diabetes then become a vehicle for autonomy, making the important role of parenting an even more difficult one than for healthy adolescents. Parents may find it difficult to let go of the control over medication, and they tread a difficult line in retaining involvement and support whilst enabling autonomy. Compas et al. (2012) refer to the need for parents to support their children in coping with their diabetes, adapting to these changing requirements in autonomy and control when transitioning from childhood into adolescence (see section below on parental coping). For both diabetes and cancer, as contrasting examples of chronic illness, Compas et al. (2012) point to secondary control coping (e.g., acceptance, cognitive restructuring, distraction), in which the individual attempts to adapt to the source of the stress, as the most useful strategy associated with better adjustment, while disengagement strategies are associated with poorer adjustment. Yet, for aspects of illness such as difficulties in maintaining control over difficult treatment regimens in diabetes, primary control coping (e.g., problem-solving) may also be useful (Compas et al., 2012). Refer back to Chapter 6 for a full description of coping responses.

PARENTAL COPING IN CHRONIC CHILDHOOD ILLNESS

There has been a significant amount of research into parental coping in childhood illness, particularly in parents coping with the diagnosis and treatment of younger children with cancer and older children with diabetes. The way a parent interacts with their child with chronic illness, and the style of support they give to them, play an important role in the child's adjustment. As with the changes in coping responses over time in children, the coping responses of parents and family also need to evolve over time, based on the developmental level of the child. The parental role in caring for a child with a chronic illness is, of course, a major source of stress. Parental stress in response to a child with a chronic illness has been divided into four domains: (i) communication; (ii) emotional functioning; (iii) medical care; and (iv) role function, using the Pediatric Inventory for Parents (PIP; Streisand et al., 2001; Table 7.3). Although devised and tested on parents of children with cancer (including leukaemia, lymphoma, neuroblastoma, osteosarcoma, Wilms' tumour, rhabdomyosarcoma, and Ewing's sarcoma), it was designed for use more generally across a range of illnesses in children (Streisand et al., 2001).

The age of the child is a significant feature in respect of parental stress and coping in a chronic illness condition. As described above in describing children's coping, contrast across ages can be seen in two examples: cancer, which generally peaks in prevalence earlier in childhood, and diabetes, which peaks in prevalence later in childhood and into the teenage years (10–14 years; the Writing Group, in Comeaux and Jaser, 2010). Both parental age and age of the child has been linked to higher levels of reported stress in parents of children with cancer, with younger parents and parents of younger children reporting significantly greater

TABLE 7.3 Sample items from the Pediatric Inventory for Parents (PIP) by scale

I Communication
Arguing with family member
Speaking with doctor
Speaking with child about his/her illness
II Emotional functioning
Trying not to think about my family's difficulties
Learning upsetting news
Feeling numb inside
III Medical care
Helping my child with medical procedures
Making decisions about medical care or medicines
Handling changes in my child's daily medical routines
IV Role function
Trying to attend to the needs of other family members
Being unable to go to work/job
Feeling uncertain about disciplining my child

All responses are on a 5-point Likert-type scale. Respondents answer two questions for each item: 'How often has the event occurred?' and 'How difficult was the event for you?'

amounts of stress than older parents or parents of older children with cancer (Streisand et al., 2001). In addition to the demographic of age, parental sex differences have also been noted, with mothers of children with cancer reporting greater amounts of stress than fathers (Vrijmoet-Wiersma et al., in Rodriguez et al., 2012), although some studies report greater similarity in high levels of distress for both parents, in some cases to the degree of a post-traumatic stress classification (Streisand et al., 2001; Dunn et al., 2012). As mentioned in Chapter 6, the degree of differentiation in the roles of mothers and fathers may account for the observed effects. Having a child with a chronic illness carries with it a burden of care and responsibility, the combined effect of which is shared in two-parent families. Many studies assume a dual parenting model, some even actively excluding divorced parents from participation (Gultekin and Baran, 2007), but the importance of the responsibility placed on the single parent is gaining interest in research (Brown et al., 2008) and, given the increased rates of lone parenting over the past half-century, some might say not before time.

Rodriguez et al. (2012) point to the implication of their study on cancer-related sources of stress for parents, and suggest that, as well as providing parents with information and problem-solving techniques, interventions need to include coping techniques specifically for dealing with the uncontrollable characteristics of their child's cancer. These might include acceptance or cognitive reappraisal to cope with anxiety about their child surviving the disease or feelings of distress when they are not able to make their child feel better.

To explore the chronic condition of T1D further, this illness provides a prime example of the need for psychosocial adaptation in parents based on the developmental needs of the child. As caregivers, parents take on a large part of the responsibility for management of this condition in younger children. The experience of T1D in adolescence, whether transitioning from a condition present since childhood or diagnosed during teenage years, the characteristics of this turbulent period of development present a conflict with the characteristics of T1D management (Comeaux and Jaser, 2010). Table 7.4 maps the challenges of chronic illness onto the recurring themes and challenges of adolescence, viewed as simultaneously linked and in conflict (see Comeaux and Jaser, 2010).

In diabetes, the role of 'autonomy' appears to be particularly salient, as adolescents seek to establish and maintain control over their condition, which involves careful monitoring of blood sugar levels and adjustment of insulin mediation (Comeaux and Jaser, 2010). For parents, getting it right over the timing and degree of responsibility given to their adolescent child for monitoring and management of their diabetes can be difficult. In other words, having diabetes heightens the normal struggle in transfer of responsibilities between parents and children during adolescence. A gradual transfer of responsibility in diabetes care, avoiding transfer at too early an age, and retaining 'supportive' and 'collaborative' involvement have been found to give better outcomes in diabetes (see Comeaux and Jaser, 2010). In a study by Wiebe et al. (2005) of 125 children with T1D aged 10–15 years, the contrasting styles of maternal 'involvement' versus 'control' were examined. For those who rated their mothers as being 'uninvolved' in their diabetes care, adherence and quality of life were poorer. This contrasted with maternal 'collaboration' in care which was linked to greater adherence and metabolic control. Considering age and sex, in the older children, greater maternal control was linked to poorer adherence and, for older girls, to poorer quality of life. The authors conclude that maternal collaborative involvement is important in coping with diabetes. As Comeaux and Jaser (2010) highlight, diabetes is of particular interest since advances in insulin medication used and the way it is delivered (use of an infusion pump versus injections) have changed the parameters of living with the condition, and early indications are that this changes the psychosocial impact

TABLE 7.4 Mapping the challenges of chronic illness onto the characteristics and challenges of adolescence

Healthy/'normal' adolescence		Chronic illness
Recurring themes	Areas of challenge	Parallel challenges
Identity	School	Increased school absences
Achievement	Sexuality	Disease-related fatigue
Autonomy	Substance abuse	Pain
Intimacy	Health behaviours	Medication regimens
	Societal attitudes	Altered methods of parenting
	Future life options	Altered social interactions
	Self-worth	

in adolescence. For these reasons, Compas et al. (2012) describe the role of parental coping in diabetes as being particularly important, even more so than in other illnesses.

Whilst I am focusing here on physical health in children, and parental involvement in relation to the impact that may have on the child, it is also worth noting that caring for a child with chronic illness may impact on the physical health of the parent(s) as primary caregivers. For example, in a comparison of 32 parents whose children had developmental disabilities and 29 parents of typically developing children, Gallagher, Phillips, Drayson, and Carroll (2009) report a poorer antibody response to influenza vaccine in the caregiving parents. This indicates a mechanism for increased viral susceptibility in the parents of the children with the chronic condition. A higher level of behavioural problems was also linked to poorer immune response. This conceptualization of parents as caregivers is an important one, as there is much research documenting the immune decline of older adults in the caregiving role but very little that documents parents in this way. This is important as it highlights the need for parental support and the reality of the spiral of effects linking parent and child health.

INTERVENTIONS IN CHRONIC CHILDHOOD ILLNESS

As discussed above, research into coping in children with chronic illness suggests that secondary control coping (e.g., acceptance, distraction, cognitive restructuring, and positive thinking) is best suited to the demands and challenges faced in dealing with chronic illness (Compas et al., 2012) since it focuses on coping through adaptation to the stressor rather than acting to change the stressor itself. Given the uncontrollable qualities of the stressors faced in connection with chronic illness, such an approach is most likely to be successful, although this does not rule out the need for primary control coping (e.g., problem-solving, emotional expression) in some circumstances, whereas disengagement coping (avoidance, denial, wishful thinking) appears not to be a useful strategy and may even interfere with successful use of other strategies in coping with chronic illness (Compas et al., 2012).

Psychosocial interventions which focus on developing specific types of coping responses in relation to stress experienced in children with chronic illness are likely to produce the best outcomes for psychosocial adaptation, as well as physiological outcome achieved either directly through the stress-reducing effects of coping and emotion regulation or indirectly through compliance with medication and attention to relevant health behaviours. Examples of interventions successfully employing such techniques include coping-skills training for adolescents with diabetes and cognitive behaviour therapy (CBT) to reduce depression in adolescents with inflammatory bowel disease using 'primary and secondary control enhancement therapy-physical illness' (PASCET-PI; see Compas et al., 2012). Such interventions are not easy to conduct, however, and difficulty in the retention of participants should not be underestimated, particularly in interventions with harder-to-reach target groups who are particularly stressed by their condition or in adolescent populations (see Chapter 3 for a discussion of methodological considerations). Reed-Knight and colleagues (2012) draw attention to this in a web-based coping skills intervention study of 31 adolescent girls with inflammatory bowel disease (IBD) and their parents. The study involved an initial one-day meeting followed by web sessions on a weekly basis over 6 weeks. The study saw a 38 per cent drop-out rate (12 of the 31 families) and the researchers point to depressive symptoms in the adolescents and to catastrophic thoughts and more parenting stress in parents who dropped out of the study. Similarly, the girls who experienced more problematic physical symptoms also participated less in the web component even if they did not drop out of the study (Reed-Knight et al., 2012).

MEDICAL PROCEDURES AND HOSPITALIZATION IN CHRONIC CHILDHOOD ILLNESS

The context of care and treatment in paediatric chronic illness requires frequent medical appointments, ongoing medication needs, possible surgery, frequent hospital stays or review of care and treatment. Diet, exercise, sleep and other health behaviours may be affected by these medical treatments or require regulation as part of the condition. In chronic illness, the hospital has been described as having a 'major health promoting role to play' for children and their families, which draws attention to the need for help not just with the physical condition but with its psychological impact (Aujoulat et al., 2006: 25). Recommendations for psychological input include: social support from peers; the provision of a supportive medical environment in which the child feels safe, and which provides some permanency with continuity of care and a nurturing environment during hospitalization; and information which explains the illness and treatment in a developmentally appropriate way, and does not withhold information from children (Aujoulat et al., 2006). These recommendations should not come as a surprise, based on the literature already reviewed in this chapter and in Chapter 6. Aside from the effects of medical treatment, hospitalization may have side-effects on everyday functioning. For example, length of hospital stay in a group of HIV-negative boys with haemophilia A or B has been associated with poorer academic achievement (Wong et al., 2004).

We simply cannot leave this topic without mentioning the use of animals in the therapeutic setting. In the past 50 years, the use of animals, particularly pet dogs, has become a widely used therapeutic tool across a range of psychological and physical health (including autism and epilepsy) conditions and applied to a range of populations and age groups including hospitalized children. Positive contact with animals has been linked to improved social and cognitive development in children. For example, establishing a bond with a pet has been positively correlated with social competency and empathy (Poresky and Hendrix, 1990). According to Grandgeorge and Hausberger (2011), in an excellent and scholarly review of human–animal relationships, animals were first brought into the therapeutic environment as early as the eleventh century, when birds were introduced to patients in a Belgian hospital, after which the use of rabbits, dogs and horses, as well as cats, followed in a variety of therapeutic settings. Starting in the 1960s, work in the US by the child psychologist Boris Levinson, often reported as the father of animal therapy, ignited an interest in the use of animals as a therapeutic tool (Levinson, 1962). Although interest in this idea was initially met with a considerable amount of scepticism, work in this area has persisted and gained considerable momentum throughout the past 50 years. The commonly recognized terms in use are animal-assisted therapy (AAT) and animal-assisted intervention (AAI), and relevant societies include the Society for Companion Animal Studies and the Pets as Therapy national charity in the UK or Pet Partners in the US. The use of trained dogs to assist the disabled, including children with disabilities, in daily activities has also gained popularity in recent years (e.g., via organizations such as Dogs for the Disabled).

The psychosocial mechanism behind the health benefit of animals as therapy appears to be via the many and varied facets of social support, driven by the fundamental need for relationships, bonding and feelings of belonging between social animals. In the therapeutic process, animals have been referred to as 'social catalysts' (Levinson, in Wells, 2011), 'social lubricants' or 'social substitutes' (see Grandgeorge and Hausberger, 2011). Indeed, evidence for the ability of human–animal contact to facilitate social interaction and alter physiological functioning, as measured by changes in the cortisol awakening response, has been demonstrated in children with autism, a condition in which ability for social interaction is limited (Viau et al., 2010). The now multidisciplinary field of animal-assisted therapy has documented a huge amount of success, but systematic and rigorous scientific testing, such as the study reported by Viau et al. (2010), has lagged behind the application of AAT, although this is partly due to the methodological difficulties involved, including ethical considerations.

One noteworthy study conducted by Kaminski and colleagues (2002) compared a child life therapy intervention (play therapy) with pet therapy (a previously used term for animal-assisted therapy) in a sample of 70 children (39 boys and 31 girls) hospitalized for a range of chronic illnesses including leukaemia, cystic fibrosis and diabetes. With the aim of addressing the lack of research on the social, emotional and physiological impact of therapy with pets, children were given a session of either play or pet therapy one evening a week during their hospital stay. The sessions were videotaped to code for characteristics of the child's response to the therapy (expressions of positive and negative affect, fearfulness, and amount of physical contact); assessed pre- and post-test by both parent and child questionnaire ratings of mood; and measures of salivary cortisol, heart rate and blood pressure were taken both before and after the session. Positive affect as reported by the parents increased from pre- to post-testing for both play and pet therapy, and there was no significant difference between the two groups on children's self-reported mood state. However, the children who received pet therapy were observed to show more positive affect and a greater level of touch or contact, and parents reported a greater increase in their child's positive affect, than those engaged in play therapy. With regard to the physiological measures, heart rate was significantly higher in the pet therapy group than the play group both before and after the intervention (possibly due to excitement about the pet therapy), but no significant group effects were found for cortisol (Kaminski et al., 2002).

A further interesting finding from this research is the response of the children to being asked the following in order to enable them to express their feelings and describe their needs more easily: 'Make believe a child in the hospital can make three wishes. What do you think the three wishes would be?' (Kaminski et al., 2002). Many of the children reported wishes about either owning or wanting to be with a pet, particularly if in the pet therapy group, and wishes to do with being ill and wanting to go home declined after both types of therapy, which the authors interpret as a positive distraction. This fits with the secondary control coping of Connor-Smith et al. (2000) and Compas et al. (2012) described above, but more research is needed which directly examines animal-assisted therapy within the context of psychological theory and models in order to understand the processes in operation fully and to build on these in future therapy. In this study, Kaminski et al. (2002) highlight both play and pet therapy as important interventions in hospital care for children. The authors conclude that both interventions decrease boredom and help create a sense of normality for children away from home, whilst the use of animals in intervention also provides distraction, 'unconditional companionship' and an increase in physical contact or therapeutic 'touch', particularly in children whose condition requires frequent hospital stays or those admitted for an extended period of time. The reciprocal benefit found in this study was that parents also felt positively towards the play and pet therapies, reporting that they felt less guilty about not being present all the time if their children were able to participate in engaging activities (Kaminski et al., 2002).

CHAPTER SUMMARY

In this chapter, I have examined the changing pattern of chronic illness in childhood and highlighted the increase in some chronic conditions as a result of new treatments for diseases which once had a much higher fatality rate. Similarly, I have looked at changes in lifestyle which predict a greater incidence of chronic illness in the future – in essence, which load the dice for future ill health – often encouraged by the ease of modern technology or sometimes unrealistic fears leading to overprotective parenting. Illness cognitions based on age and experience are important in adaptation to chronic illness, but neither the coping abilities of children nor the impact on the family (parents and siblings) should be underestimated. The interplay between hospitalization, medical procedures and ongoing care provided at home are an important part of the impact of chronic illness on the child and their family, and interventions to facilitate coping in these different settings have been outlined, including the increasingly recognized role of animal-assisted therapy. This chapter has covered the psychosocial aspects of long-term illness and chronic illness characteristic of conditions which can be 'cured'. In Chapter 8, we go on to consider issues relating to 'cure' and survivorship, the role of palliative care and, despite significant medical advances, issues relating to terminal illness in childhood.

KEY CONCEPTS AND ISSUES

- The difficulty of defining chronic illness
- Illness prevalence
- Illness incidence
- Nature deficit disorder (NDD)
- The multifaceted biopsychosocial impact of chronic illness
- Family support/resilience
- Visible versus unseen conditions
- Illness cognitions
- Primary and secondary control coping
- Person-specific and situation-specific factors as stress moderators
- Illness-specific stressors
- Parental stress
- Health behaviours
- Animal-assisted therapy (AAT) and animal-assisted intervention (AAI)

FURTHER READING

For an excellent, up-to-date and extremely well-written review of coping in children and adolescence:

Compas, B.E., Jaser, S.S., Dunn, M.J. and Rodriguez, E.M. (2012) Coping with chronic illness in childhood and adolescence. *Annual Review of Clinical Psychology*, 8: 455–80.

Although written over 20 years ago, this book contains a wealth of information about chronic disease in childhood which is still very relevant. The more dated aspects give insight into prevalence rates, terminology, coping and medical care in childhood illness where there is variation over time, and provide an important contrast to the current decade:

Eiser, C. (1990) *Chronic Childhood Disease: An Introduction to Psychological Theory and Research.* Cambridge: Cambridge University Press.

A review article covering the assessment of stress and coping measures in children:

Blount, R.L., Simons, L.E., Devine, K.A., Jaaniste, T., Cohen, L.L., Chambers, C.T. and Hayutin, L.G. (2008) Evidence-based assessment of coping and stress in pediatric psychology. *Journal of Pediatric Psychology*, 33(9): 1021–45.

A fabulous text which provides psychological interventions across a range of chronic illnesses in children, with a chapter devoted to each, including cancer, diabetes, asthma, sickle cell disease, juvenile arthritis and cystic fibrosis:

Drotar, D., Witherspoon, D.O., Zebracki, K. and Cant Peterson, C. (2006) *Psychological Interventions in Chronic Childhood Illness.* Washington: American Psychological Association.

For an up-to-date, easily accessible read with excellent references on the topic of animal-assisted therapy:

Wells, D. (2011) The value of pets for human health. *The Psychologist*, 24(3): 172–6.

USEFUL WEBSITES

If you think I am exaggerating the media storm generated by nature deficit disorder and the National Trust report, try typing these terms into Google and see how many hits appear. If this is too much to read, here is the BBC website which summarizes the report: www.bbc.co.uk/news/science-environment-17495032

The report itself makes for an interesting read and is beautifully illustrated: www.nationaltrust.org.uk/document-1355766991839

ANIMAL-ASSISTED THERAPY/ANIMAL-ASSISTED INTERVENTIONS

The Society for Companion Animal Studies: www.scas.org.uk

Pets as Therapy (UK): www.petsastherapy.org

Pet partners (US): www.deltasociety.org

Dogs for the Disabled: www.dogsforthedisabled.org

TERMINAL ILLNESS AND SURVIVORSHIP ISSUES

8

This chapter will consider psychosocial issues in the palliative care of children and survivorship following life-threatening illness, whether the illness is of an acute or chronic nature. Particular reference is made to age-specific cognitive and behavioural differences from the younger child to the older teenage years. As in previous chapters, our focus is on the life-course perspective, with consideration of the effects of survivorship extending into adulthood.

CHILDHOOD PALLIATIVE CARE AND TERMINAL ILLNESS

Death during childhood in the modern developed world is viewed as comparatively rare (Rushforth, 1999); rare, that is, compared to the plagues of previous centuries or to death from malnutrition and diseases such as AIDS in the developing world. Statistics from the

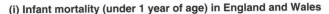

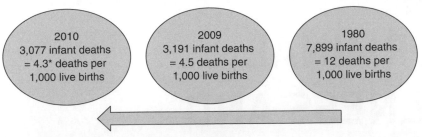

* Lowest ever recorded rate in England and Wales

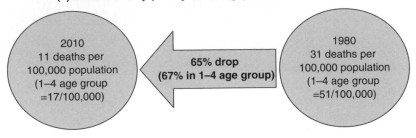

FIGURE 8.1   Child and infant mortality rates in England and Wales
Source: ONS (2012).

US Center for Disease Control and Prevention (CDC) reported mortality rates in 2009 at 26.1 deaths per 100,000 population for children aged 1–4 years, and 13.9 deaths per 100,000 population for children aged 5–14 years (CDC, 2010). This is substantially higher than the latest figures for the UK. Child mortality rates for England and Wales are given in Figure 8.1 (ONS, 2012). In the US, for figures up to 2009, the leading causes of death in children aged 1–4 years were accidents (i.e., unintentional injuries) and congenital malformations, deformations and chromosomal abnormalities (CDC, 2010). For children aged 5–14 years, the leading causes of death in the US are attributable to accidents and cancer (CDC, 2010). Similarly, based on 2010 data from the UK, congenital conditions and cancers are reported as the most common causes of death in children under 16 years of age (ONS, 2012).

CHILDREN'S UNDERSTANDING OF DEATH

Knowledge and awareness of how children understand and make sense of death are important in relaying appropriate information and providing adequate support for children facing the possibility of their own early mortality. Children have many sources of learning about death, through bereavement of their own family and friends, as well as through the experience of the death of a pet (Rushforth, 1999). In line with the Piagetian stage modelling described in Chapters 2 and 6, classic work in the 1970s and 1980s proposed a cognitive staging process of understanding for children facing their own death. An example of early landmark work in this area by Bluebond-Langer (in Rushforth, 1999) conceptualised a series of stages that children progress through when facing death, which include:

1 Recognition of an illness as 'serious'.
2 Understanding the importance of treatments.
3 Recognition of the illness as 'irreversible' together with an understanding that the medication and treatment will not be able to cure them. (Rushworth 1999: 689)

Rushforth (1999) built on this staging model to incorporate a number of other important variables relating to the child's experience, which impact on the process. These include illness duration, remission experience, and the experience of others with similar conditions. Rushforth points out the importance of medical staff being aware of the child's level of understanding and their readiness to hear more details about the condition and its implications. In particular, she emphasizes the qualities of care which incorporate 'honesty', addressing the child's questions directly, and 'hope', not necessarily for a cure if this is unrealistic but for 'comfort', developing the quality of life by living well in the time left and setting goals within the available time frame.

The central question of relevance here is: at what age can children understand the concept of death? This is a concept that many people struggle with at any age. A baseline of approximately 9 years of age has been suggested by some researchers as the earliest time that children are able to take on board the concept of death, with a fuller understanding not developing until the adolescent years (Meadows, in Rushforth, 1999). Himelstein et al. (2004: 1753) state that full maturity in understanding death can only be reached when there is integration of the following concepts: (i) 'irreversibility'; (ii) 'finality and non-functionality'; (iii) 'universality'; and (iv) 'causality'. The importance of understanding a child's developmental level is highlighted by Himelstein et al. (2004) in considering communication with children facing death. They point out the need for communication not only at a verbal level but also through non-verbal routes such as body language and symbolic expression of emotion via play, drawing, writing and music. Himelstein et al. (2004) present a more detailed breakdown of age-specific stages in development as applied to the concept of death: with understanding beginning during the ages of 2–6 years and dominated by magical thinking and the belief that death is temporary and reversible; moving onto concrete thinking at 6–12 years, in which death is seen as personal, and adult concepts begin to emerge, accompanied by an interest in the physical aspects of death; progressing to 12–18 years when self-reflective thinking is possible and non-physical explanations of death are explored. The idea is that these developmental stages for conceptualizing death develop in parallel with spiritual beliefs and understanding, and together suggest the basis for appropriate interventions (Himelstein et al., 2004).

As Rushforth (1999) points out, a child's understanding of death will always be 'complex', influenced by a range of factors such as media images (portrayal of immortality in children's films and programmes), and cultural and religious beliefs, but 'never wrong'. She lists three important summary points regarding a child's understanding of death: (i) that it 'becomes more sophisticated with age'; (ii) that it is 'accelerated by education'; and (iii) that it is 'undoubtedly influenced by experience' and concludes that the 'greatest disservice' can be done by trying to protect children from information we believe may be harmful. Children have an elaborate imaginative world and trying to protect them by avoiding important issues related to their own survival may only lead them to make up their own version of events as they try to make sense of the situation, which could be inaccurate or even more harmful (Rushforth, 1999).

Himelstein et al. (2004) present an excellent comparison of myths and realities relating to grief and issues around death and dying, as experienced by children and adolescents. They challenge popular myths or traditional views and stereotypes about childhood grief and exposure to death. Rather than representing children being unable to grieve for loved ones and, in the case of children who are themselves dying, being 'unaware' of this, this more current work emphasizes the importance of facilitating and supporting the grieving process for children and adolescents. Himelstein et al. (2004) point out that, whilst being 'developmentally distinct', children and adolescents are very much able to grieve, and even young children appear to be aware of impending death. As they illustrate, it is often adult denial and inhibition about dealing with issues of death and dying in childhood that prevents appropriate care and support in the grieving process.

PALLIATIVE CARE

There has been considerable debate in the adult literature surrounding the relationship between hospice and palliative care, leading to substantial developments in policy and practice in recent years (for example, see the National Cancer Research Institute website: www.ncri.org.uk). Such debates and issues extend into the paediatric literature. Whilst there is similarity between adult and child palliative and hospice care needs and services, there are also significant differences related to stage of life and associated school and family involvement in childhood illness (see Association for Children's Palliative Care documents). The Association for Children's Palliative Care (ACT) provides palliative care pathways specifically for neonates, children and their families and young people, as well as pathways for transition to adult services in England (see www.act. org.uk). An excellent review by Himelstein (2006) distinguishes between palliative care and hospice care by describing paediatric palliative care as being 'further upstream' (2006: 163) in terms of provision of care than the paediatric hospice setting. In other words, hospice care falls under the umbrella of palliative care, but with a greater focus on specialized care towards the latter stages of terminal illness, although not exclusively,

TABLE 8.1   Four categories of condition for palliative care with examples

Category of condition qualifying as needing palliative care services	Examples of condition
1. Life-threatening condition for which curative or life-prolonging treatment is possible but may fail. Access to services may be necessary during an acute crisis when threat to life is of short duration. Need for services ceases when long-term remission reached or treatment successfully cures condition.	Malignancy (cancer) which is advanced, progressive or has a poor prognosis; complex and severe congenital or acquired heart disease, liver or kidney failure.
2. Requires long periods of intensive treatment with the aim of prolonging quality of life but where premature death is inevitable.	Human immunodeficiency virus (HIV+); cystic fibrosis; severe gastrointestinal disorders; renal failure when dialysis and/or transplantation not possible; chronic or severe renal failure; Duchenne muscular dystrophy.
3. Progressive conditions where treatment is exclusively palliative from diagnosis (i.e., no curative treatment option). May extend over several years.	Mucopolysaccharidoses; progressive metabolic disorders; Batten disease; some chromosomal abnormalities such as trisomy 13 (Patau syndrome) or trisomy 18 (Edward's syndrome).
4. Irreversible, non-progressive conditions causing severe disability which result in vulnerability to health complications and likelihood of premature death.	Severe cerebral palsy; extreme prematurity; severe neurologic symptoms following infectious disease; hypoxic/anoxic brain injury; severe brain malformations.

Source: Based on Himelstein (2006: 163) and www.togetherforshortlives.org.uk

and may include respite care. The broader focus of palliative care in children is defined as 'not about dying' but instead 'about helping children and families to live to their fullest while facing complex medical conditions' beginning from diagnosis onwards. It is seen very much as a style of multidisciplinary care which needs to be provided through any number of health-care services, institutions, and professionals, as well as supported through non-professional family and community care. It includes care provided across a range of conditions which have the potential of being terminal, even if the eventual outcome is not death. Palliative care has been classified into four distinct but sometimes overlapping groups, as shown in Table 8.1 (for a full account of the principles of paediatric palliative care and the different categories of conditions included, see Himelstein, 2006).

Himelstein et al. (2004) identify what they term five main 'spheres' or aspects of palliative care for children which fit well with a biopsychosocial focus. These aspects relate to physical, psychosocial, spiritual and practical concerns, as well as the planning of future care. Within the psychosocial aspects of care, they include the identification of fears and anxieties in the child and their family, as well as understanding the child's style of coping and communication as important for formulating a plan for paediatric palliative care. To focus first on physical symptoms, children and their families are required to cope with a range of unpleasant and often severe symptoms, whether caused by the condition itself or by the treatments necessitated by the condition. Himelstein et al. (2004) describe the major symptom characteristics in children, across the four different categories of conditions requiring palliative care, as categorized into pain and non-pain symptoms. As pain is highly relevant to child health psychology in both palliative and non-palliative care, an entire chapter is devoted to it (see Chapter 9). From what has been covered in previous chapters, it should be obvious by now that such physical symptoms can be influenced by psychosocial approaches, and this is recognized by Himelstein et al. (2004) in the inclusion of both pharmacological and non-pharmacological approaches to the treatment of physical pain symptoms. Non-pain symptoms are categorized into ten groupings: (i) dyspnoea (breathing difficulties); (ii) nausea and vomiting; (iii) constipation; (iv) gastro-oesophogeal reflux; (v) anorexia and cachexia (severe weight loss); (vi) pruritis (itching); (vii) bone marrow failure; (viii) urinary retention; (ix) fatigue; and (x) neurological symptoms (see Himelstein, 2006, for detail).

As well as dealing with issues of death and dying and assessing resources for bereavement, the psychosocial aspects of palliative care identified in this model by Himelstein et al. (2004) are of particular relevance for our focus in this chapter. They involve identification of concerns and fears, and coping and communication styles for both the child and their family, in order to tailor and develop an appropriate intervention plan. Policy and practice in the developed world now works towards implementing gold standards in palliative care as set out in such types of model, and significant advances have been made in palliative care in the past decade. The importance of such services is undisputed, but implementing consistent high-quality care is not always straightforward. The child's family are intimately bound up in the delivery and receipt of care for the child with palliative care needs. Based on the earlier definition of palliative care starting at the point of diagnosis, and just as the delivery of care and appropriate disclosure to children is required by the family and medical profession, so style of disclosure about a life-limiting condition to parents by medical professionals is also important. This is highlighted in a study by Davies and colleagues (2003), who conducted a qualitative analysis of interviews with a UK sample of parents (including couples and single mothers). The sample included the parents of 30 children diagnosed with a life-limiting condition (40 per cent of the sample with severe cerebral palsy, others with genetic disorders such as Hallervorden–Spatz disease, metabolic leukodystrophy, Sanfillipo syndrome, and muscular dystrophy). Parents described their experiences of paediatrician communication surrounding diagnosis. Many of the parents in this study reported positive paediatrician experiences around communication of their child's life-limiting condition, and pointed to the relief they felt at having

BOX 8.1

Sensitive and insensitive paediatrician experiences

Source: R. Davies, B. Davis and J. Sibert (2003) Parents' stories of sensitive and insensitive care by paediatricians in the time leading up to and including diagnostic disclosure of a life-limiting condition in their child. *Child: Care, Health and Development*, 29(1): 77–82.

Contrasting case examples of sensitive and insensitive paediatrician experiences (Figure 8.2) by parents of children diagnosed with a life-limiting condition:

Case 1 Sensitive and family-focused care	Case 2 Insensitive care
First meeting with parents following referral from GP: *Mother*: He said he thought there was something wrong just by looking at E and he said he would do some blood tests and he would get the tests back in six weeks. We had to take E in for these tests and they had to wrap him up in almost a straight jacket, and we took him onto the children's ward and he (the paediatrician) really filled up and he said 'It's a shame'. Diagnosis was given as promised six weeks later of MPS. *Mother*: And he had obviously planned what he was going to say and I made it quite difficult for him really, he was so lovely and we just went to pieces didn't we? (Looking at husband who nods in response.) Paediatrician visited the family at home the next day. On a later occasion parents confided about how their caring responsibilities were putting a strain upon their relationship and the mother's reluctance to take up respite at a children's hospice. *Father*: I told him ... He said (paediatrician) 'Respite is the most important thing it will either make or break a marriage. The ones who don't accept help go under. Parents accepted respite that has helped them as a family. Later on in the same interview when discussing their child's medical care and this paediatrician: *Father*: He's a good bloke. *Mother*: He's like our friend. *Parents of child diagnosed with Sanfilippo syndrome (MPS III)*	Parents given child's diagnosis during the middle of a ward round: *Father*: I thought it was absolutely appalling. It was very blunt. I mean I think the way it was done took a long while for it to sink in because it was blunt. I know it sounds a bit of a contradiction but it was told in a very matter of fact way with no feeling. The bedside manners were appalling. The facts were laid out as black and white and as plain as they could be. They called us in and said 'Right we've had the results, and she has severe brain damage which means M will never walk, she will never talk, she will never be able to do anything for herself' and that was it ... (pause as father became distressed and tearful). *R*: (stunned and searching for words) Oh Gosh, and just left the two of you there? *Father*: Yes, and the nurse came in and she was very good but this particular consultant, his manner was all ... I think that was partly the reason he did it because he didn't want to break down. He was trying to protect himself I think as much as us but in doing so ... that's something we (as parents) have talked about a lot. *Mother*: And then they were off doing the ward round. They prescribe drugs and then they are off and they know they have left sheer and utter devastation to the family. *Parents of a child diagnosed with severe cerebral palsy and spastic quadriplegia*

FIGURE 8.2   Experiences of sensitive and insensitive paediatrician care

Source: Davies et al. (2003: 79–80).

a diagnosis after years of their concerns being disregarded and ignored, even though they then had to cope with their child's limited future. Others, however, reported examples of insensitivity in the way they were treated around diagnosis. This study is particularly interesting in its focus on delayed diagnosis, in some cases by several years, despite parental suspicions and frequent insistence that something was wrong. Preconceptions of the paediatrician relating to the social class of the parents also appeared to influence the degree to which the parents' concerns and observations of their child were listened to or ignored, with examples of working-class parents experiencing dismissive responses.

Davies et al. (2003) point to a dichotomy in the way in which paediatricians interacted with parents. When delivering appropriately sensitive treatment, some were 'humanistic', good communicators who were able to retain professionalism as well as being able to empathize with parents (Davies et al., 2003). Insensitive paediatricians, on the other hand, were 'technocratic', poor communicators, who were 'unwilling or unable to enter the life world of parents' (Davies et al., 2003: 81). Contrasting case examples from this study are given in Box 8.1.

The study by Davies et al. (2003) highlights the vital role of providing sensitivity in listening to and acting upon parental concerns and in disclosing diagnostic information in life-limiting conditions. Insensitivity around diagnosis only adds to the stress experienced by parents in children with chronic conditions and is accentuated in terminal or life-limiting conditions. Research findings from the different perspectives covered above serve to highlight the importance of the reciprocal nature of the relationships between parent, child and paediatrician in the provision of palliative care and also in survivorship, as illustrated in Figure 8.3.

Before moving from this topic of palliative care to consider issues in survivorship, it is important to consider palliative care at the other end of childhood, the post-teenage years, when the process of transition from child and adolescent services to adult services is necessitated. In a review of palliative care during transition, Doug et al. (2011) point out that, due to an increase in life expectancy with medical advances, there are a greater number of patients with life-threatening or life-limiting conditions who survive to the point of adulthood and require transfer to adult health-care services. They highlight the increased interest in this topic of transition in medical care and point out that the literature, whilst focusing on chronic illness and disability, has to some degree ignored the transition relevant to those requiring palliative care services. Although they found a lack of outcome data to limit their ability to assess this process, they point to a number of factors which may facilitate and a number of barriers which may hinder a successful transition. These are based on the need for information, communication, and planning/coordination within the context of a multidisciplinary team. In particular, services for transition of care in cases of cystic fibrosis and cancer were found to be particularly well documented in the literature, yet a systematic assessment and evaluation of the process is called for by these authors (see Doug et al., 2011).

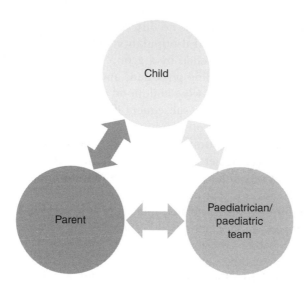

FIGURE 8.3 Importance of the reciprocal nature of communication in relationships between parent, child and paediatrician in the provision of palliative care

THE CHALLENGE OF SURVIVING CHILDHOOD ILLNESS

As I noted in Chapter 7, a large proportion of the literature examining the experience of chronic illness in childhood has focused on cancer, particularly acute lymphoblastic leukaemia (ALL), a condition which, before the advent of new treatments in the 1960s and beyond, was associated with a significantly lower survival rate than the 90 per cent figure now reached. The acute illness origins of this disease and its chronic characteristics have already been discussed (Chapters 6 and 7). Here we consider the issue of survivorship and, whilst reference will be made to a variety of conditions, childhood cancer contributes, not surprisingly, the lion's share of research in this area since survival rates for cancer have increased significantly in comparison with other conditions. Before we can do this, however, issues relating to the terms 'in remission', 'cured' and 'long-term survivor' first need addressing. 'In remission' refers to a state when cancer has responded to treatment and no signs or symptoms of the disease are evident. Depending on the type of cancer, after a relapse-free period of between 2 and 10 years following diagnosis, the term 'cured' is considered an acceptable and preferred term, particularly for use with patients, whereas the status of 'long-term survivor' is suggested as being more helpful to medical professionals in planning care and in scientific research (Haupt et al., 2007). When in remission, the remission rate can be used as a calculation of the probability of the cancer not recurring, whereas once a state of 'cure' is reached, the mortality rate for that child 'from their original disease' is no different to the all-cause mortality rate for a peer of the same age from the general population (Haupt et al., 2007). Based on the Erice statement, an agreement reached by a group of European and North American paediatric cancer specialists (including physicians and psychologists), parents and survivors, the use of the term 'cure' following childhood cancer has been defined as referring to the original disease only, and not to subsequent disability or side-effects resulting from treatment (Haupt et al., 2007). In consideration of the long-term goal of addressing the cure and planning long-term continued care for paediatric cancer survivors and their families, the Erice group (Haupt et al., 2007) use the following overview statement on which their ten points of recommendation are made: 'The long-term goal of the cure and care of the child with cancer is that he/she become a resilient, fully functioning, autonomous adult with an optimal health-related quality of life, accepted in the society at the same level of his/her age peers' (Haupt et al., 2007: 1779).

Based on this description of the goal for cancer survivorship, I consider the experience of survivorship following childhood illness, from a biopsychosocial perspective. As in earlier chapters when considering long-lasting effects of childhood stress on physical health outcomes (see Chapter 5), here we consider the long-term influences of childhood illness both as a survivor during childhood and through into adult life. These effects may include biological (or physical) and psychosocial (or emotional) outcomes for the survivor. Such outcomes have significant impact on the family (parents and siblings) and are consequences of the cured disease or its treatment, rather than being caused by the direct effect of an ongoing original illness. The focus here is on children who have survived an illness which had the potential to be fatal, and issues of survivorship may relate to either chronic or acute conditions. Although the majority of work in this area examines cancer or other conditions of chronic duration, there are a handful of studies that have looked at the long-term impacts of acute infection and these are also highlighted.

Survivorship outcomes (i.e., long-term effects of childhood illness) have been addressed in a number of different but overlapping categories in the literature. Some of the earlier work preferred the use of the more collective term 'quality of life' to refer to a range of biological and psychosocial effects of survivorship. 'Quality of life' is an important term in survivorship as it focuses attention towards the holistic needs of patients beyond treatment of the initial illness, and keeps it firmly within a biopsychosocial framework (for a World Health Organization definition of quality of life, see Chapter 1). As with many useful terms, however, its overuse has led to a multitude of meanings and lack of specificity. Synonymous terms include 'well-being' or 'happiness', and measurement of quality of life can extend from simple assessments of depression to complex dedicated quality of life scales. Without getting into this debate, it is worth being aware of such issues of terminology and the need for clarification when considering research findings. There have been some excellent studies which have used the 'quality of life' terminology, and these are included in reviewing this literature, but, where possible, specific aspects of biopsychosocial functioning have been focused on, with the understanding that they all contribute to overall quality of life.

By far and away the clearest, most concise and insightful paper which addresses quality of life in survivors is by Quinn and colleagues (2012). This is a qualitative study assessing thematic gaps in quality of life assessments when applied to young adult survivors of childhood cancer (termed YASCC by Quinn et al.). These authors separate late effects of cancer and treatment into physical and psychological, and point to a shift in assessment from 'quality of life' to 'quality of survivorship' which is perhaps a much more useful and descriptive term for quality of life in the survivorship context. They also point to the move away from identification of needs in a cross-sectional manner towards a monitoring of the quality of survivorship over time, acknowledging that there may be changes over time. Such monitoring can capture transitions between the status of 'child to adolescent', 'adolescent to young adult' and 'patient to survivor' (Quinn et al., 2012: 111, 112).

In this chapter, I refer to five main categories under which survivorship effects or outcomes have been considered, unpacking the more general quality of life terminology, but with this 'quality of survivorship' focus in mind. These effects are interconnected at a biopsychosocial level and to varying degrees across a range of conditions, types of cancer and individual differences in their influence on health. They can be categorized as: (i) physical, medical, or late effects; and psychosocial effects based on (ii) cognitive; (iii) emotional; (iv) social; and (v) behavioural functioning. Each of these types of outcome and their interactions are important in survivorship of acute or chronic illness and, as such, they are vital within health psychology theory and practice: for example, in promoting adaptive psychosocial coping, communicating risks which encourage the fostering of appropriate health behaviours to minimize late effects, and harnessing resilience observed in benefit-finding and positive growth. With this in mind, we consider each of these five categories in turn, before going on to consider interventions based on these outcomes.

PHYSICAL, MEDICAL OR LATE EFFECTS IN THE SURVIVAL OF CHILDHOOD ILLNESS

The effect of advances in treatments, leading to a cure in conditions that would otherwise be terminal, naturally means an increase in the number of survivors into childhood, adolescence and adulthood. Yet the benefit of survivorship may bring with it the additional morbidity of late effects of disease and treatment, particularly following childhood cancer, and these effects may in themselves be fatal. Late effects following childhood cancer can include a range of physical problems or impairments which may appear within a few years after the initial condition is 'cured' or up to several decades later (Alvarex et al., in Hess et al., 2011). These can include neuromuscular functioning and reduced muscle growth; a compromised immune system; cardiovascular functioning; dental problems; hypothyroidism; breast cancer; fatigue, memory and concentration; pain; disability; and obesity (Wallace et al., 2001; Clanton et al., 2011; Hess et al., 2011; Lu et al., 2011; Green et al., 2012; Johannsdottir et al., 2012; Ness et al., 2012; Quinn et al., 2012) which may be associated with increased likelihood of hospitalization (Kurt et al., 2012). Infertility and also congenital anomalies have also been viewed as possible late effects (Hess et al., 2011). Whilst fertility is accepted as a potential physical late effect, evidence of increased congenital disorders in children of survivors has been reported as inconclusive. A recent report from the Childhood Cancer Survivor Study (CCSS) cohort states that children of cancer survivors (men or women) are no more likely to be born with congenital anomalies (Signorello et al., 2012). The CCSS is an ongoing large-scale cohort study of over 14,000 cancer survivors, all of whom were diagnosed with cancer before the age of 21 years (1970–1986) and who survived 5 years from diagnosis, drawn from 25 participating institutions across North America (Robison et al., 2002). One of the distinguishing features of this study is that the siblings of these survivors are also recruited into the study for comparison.

Remarkable in the size of the healthy control group used, a study by Dowling et al. (2010) compared 410 adult survivors of childhood cancer in the US with 294,641 individuals who had not experienced cancer. This study is also interesting as it includes a considerable proportion of participants who were over the age of 40 years (38.12 per cent in the cancer survivor group and 56.12 per cent in the control group) whereas many studies of survivorship concentrate on early adulthood in the twenties and into the thirties age group only. Dowling et al. (2010) conclude that, across a range of conditions, the adult survivors reported poorer health outcomes and also more functional limitations associated with their health than the non-cancer group. Figure 8.4 gives an extensive list of late effects in childhood cancer and the proportion of survivors reporting them (Michel et al., 2009).

As Hess et al. (2011) point out, in order for survivors of childhood illness to be responsible for their health, they need to be sufficiently informed and aware of their disease, the treatments received, and the possibility and seriousness of late effects. However, parental concern for, and protection of, their child who had cancer during the first few years of life may, for example, lead them to avoid discussion of the illness in order to try to minimize its impact and avoid memories of the stressful or traumatic diagnosis and treatment. This could increase risk for the impact of late effects through delay in seeking medical attention, not engaging in appropriate health behaviours, or failing to acknowledge possible genetic risks when considering having children. Some of these effects were considered in a Norwegian study by Hess et al. (2011) of 128 adult survivors of childhood malignant lymphoma (Hodgkin's and non-Hodgkin's) with a mean age 14 years at diagnosis and 32 years at time of study assessment. Most of the participants could accurately recall their diagnosis and treatment. However, only 34 per cent of survivors in the sample were aware of the risks of late effects and able to name at least one of them. Neither the child's age at diagnosis (age range in this study was 0–18 years) nor their educational level was associated with their knowledge of late effects. The remaining 66 per cent of survivors highlight the need for increased awareness of late effects.

It is not only survivors who underestimate future late effects of cancer treatment. Medical documenting of late effects is also significantly underestimated when compared

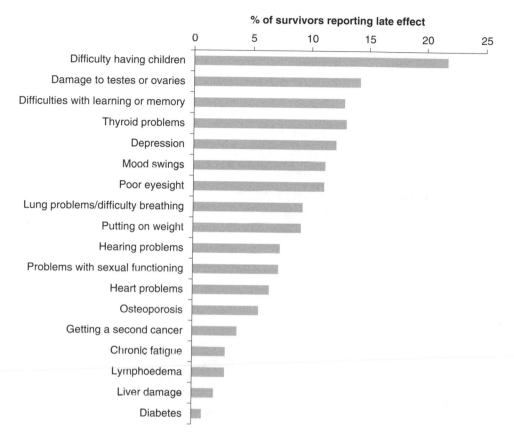

% of survivors reporting late effect

FIGURE 8.4 Proportion of survivors reporting different late effects

Source: Michel et al. (2009: 1618, fig. 2).

to the number of actual experienced late effects reported by parents and adult survivors, and, consequently, the range of services available to address these needs may be inadequate (Taylor et al., 2010). This indicates a hidden morbidity and underestimated need with respect to late effects in survivors of childhood cancer.

The issue of long-term follow-up into adulthood is vital, therefore, in survivors of life-threatening conditions, particularly as seen in cancer survivors, in order to promote awareness of late effects, as well as to enable early detection of any cancer recurrence, and to document mortality and morbidity rates of different treatments adequately (Wallace et al., 2001; Eiser et al., 2006). As shown in Figure 8.5, over 80 per cent of a total of 141 survivors (aged 18–45 years) in the UK wanted to discuss late effects at their clinical consultation, but this need was met for less than 60 per cent (Michel et al., 2009). As Michel et al. (2009) point out, although what they term 'consultant-led' follow-up appointments in clinic were popular with adult survivors of childhood cancer, given the increase in survivor

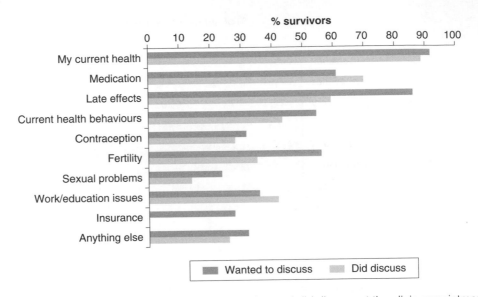

FIGURE 8.5   Frequency of topics survivors wanted to and did discuss at the clinic appointment

Source: Michel et al. (2009: 1619).

numbers, this style of follow-up may not be possible, and alternative follow-up services suited to the needs of the survivor will need to be developed. With regard to non-cancer conditions, a Swedish study of acute encephalitis (inflammation or infection of the brain) found persistent or long-term symptoms (including headache, fatigue and irritability) in up to 60 per cent of childhood survivors (sample $n = 71$) as reported by parents 3–8 years after onset of this condition (Fowler et al., 2010).

THE PSYCHOSOCIAL EXPERIENCE IN THE SURVIVAL OF CHILDHOOD ILLNESS

COGNITIVE FUNCTIONING EFFECTS IN SURVIVORSHIP

A significant effect of cancer treatment such as chemotherapy and, in particular, cranial radiotherapy is the long-term impact on neurocognitive functioning in adult survivors, the different aspects of which have been reported across a number of studies. For example, in a US study, Kadan-Lottick et al. (2010) compared 5,937 adult survivors of non-central nervous system cancers (including ALL, myeloid leukaemia, Hodgkin's disease, non-Hodgkin's lymphoma and neuroblastoma) with 382 siblings without cancer, from the CCSS cohort. They report a 50 per cent higher frequency of neurocognitive deficits across measures of task efficiency, memory and emotional regulation. Factors associated with increased frequency of deficits within the cancer group were diagnosis before the age of 6 years, being female, having received cranial radiation therapy, and hearing impairments (Kadan Lottick et al., 2010). Other studies have also reported sex differences in neurocognitive functioning seen early on in child survivors of cancer. For example, Jain and colleagues (2009) found sex differences in childhood cancer survivors on assessment of attention and executive control. They were able to distinguish between girls' and boys' neurocognitive impairments in a sample of 103 survivors of ALL (average age of approximately 3 years at diagnosis and 11 years at study follow-up). Girls performed more poorly than boys on cognitive tests requiring ability of the anterior attention system ('shifting attention') and subcortical attention system ('sustained attention') and boys performed more poorly than girls on tests of anterior control ('inhibition' and 'working memory'; Jain et al., 2009).

PSYCHOLOGICAL/EMOTIONAL EFFECTS IN SURVIVORSHIP

The psychological morbidity associated with childhood cancer has been reported in a number of studies, in both child and adult survivors. Just as physical late effects are prevalent following childhood cancer, so are psychological late effects, to the degree of experiencing post-traumatic stress symptoms (PTSS) or being clinically classified as having post-traumatic stress disorder (PTSD) (Taylor et al., 2012). In a UK study of 118 survivors of childhood cancer, aged 16–35 years at follow-up at least 2 years post-treatment, a prevalence rate of 13.9 per cent was reported for PTSD, which the authors comment is comparable with US figures (Taylor et al., 2012). Both PTSS and PTSD were related to the number of physical late effects reported, particularly by female survivors, and PTSS also predicted self-efficacy scores, highlighting the importance of psychological screening and the need for care that attends to both psychological and physical late-effect needs of cancer survivors (Taylor et al., 2012).

In the CCSS cohort, which compared cancer survivors with non-cancer siblings in the US and Canada, survivors were found to have four times the risk for PTSD (Stuber et al., 2010). When considered separately, siblings of survivors from this cohort study have been reported as 'psychologically healthy' but, in a relatively small subsample (3.8 per cent), psychological symptoms of distress and depression have been noted (Buchbinder et al., 2011). Risk factors for distress and depression in the sibling were linked to the psychological distress and physical health problems in the survivor. In particular, being a younger sibling was associated with more distress and being a male sibling (i.e., a brother) of a cancer survivor, rather than a sister, was linked to greater depression (Buchbinder et al., 2011). A recent report from the CCSS cohort also highlights the relevance of physical appearance in long-term psychological adaptation (Kinahan et al., 2012). Scarring and disfigurement (to chest or abdomen; head or neck; arm or leg) and 'persistent hair loss' were found to be associated with psychological symptoms such as depression, anxiety and somatization in adult survivors of childhood cancer, and link to overall quality of life (Kinahan et al., 2012). Similarly, in the Swedish study by Fowler et al. (2010) of acute encephalitis survivors mentioned above, as well as physical and cognitive symptoms, irritability and personality changes were reported by the parents.

LINKING PSYCHOLOGICAL COPING RESPONSES AND NEUROCOGNITIVE FUNCTIONING

An exciting area of research has emerged in recent years which links deficits in psychosocial coping and resulting difficulties in emotional and social functioning with specific parts of the brain involved in executive functions such as working memory, planning and emotion regulation. Most notably, these brain regions include the prefrontal cortex and the anterior cingulate cortex, and damage to these areas during development in childhood may result in neurocognitive deficits. In terms of coping, this is important as working memory appears to play a crucial role in coping with stress. Since ALL frequently occurs at a young age in childhood, and treatment involves intensive chemotherapy, including synthetic glucocorticoids such as dexamethasone, there is potential for damage to the

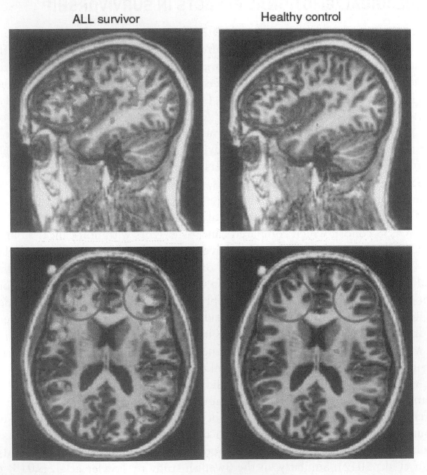

FIGURE 8.6   fMRI scans of ALL survivors versus healthy controls

Source: Robinson et al. (2010: 587, fig. 0).

developing brain (see Compas, 2006). To examine this relationship, Campbell et al. (2009) compared 30 children and adolescents aged 10–20 years, who had previously received treatment for ALL, with their healthy counterparts (age- and sex-matched controls). They measured aspects of executive brain function, including working memory; assessed how participants coped with social stress from their peers (e.g., being teased or falling out with a friend); and recorded emotional and behavioural difficulties experienced. The ALL group were found to score more poorly on working memory than the control group, and stronger relationships were found between executive functions and coping or emotional and behavioural difficulties. Most interestingly, for the ALL group, secondary control coping mediated the relationship between executive functions such as working memory and behaviour problems, lending support to the notion that the ability to make use of secondary control coping is determined by adequate functioning of executive control areas of the brain. Consequently, damage to these brain regions via chemotherapy treatment may explain why some ALL children may experience difficulty eliciting these secondary control coping responses and this may result in emotional or behavioural problems (Campbell et al., 2009). There is certainly evidence that parents experience significant difficulty dealing with the emotional and behavioural difficulties exhibited by their children (including anger and aggression, confusion and depression, and volatility in switching from one emotion to the other) when receiving corticosteroid medication during the continuation phase of treatment (McGrath and Rawson-Huff, 2010). Further research has begun to clarify these effects using functional brain imaging (fMRI) techniques and suggests that in ALL survivors these brain regions may 'compensate' for neurocognitive damage by focusing greater amounts of energy (oxygen) to those brain regions in order to perform cognitive tasks involving working memory (Robinson et al., 2010), as shown in Figure 8.6.

BOX 8.2

Capturing coping cognitions on film or simply 'modern-day phrenology'?

Effectively, brain scans of the type reported in Robinson et al. (2010) could be said to be providing a physical illustration of the cognitive concept of coping. This is an attractive if not compelling idea, that an abstract notion such as how children cope with stressful events such as illness could be captured in a structural representation. Yet others might question the utility of fMRI research in the context of identifying psychological concepts, and some staunch critics may even view it as 'modern-day phrenology' or 'neuromania' (Dobbs, 2005; Tallis, 2011). These caveats aside, as in all research, if driven by sound theory and rationale, and not overinterpreted, then perhaps there is something to be gained from this perspective on coping and neurocognitive functioning in survivors of childhood cancer. The debate continues. What do you think?

As Compas (2006) describes, since chemotherapy includes large doses of synthetic gluco-corticoid, the effects of chemotherapy treatment 'mimic' a high-stress glucocorticoid effect on the brain. Thinking back to Chapter 5, in which we covered hypercortisolaemic states in childhood, the implications for coping research are enormous. Whatever the root of the increased glucocorticoids to the brain, psychological coping may be influenced not just by the choice of coping strategy but by the ability of the brain to process that strategy: in other words, a two-way process is occurring.

SOCIAL EFFECTS IN SURVIVORSHIP

Social effects are intricately linked to psychological states. The psychosocial impact of surviving childhood cancer is described by Crom (2009), who movingly portrays the often ignored personal experiences of survivors. Drawn from discussions at a US summer camp for young adult survivors (aged 18–25 years) of brain tumours during childhood, three salient themes are reported: (i) the experience of social isolation, loneliness and bullying; (ii) an awareness of limitations and feeling that there is an outside perception that they are 'deficient' or 'less'; and (iii) an ability to be able to express their personal and social concerns and fears fully in an 'articulate' and 'insightful' way, and to support one another.

Social functioning, particularly in relation to marriage, employment and health insur-ance cover, has also been found to be poorer in adult survivors of childhood cancer than in the general population or compared to non-cancer siblings of survivors. For example, Crom et al. (2007) report that cancer survivors in the US who received radiation as part of their treatment were less likely to be married and less likely to be in full-time employment; insurance rates were higher; and more difficulty was experienced in obtaining health care due to unemployment. Neurocognitive and related physical and emotional impairments have been linked to a significantly higher rate of unemployment (up to eight times higher) in adult survivors of childhood cancer, compared to survivors without these deficits, and the effect is particularly damaging for women (Kirchhoff et al., 2011). The authors rec-ommend screening and intervention to increase employment prospects in survivors expe-riencing neurocognitive and related problems.

In the CCSS cohort, whilst divorce rates were comparable to that of sibling controls, survivors were reported to have a significantly lower likelihood of marrying even after controlling for age, gender and race (Janson et al., 2009). As in the Crom et al. (2007) study, having received cranial radiation treatment was associated with being unmarried and, furthermore, physical factors such as short stature, cognitive deficits and physical functioning were found to mediate the relationship between cranial radiation and marital status (Janson et al., 2009). Similarly, social factors, including reproductive rates, were examined in a study of 247 young adult survivors of childhood cancer (aged between 19 and 34 years), identified from national cancer registries, across five Nordic countries (Norway, Denmark, Sweden, Finland and Iceland) compared with 1,814 controls from the general Norwegian population (Johannsdottir et al., 2010). They found similar levels of academic education between survivors and controls, but significantly fewer survivors than controls were employed and significantly more were in receipt of social benefits. Marital status was comparable across the groups, but controls were significantly more likely to have children (Johannsdottir et al., 2010). In a review of social outcomes reported in the CCSS studies, Gurney et al. (2009) also highlight the needs of survivors for special education services, particularly the social impact of treatment with implications for hearing loss, and that, whilst educational attainment at high school (senior school in UK) may be similar, fewer survivors attend higher education (i.e., college, university) than comparison groups.

In the quality of survivorship study by Quinn et al. (2012) referred to above, three themes were identified which have been previously ignored in traditional quality of life measures that did not focus on the specific needs of young adult survivors of childhood cancer (YASCC) and these relate largely to psychosocial needs. To obtain these data, Quinn et al. (2012) conducted in-depth interviews, either individually or via focus groups, with young adults aged 21–30 years (all of whom had been diagnosed with cancer before the age of 18 years, and a minimum of 2 years since the end of treatment). The three themes identified as absent from current instruments and relevant to the life transition made by YASCC were: (i) 'perceived sense of self' (issues relating to identity and 'normalcy'); (ii) 'relationships' (including behaviour and regulation of emotion, relationship with parents, problems establishing romantic relationships and appearance concerns); and (iii) 'parenthood' (feelings of 'loss' in connection with normal expectations about becoming a parent because of physical and psychological long-term effects, including concerns over the transmission of congenital abnormalities and infertility). This second of Quinn et al.'s (2012) themes, the

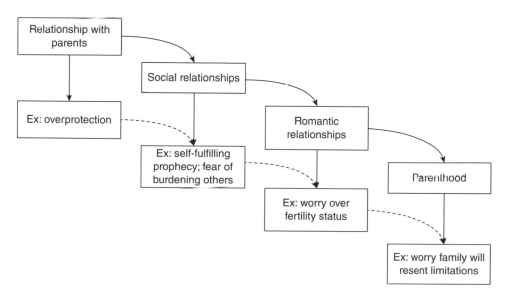

FIGURE 8.7   Impact of cancer diagnosis on relationships

Source: Quinn et al. (2012: fig. 1).

impact on social relationships, is illustrated in Figure 8.7. It shows the pervasive influence of the experience of cancer on social relationships in young adults and the need to include such aspects of psychological late effects in assessment and intervention.

The parental influence referred to by Quinn et al. (2012) is also highlighted by Eiser and colleagues (2004) who applied regulatory focus theory (RFT) to parenting styles in parents of adolescent survivors of ALL and central nervous system (CNS) tumours. Distinguishing between prevention-focused parenting (defined as 'an overly protective concern with possible mishaps and illness recurrence') and promotion-focused parenting (defined as 'encouraging expectations of recovery and normal life'), prevention-focused parenting was found to be associated with poorer quality of life as rated by the parents and adolescent survivors (Eiser et al., 2004: 123). Independently of parenting focus, ALL survivors had higher quality of life scores than survivors of CNS tumours. This study emphasizes the need for encouraging promotion-focused parenting, and offers a starting point for addressing relationship needs in survivors who have experienced more of a prevention-focused parenting style.

BEHAVIOURAL OUTCOMES OF SURVIVORSHIP

One of the behavioural effects that perhaps comes to mind most readily when considering the effect of surviving childhood cancer is behavioural adaptation within the school environment. Given the physical, psychosocial and neurocognitive impacts described, both the peer environment and academic performance present potential hurdles and difficulties for children and adolescents. In comparison with population norms, child survivors of brain tumours (aged 6–16 years and at least 2 years post-treatment) have been reported to score more highly on behavioural problems such as hyperactivity or inattention, as well as emotional symptoms and social difficulties with peers (Upton and Eiser, 2006). For IQ and quality of life, Sheppard et al. (2005) report some very positive psychosocial outcome effects in a sample of 54 children aged 8–16 years who were survivors of childhood retinoblastoma (Rb). Using a combination of parental interview and questionnaire assessment, they found children to have adapted well in school, showing age-appropriate performance on IQ tasks, particularly on verbal IQ. Interview data were particularly positive, although questionnaire reports from mothers did not entirely support these positive findings, with lower quality of life scores for psychosocial and physical aspects compared with population norms. Of particular concern, raised in interview, was being teased due to various forms of facial appearance (74 per cent), a particular feature of this condition and its treatment in addition to visual difficulties. Specifically, facial symmetry was a source of concern for over 20 per cent of the sample. Further work from this research group highlights the need for support to mothers of Rb survivors in helping them to communicate information to their children about the future health risks of the disease, including genetic risks and secondary cancers as a result of the treatment (Clarke et al., 2008). Given the reported latency period for development of a secondary cancer being as long as 50 years after first diagnosis for over half of childhood Rb patients (Roarty et al., in Clarke et al.,

2008), open communication is seen as vital in helping children form knowledge about their disease history which may influence subsequent health behaviours and, ultimately, interact with their future health status.

In survivors of conditions other than cancer, Jacobs and colleagues (2004) report a study of 19 children previously admitted to hospital with acute disseminated encephalomyelitis (inflammation of the brain and spinal cord), ten of whom were under the age of 5 years at the time of admission. Compared to controls matched for age and socioeconomic status, the children under the age of 5 years at diagnosis had greater cognitive and social problems, particularly those related to behavioural and emotional difficulties (Jacobs et al., 2004). Sumpter and co-workers (2011) point out the need for increasing parental awareness of the long-term consequences of acute childhood meningitis as advised by current UK clinical guidelines. In their study of 112 survivors of childhood meningitis (aged 5–16 years), parents and teachers completed self-report questionnaires rating the children across a number of psychosocial adjustment variables. Children were at least one year post-discharge from hospital and on average 8 years post-illness. Sumpter et al. (2011) report clinically significant behavioural difficulties and a reduced quality of life in these children; also, learning disability, hearing and visual impairments, and socioeconomic status each predicted behavioural and quality of life outcomes. The authors point to the need to be aware of such emotional and behavioural difficulties during stressful life transitions such as starting school (see Chapter 5 for the methodological significance of school transition).

HEALTH BEHAVIOURS

The impact of psychosocial factors may also underlie physical health effects through health behaviours. For example, presenting a multifactorial model of the increased risk of obesity in survivors of childhood cancer, Green et al. (2012) highlight the mediating effects of cancer-related anxiety, cancer-related pain and an inactive lifestyle in the relationship between physical functioning and obesity in over 9,000 participants from the CCSS cohort. They point out the need for interventions which address various therapeutic routes to reducing anxiety and depression in order to reduce obesity in adult survivors of childhood cancer. The use of behaviour-change strategies which address anxiety reduction and increase motivation is recommended (Green et al., 2012). Similarly, the health behaviour of sleep has been found to underlie fatigue and neurocognitive function in cancer survivors, leading to the suggestion to include advice about 'sleep hygiene' (the current term for good sleep practices) amongst survivors (Clanton et al., 2011).

Smoking is a known risk factor for cancer and has been reported as less prevalent amongst adult cancer survivors diagnosed in childhood compared with the general population (for review, see Clarke and Eiser, 2007). Based on data from the British Childhood Cancer Survivor Study (BCCSS), the smoking prevalence rate in survivors has been reported as a third lower, and in survivors who do smoke, the number of cigarettes consumed per day is on average 1.5 fewer than in the general population (Frobisher et al.,

2008). A number of sociodemographic variables influenced the prevalence rate of smoking in these adult survivors, including age at diagnosis, with greater prevalence of smoking if the cancer was diagnosed between the ages of 10 and 14 years, compared to a younger age at diagnosis, identifying this diagnostic age group as in need of targeting for smoking prevention (Frobisher et al., 2008).

Findings from the CCSS cohort highlight the increased likelihood of neurocognitive and emotional problems leading to poorer health behaviours, particularly adherence to recommendations related to physical activity or dental care, and avoidance of health-screening procedures such as having a mammogram, bone density or skin examination (Krull et al., 2011). A later analysis from this group points to a number of health behaviour problems during adolescence resulting from psychological late effects of cancer which may increase the risk of adverse health outcomes in adulthood (Krull et al., 2011). In this particular analysis, participant data from cancer survivors and control siblings were compared across two time points: first, as adolescents (aged 12–17 years), and then as adults approximately 7 years later. Significant differences were found between survivors and siblings for attention deficits, antisocial behaviours, depression/anxiety, headstrong behaviour, and social withdrawal. As young adults, fewer survivors achieved a normal body mass index (BMI) than in adolescence, and social withdrawal increased their risk of being overweight or obese, as did adolescent depression or anxiety and the use of stimulant medication. Adolescent social withdrawal was also linked to adult physical inactivity (Krull et al., 2011).

POSITIVE OUTCOMES IN SURVIVORSHIP

There is increasing interest in exploring positive outcomes following life-changing events for adults and children. Just as in chronic illness where children and adults cope well, with some showing resilience in the face of the stress of childhood illness, most survivors are described as being 'relatively well adjusted' and some show 'extraordinary adjustment' (Haupt et al., 2007). Positive psychological outcomes following childhood cancer (leukaemia, central nervous system or solid tumour) have been reported in child survivors of cancer aged 12–15 years in the form of 'benefit-finding'. 'Post-traumatic growth' was also seen in the parents, although no association was found linking positive outcomes between parents and children (Michel et al., 2009). Implications for counselling to facilitate adaptation through benefit-finding are suggested by the authors.

The significance of finding meaning in traumatic events, benefit-finding and post-traumatic growth links with coping theory and to a reduction in psychological and physical morbidity which may have consequences for mortality within the biopsychosocial approach discussed throughout these chapters. For example, in an interesting mixed methods study by Devine and colleagues (2010), the experience of post-traumatic growth (PTG) was examined in a group of 60 young adult survivors with a mean age of childhood diagnosis at 9 years and adult study participation at 20 years. Survivors had experienced a range of chronic illnesses in childhood, including asthma, epilepsy, diabetes, cancer, Crohn's disease, juvenile rheumatoid arthritis, lupus, rheumatic fever, haemophilia, Lyme disease, measles and gastro-oesophageal disease. Approximately half of the participants were still experiencing symptoms of the illness and half were termed 'recovered'. This recovered group reported more PTG (empathy, self-efficacy and life appreciation), particularly if the illness had been more severe. Qualitative analysis of written, open-ended questions found additional themes, including a positive 'shift' in their life focus which involved 'development of insight' and cognitive reframing of the traumatic experience of chronic illness (Devine et al., 2010). Recent data from the CCSS cohort also show evidence of perceived positive impact, as measured by an inventory of posttraumatic growth, in adult survivors of childhood cancer in comparison with siblings (Zebrack et al., 2012). The experience of positive impact was linked to demographic factors such as race and gender, with women and those of non-white ethnicities reporting greater positive impact. Medical characteristics of the cancer also influenced positive impact ratings, with greater positive impact reported in those who had received at least one intense therapy, where the cancer had reoccurred or where there was a further malignancy. Being older at diagnosis and a shorter amount of time since diagnosis were also associated with more positive impact (Zebrack et al., 2012).

PSYCHOSOCIAL INTERVENTIONS FOR SURVIVORS OF CHILDHOOD CANCER

As can be seen from the studies reported above, listing a range of physical and psychological effects in adult survivors of childhood illness, particularly cancer, there is scope for greater follow-up and potential for intervention across both childhood and adulthood to reduce the risk of negative outcomes. Early intervention focused on health promotion is indicated as the most beneficial in this respect. Intervention studies have utilized a variety, and frequently a combination, of popular health psychology models to design and increase the effectiveness of interventions. Key areas for intervention are in encouraging attendance at follow-up appointments, in increasing awareness of late physical and psychological effects, and in increasing engagement in health behaviours which might reduce the likelihood or severity of late effects. For example, Eiser and colleagues (2000) drew on the stages of change model (see Chapter 1) to encourage readiness for behavioural change in a sample of 263 young adult survivors of childhood cancer (average age 21 years) in the UK. They developed a successful intervention using an information package consisting of a booklet designed specifically for young adult survivors aged 16 years and upwards, issued by their doctor during a routine care appointment, along with further information about the treatment received and relevant information sheets. After participating in the intervention, survivors reported an increase in self-efficacy, an increase in self-perception of their vulnerability in respect to future health, and a greater readiness to change their health behaviours (Eiser et al., 2000).

Using a written booklet to convey similar information, but in an age-appropriate style written specifically for 10–16-year-old survivors of childhood cancer, Absolom and colleagues (2004) were also able to increase positive attitude towards clinic follow-up appointments and to promote readiness for health behaviour change in a UK sample of 20 adolescent cancer survivors (leukaemia/lymphoma; CNS or solid tumours). This study also utilized the concepts of 'central' and 'peripheral' processing taken from the 'likelihood elaboration model' (Petty et al., in Absolom et al., 2004), which is designed to influence persuasion and attitude change. Central processing is considered preferable to peripheral processing as it involves the individual engaging more directly with the material and requires them to grapple with the content. Absolom et al. (2004) found that survivors who engaged in central processing ascribed greater importance to the information provided in the booklet and showed greater readiness for health behaviour change. A study by Michel et al. (2011) used the 'health belief model' to structure their assessment of reasons given by young Swiss adult survivors of childhood cancer for attendance or non-attendance at follow-up clinic appointments. Their findings highlight the importance of addressing barriers to attendance (e.g., the fear of negative late effects being discovered at appointments or the belief that regular follow-up was not necessary) in order to increase attendance at follow-up visits.

Specific lifestyle and health behaviour change has also been addressed in adolescent and young adult groups of cancer survivors. For example, Mays et al. (2011) used a group-based interactive workshop of half-day duration, theoretically informed by elements of the 'health belief model', the 'transtheoretical model' and social cognition theory (see Chapter 1) to increase sun-safety practices as well as other health behaviours of relevance to adolescent survivors of cancer. In particular, they sought to increase awareness, reduce barriers/increase benefits and increase self-efficacy, all viewed as mediators of health behaviour change. Compared to waiting-list controls, survivors undergoing the intervention significantly improved their sun-safety practices (Mays et al., 2011). This work is important as it shows both the application of theory but also the relevance of this application to a health behaviour associated with reducing the risk of secondary cancers. Other studies have focused on the need for greater attention to follow-up care and the importance of health behaviours such as smoking (see Eiser, 2007) and physical exercise (Belanger et al., 2011) in young adult survivors. Gender has also been identified as an important consideration in the success of health behaviour change programmes in adolescent survivors, with women showing greater change (Hudson et al., 2002).

In anticipation of known survivor difficulties, other studies have addressed specific deficits, such as neurocognitive functioning in children with cancer whilst the child is still receiving treatment. Moore Ki and colleagues (2012) randomized a group of 32 US children (average age 6.6 years) undergoing standard treatment without cranial radiation therapy for leukaemia to either an interactive multi-modal mathematics intervention (40–50 hours per participant, delivered in person over 1–2 hours each week) or regular care control. The intervention group scored significantly higher on applied maths tasks immediately post-intervention and showed an improvement in working memory at follow-up one year later, compared to controls (Moore Ki et al., 2012). The authors point to a need for an easily available 'virtual' method for delivery for such an intervention.

IMPLICATIONS FOR THE LIFE-COURSE PERSPECTIVE

Before leaving the topics of terminal illness during childhood and the long-term effects of survivorship covered in this chapter, it is worth taking a step back to consider where these themes fit within the broader and recurring themes discussed throughout this book: in particular, the theme of stress and the transactional theory of stress and coping model proposed by Lazarus and Folkman (1984), widely accepted as the guiding principle in health psychology, in conjunction with the psychobiological theory of allostasis and allostatic load (Sterling and Eyer, 1988; McEwen, 1998b; see Chapters 2 and 5). Facing death and dealing with palliative care can be placed at one end of the severity spectrum of coping with stressful experiences. Even if survival is the eventual outcome, the 'threat' of premature death is the challenge that both the parents and child are coping with in addition to a multitude of other associated stressors, including treatment and its side-effects. The transactional theory uses the terminology of 'real' versus 'perceived' threat. In some conditions and circumstances, the threat to life is more certain, whereas in others it is possible but the chances of survivorship are greater. The transaction between threat and resources to cope with the threat are vital considerations in providing appropriately tailored care for children and their families facing the threat of survival and the short- and long-term impact of illness.

CHAPTER SUMMARY

In this chapter, we have considered the meaning of palliative care in the context of life-threatening or life-limiting illness in childhood. We then explored the physical and psychosocial effects of surviving childhood illness for patients and their families at different life stages, from child and adolescent through to adult survivor. The link between physical and psychosocial and between cognitive, emotion, social and behavioural effects was approached from a biopsychosocial perspective using evidence from research across a range of methodologies from qualitative interviewing to MRI scanning. This evidence was then used to consider psychosocial interventions which make use of a variety of theories and models to influence health behaviours as routes to improving both physical outcome and quality of survivorship. As can be seen from this brief review of the major themes, there is a large and growing, theoretically informed, applied research interest in palliative care and survivorship in childhood illness. This area offers significant potential for health psychology practice within multidisciplinary medical settings. In Chapter 9, we go on to consider specifically the experience of pain in the context of acute and chronic illness in childhood and adolescence.

KEY CONCEPTS AND ISSUES

- Complexity of the child's understanding of death
- Definition of palliative care
- Quality of life/quality of survival

- Life-limiting conditions
- Humanistic versus technocratic communication style
- Survivorship
- Young adult survivors of childhood cancer (YASCC)
- In remission, cure and long-term survivorship
- Late effects
- Neuromania
- Benefit-finding and post-traumatic growth (PTG)

FURTHER READING

Clear, useful and insightful coverage of terms used in survivorship, statistics for different ages, and an excellent concise and informative literature review in this area, as well as quality of life/survivorship instruments, which are the original focus of the paper:

Quinn, G.P., Huang, I.C., Murphy, D., Zidonik-Eddelton, K. and Krull, K.R. (2012) Missing content from health-related quality of life instruments: interviews with young adult survivors of childhood cancer. *Quality of Life Research* (EPub date: 31 January).

An early paper by Robison which describes the Childhood Cancer Survivorship Study (CCSS) cohort and registry:

Robison, L.L., Mertens, A.C., Boice, J.D., Breslow, N.E., Donaldson, S.S., Green, D.M. and Zeltzer, L.K. (2002) Study design and cohort characteristics of the Childhood Cancer Survivor Study: a multi-institutional collaborative project. *Medical and Pediatric Oncology*, 38(4): 229–39.

In-depth coverage of the effects of childhood cancer on the child and their family:

Eiser, C. (2004) *Children with Cancer: The Quality of Life.* New Jersey: Lawrence Erlbaum.

An insightful and moving text which incorporates therapeutic interventions in life-threatening illness, including chapters on grief and death:

Sourkes, B.M. (1995) *Armfuls of Time: The Psychological Experience of the Child with a Life-threatening Illness.* London: Routledge.

USEFUL WEBSITES

The National Cancer Survivorship Initiative (NCSI) UK (survivors of childhood and young people's cancers, a partnership between Macmillan Cancer Support, the Department of Health and the NHS): www.ncsi.org.uk

NCSI initiative published March 2013: Living With and Beyond Cancer: Taking Action to Improve Outcomes, Department of Health: https://www.gov.uk/government/publications/living-with-and-beyond-cancer-taking-action-to-improve-outcomes

Together for Short Lives, which now incorporates the Association for Children's Palliative Care (ACT) and Children's Hospices UK: www.togetherforshortlives.org.uk

Provides two useful documents:

1 Children and adults' palliative care: a comparison
2 Children's palliative care definitions

The Childhood Cancer Survivor Study (CCSS) website, which includes a tab for an impressive list of research publications to come out of this study: http://ccss.stjude.org

THE EXPERIENCE OF PAIN IN CHILDHOOD

9

Covered in this chapter

- The biopsychosocial approach to the experience of pain
- The pain experience in children and analgesic management of pain
- The prevalence of pain and disability in children
- Cognitive, behavioural and emotional factors in coping with pain
- The role of early life pain experience on subsequent pain
- Psychosocial interventions in acute and chronic pain

In this chapter, I explore the biopsychosocial experience of pain and how children cope with pain, from neonates and infants through to the experience of pain in adolescence. To begin with, I consider the prevalence of pain in children and the context of pain relief through pharmacological intervention. I then compare the characteristics of the experience of acute pain (e.g., dental pain or pain from an acute traumatic injury such as a car accident) with the characteristics of chronic pain experienced in chronic conditions (e.g., juvenile arthritis or sickle cell disease). In particular, I focus on how children cope with acute and chronic pain and how this may change over time, with age and experience, and consider both adaptive coping and maladaptive coping responses such as catastrophizing. Also considered are the assessment of pain, differences between children and adolescents in the expression of pain, and the role of sex differences in pain. I then draw on this knowledge to examine psychosocial interventions to reduce the experience of acute and chronic pain in children. Whilst reading this chapter, keep in mind the concepts of stress, coping, acute and chronic definitions and lifespan issues already covered in previous chapters. For those who like more of a challenge, think about what parallels might exist between the research areas of pain and stress, between coping under conditions of acute and chronic stress and adaptation in acute and chronic pain, and where the pain experience in childhood fits with the theory of allostasis and concept of allostatic load across the life course (to be fair, I did say for those who like more of a challenge).

THE BIOPSYCHOSOCIAL APPROACH TO THE EXPERIENCE OF PAIN

DEFINITIONS, THEORIES AND MODELS: FROM 'BELFRY' TO 'GATE' AND BEYOND

Before we can explore the labyrinth of research pathways which support and inform the experience of pain, we first need to define exactly what is meant by the experience of pain. It is important to be able to distinguish between terms such as 'nociception', 'pain', 'acute pain', 'chronic pain' and 'recurrent pain'. These are defined in Box 9.1.

The description of pain in its most basic form, as understood in the days of philosopher René Descartes (1664), was pain as a physical response (this was at least the working theory of the philosophers and physiologists of the time, although I suspect that the average man or woman in the street was well aware that their pain experience was influenced by a range of psychosocial factors even though the word 'psychosocial' had not been coined). Descartes (1984) used the classic metaphor of a bell in a bell-tower, the rope from the bell being the nerves of the spinal cord linking the site of the noxious stimuli directly up to the brain or 'bell-tower' in which the experience of pain was registered. Descartes' ideas informed 'specificity theory' (led by key figures in the field such as Muller and von Frey in the nineteenth century), which views pain as being the product of one-way communication between pain receptors in the skin and the pain centre located in the brain via specific pain receptors (Melzack and Wall, 2008): in other words, a direct sensory modality for pain from specific tissue sites in the skin to the brain. However, specificity theory failed to account for differences in pain across individuals or to provide an explanation for various types of clinical pain (Melzack and Wall, 2008). Later theories in the late nineteenth and early part of the twentieth century were based on 'pattern theory' (the key figure being Goldschneider), which views different sensory modalities (e.g., touch, heat) as being capable of contributing to a pattern of overall intensity or 'summation' which triggers the pain experience (for a full account and evaluation of these theories, see Melzack and Wall, 2008). Both these theories are still prevalent within the medical model of pain but, as Melzack and Wall (2008) point out, although both make important contributions to the understanding of pain, they fail to account for affective, motivational (termed 'sensory motivational' and 'motivational affective') and cognitive processes which

BOX 9.1

What is pain? Some useful terms and definitions

Nociception: 'the neural mechanism by which an individual detects the presence of a potentially tissue-harming stimulus. There is no implication of (or requirement for) awareness of this stimulus' (Jaggar, 2005: 3).

Pain is 'a complex, multidimensional phenomenon' (Schechter et al., 2003: 15), defined as 'an unpleasant sensory and emotional experience associated with actual or potential tissue damage, or described in terms of such damage' (International Association for the Study of Pain). Jaggar (2005: 3) notes that 'perception of sensory events is a requirement, but actual tissue damage is not'.

Acute pain: 'the term generally ascribed to pain associated with a brief episode of tissue injury or inflammation, such as that caused by surgery, burns, or a fracture. In most cases, the intensity of pain diminishes steadily with time over a period of days to weeks' (Schechter et al., 2003: 14). Acute pain is pain that lasts less than 12 weeks (British Pain Society).

Chronic pain: 'conditions of persistent or of nearly constant pain over a period of 3 months or longer' (Schechter et al., 2003: 15). It is pain which lasts longer than 12 weeks or if the pain is following trauma or surgery then 'after the time that healing would have been thought to have occurred' (British Pain Society). Chronic pain conditions include chronic arthritis and sickle cell disease.

Recurrent pain: pain which is intermittent across time and can be intense but is not persistent or constant. It can occur in the absence of psychopathology or 'signs of a specific organic disease' (Schechter et al., 2003: 15). Recurrent pain examples include headache, abdominal pain, chest pain and limb pains. Occurrence is common in school children (occurrence rate = 5–10 per cent; Schechter et al., 2003: 15).

Neuropathic pain: persistent pain 'in the central or peripheral nervous system in the absence of on-going tissue injury' (Schechter et al., 2003: 15).

Somatoform pain disorder: 'persistent pain as a manifestation of psychiatric disease' (previously, psychogenic pain or hypochondriasis; Schechter et al., 2003: 15).

influence the pain experience. Interestingly, they put in the limelight the frequently overlooked philosopher and psychologist Henry Rutgers Marshall who, ahead of his time in the late nineteenth century, argued against these two dominant theories, in his own 'affect theory', for the inclusion of 'emotional quality' as a central component of the pain experience.

Building on these biological theories and early ideas of affective aspects of pain, Melzack and Wall (1965) revolutionized pain theory, and subsequently the clinical practice of treating pain, with their 'gate control theory' of pain, which was followed by Melzack's later concept of the 'neuromatrix' (Melzack, 1999a). Figure 9.1 shows

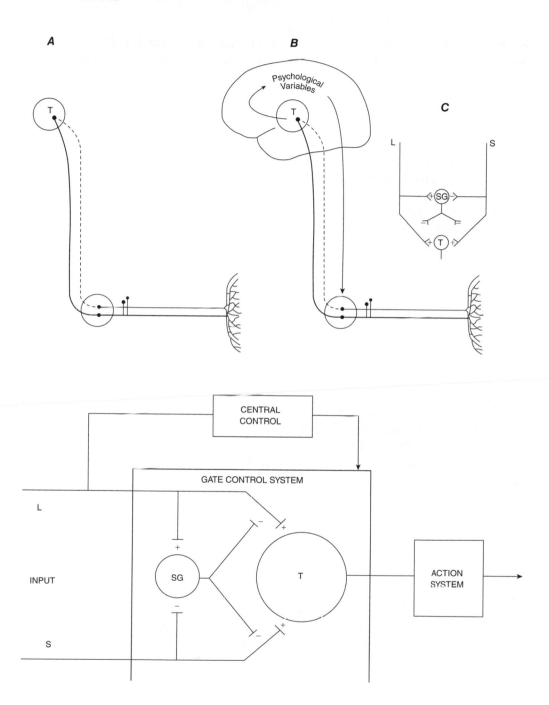

FIGURE 9.1 Evolution of the 'gate control theory'
Source: Melzack (1999a).

the original 1965 schematic diagram of 'gate control theory' (pictured along the bottom of the diagram) as well as the earlier and more basic diagram of Noordenbos's (A), and Melzack's (B) and Wall's (C) later sketches, which progressively inspired it (Melzack, 2001).

In terms of metaphors, then, it took 300 years to move from the metaphor of the belfry to one of a gate (albeit, an electrical circuitry 'gate' rather than the more colourful metaphor this perhaps conjures up today). So what does this now well-accepted 'gate control theory' of pain tell us? At the core of this theory is the idea that the experience of pain is more than merely sensory perception. It simultaneously involves both a biological feedforward action and a psychophysiological feedback action, the product of which determines the degree that the 'gate' is open and hence the amount of pain perceived. The first of these, the feedforward action, operates from the pain receptors located in the skin and bodily organs linking to a series of 'gates' in the substantia gelatinosa (SG) which lies within the dorsal horn throughout the spinal column. The SG initiates the production of substance P which activates the T fibres, thus 'opening' the 'gate'; the degree to which the gates are open depending on the combined amount of excitatory and inhibitory information being transmitted across three types of nerve fibres: (i) the A delta fibres (associated with sharp pain); (ii) the C fibres (associated with dull, throbbing pain); and (iii) the A beta fibres which respond to touch and gentle pressure. These impulses are then transmitted to the pain centres of the brain. The A delta fibres and C fibres (both 'S' in Melzack and Wall's original 1965 diagram) relay pain information on this feedforward part of the system, opening the gate, whilst activation of the A beta fibres ('L' in Melzack and Wall's original 1965 diagram) has the opposite effect of closing the gate via a feedback mechanism which loops from the brain directly back to the gate mechanism. This explains why gently rubbing the site of injury reduces the experience of pain, since the A beta fibres transmit information more quickly than the C fibres (Morrison and Bennett, 2012). Simultaneously, our cognitive and emotional response systems are activated in the brain (central control box), and these activate nerves that relay information down through the spinal column to the gates receiving feedforward impulses. The thalamus and cortex of the brain detect A fibre nociception and are associated with planning and action (e.g., motivating an individual to get away from the pain), whereas the limbic system, hypothalamus and autonomic nervous system detect C fibre activation and enable an emotional response to the pain. Operating via the release of hormones such as endorphins (naturally occurring pain relievers), this psychophysiological feedback can open the gates further or close the gates depending on the characteristics of the emotions and cognitions; for example, anxiety may add to the degree that the gate is open, whereas relaxation may contribute to closing the gate (Morrison and Bennett, 2012). Endorphins (natural pain relievers) act to reduce the effectiveness of substance P (neurotransmitter which enables pain to be transmitted across nerves; Kalat, 2001) at the level of the brain and SG in the spinal cord (Morrison and Bennett, 2012). Pharmacological pain medication can act to close the gate by interrupting both feedback and feedforward mechanisms. A modern representation of this feedforward and feedback system is shown in Figure 9.2 which illustrates the ascending and descending pain pathways from the spinal cord to the brain. It is in these descending pain pathways that the psychological factors of affect, motivation and cognition are able to act to moderate the sensory perception of pain or, in Melzack's own words, the 'brain processes can select, filter and modulate pain signals' (Melzack, 1999a: S122). Melzack considered the gate control theory as revolutionary in prioritizing the central nervous system (CNS) as 'an essential component' in the experience of pain.

Melzack (1999a) added to this 'gate control theory' of pain in order to explain more complex pain experiences which the original theory was unable to accommodate, such as cases of phantom limb pain in which patients who had had a limb amputated still experienced significant chronic pain in the non-existent limb. Of course, the limb was no longer able to transmit the sensory information generating the pain, so what Melzack cleverly deduced was that the neural networks responsible for the pain experience were still in existence in the brain, acting as stimuli to produce the pain, even though the route for the sensory stimuli to produce the patterns no longer existed. Effectively, the brain processes are acting 'in the absence of any inputs' (Melzack, 1999a: S123). Melzack referred to the 'body-self' as an individual's distinct awareness of themselves in relation to their environment, and this body-self involves numerous dimensions (e.g., sensory, affective, evaluative, and postural) with underlying brain processes that are genetically 'built-in' but capable of

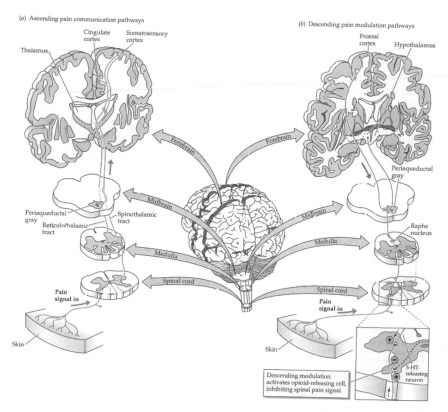

FIGURE 9.2   Ascending and descending pain pathways

Source: Rozenzweig et al. (2002: 240).

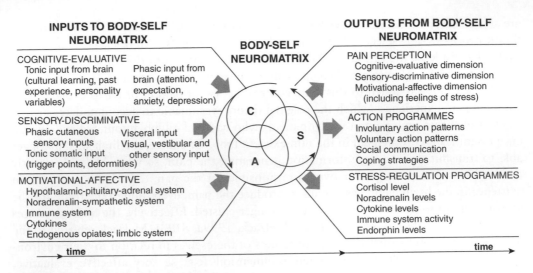

FIGURE 9.3　The body-self neuromatrix

Source: Melzack (2001: 1382, fig. 1).

modification via experience (Melzack, 1999b: S123). The 'neuromatrix', then, was defined as 'the anatomical substrate of the body-self' (Melzack, 1999b: 881) and is composed of 'a large, widespread network of neurons that consists of loops between the thalamus and cortex and limbic system' (Melzack, 2001: 1379). Melzack did not stop there; he further defined the individual pattern of nerve impulses in the neuromatrix as the 'neurosignature', (Melzack 1999a: S123, S125) and this neurosignature from the body-self neuromatrix projects into the 'sentient neural hub' (Melzack 2001: 1379) in the brain at which point awareness of the pain experience occurs. Figure 9.3 shows Melzack's illustration of the neuromatrix with body-self inputs and outputs.

The neuromatrix not only further places psychological factors associated with affective, motivational and cognitive components firmly within the pain experience, but it opens up the floodgates (no pun intended) for understanding how the powerful effects of these psychological components may influence the sensory experience of pain. It also provides an explanation for chronic pain conditions where there is no identifiable physical damage or sensory input (e.g., phantom limb pain, chronic musculoskeletal pain, fibromyalgia, or complex regional pain syndrome), but where the pain gates appear to be permanently 'open' or in a state of constant heightened 'vigilance' (Melzack, 2005). Importantly, these theories widen the scope for development of non-pharmacological psychosocial interventions to modulate the pain experience.

To move from this general understanding of pain theories and models to the experience of pain in children, the concept of the neurosignature of the neuromatrix is particularly pertinent since, in the early years of life, this neuromatrix or patterning of response is only just forming. Genetic make-up is an important underlying influence on the neuromatrix, but it also becomes shaped and defined by the psychosocial environment and by previous pain experience (Melzack, 1999a, 2001). As with stress, understanding pain experience in childhood provides not only a useful theoretical and clinical insight into managing pain in children but also informs the nature of the pain experience from a life-course perspective. Before we continue with relating these theories to pain in children, there is one more aspect of this biopsychosocial approach to pain that we need to piece together and that is the relationship between pain and stress at both the sensory and the psychosocial level.

LINKING PAIN AND STRESS

Just as the experience of illness is stressful, pain is also stressful and activates stress response pathways. The term 'pain stress' has even been used in the literature on pain (Di Gioia et al., 2011). We have already mentioned the activation of emotional responses in pain, via the limbic system, involving the hypothalamus and autonomic nervous system, which is part of the stress response system associated with the hypothalamic-pituitary-adrenal (HPA) axis and central nervous system. It is this second part of the stress response system that is particularly implicated in pain, but it is worth remembering that the more immediate adrenalin-producing 'flight, fight or fright' response of the sympathetic adrenomedullary (SAM) system, associated with peripheral nervous system response, is also activated. This dual action stress response system is described in Chapter 2 and referred to throughout this book.

Melzack (1999a) himself specifically acknowledged the role of stress in pain, via activation of the SAM system and stimulation of the locus coeruleus in the brainstem and via activation of the HPA axis and stimulation of the hypothalamus in the brain, setting off a cascade of endocrine responses resulting in the production of cortisol. In fact, Melzack (1999a) highlights the importance of the stress response system in pain, pointing out that: 'By recognising the role of the stress system in pain processes, we discover that the scope of the puzzle of pain is vastly expanded and new pieces of the puzzle provide valuable clues in our quest to understand chronic pain' (1999a: S124).

Melzack argued that when an individual incurs physical injury or insult, they do not just experience pain but at the same time the body's stress response system is activated (see Chapter 2) as a result of disruption to the 'homeostatic regulation systems' in the brain (Melzack, 1999a: S123). Both pain and stress are biological response systems and their interplay is implicated in a number of chronic pain conditions. As with pain, activation of the stress response, whether by physical injury, infection, pathology or psychological insult, creates an attempt by the brain to try to redress the homeostatic balance through 'neural, hormonal and behavioural activity' (Melzack, 1999: S124).

In particular, Melzack (1999a, b, 2001) highlights the stress hormone, cortisol, as central to the link between pain and stress. As discussed in Chapter 2, cortisol is essential to life and is no more apparent than after injury when survival depends on its production in order to mobilize energy. However, continued release of cortisol over a prolonged period of time can lead to disruption of the immune system with associated alteration in cytokine profile, resulting in hypercortisolaemic states (chronically high cortisol) seen in Th2 over-activation and may subsequently lead to hypocortisolaemic states (chronically low levels of cortisol) seen in Th1 under-activation. Such states are associated with the deleterious effects of muscle weakness and destruction of bone and tissue. Examples of this are seen in inflammatory chronic pain syndromes characterized by hypocortisolaemic states, such as rheumatoid arthritis, and have also been observed in musculoskeletal conditions (Turner-Cobb et al., 2010). Melzack (1999a) also links sex differences in pain to increases in cortisol via oestrogen, which induces cytokine release, and an increase in chronic pain conditions with age, due to the over-production of cortisol damaging the hippocampus and setting off a vicious spiral which further reduces the ability of the brain to control cortisol release.

Receiving increasing attention in pain research is the focus of the social context of pain and the interaction of this context with individual factors and what these bring to the pain experience. The social context can include relationships, social support, family environment, and previous experience with pain, and individual factors include demographic variables such as age and sex (for an excellent review, see Gatchel et al., 2007). In modern conceptualizations and application of the biopsychosocial perspective to pain, the focus is shifting to consider these factors not only as integral to the model but as being involved as precursors of the pain experience. In other words, it is not just that psychosocial factors are involved in the feedback from the brain to pain perception, but that they are already in place, ready and waiting, as the individual brings these to the situation before the pain experience hits, thus having a huge influence on the outcome. When considering pain in children, we are considering a neural network under development, the early social context beginning to play out on the experience of pain and the experience of pain shaping future responses. That the social context is so influential in the pain experience means that there is enormous potential for psychosocial intervention to influence the psychobiological experience of pain.

Hence, it is essential to consider a life-course perspective when attempting to understand the biopsychosocial model of pain, as well as the effect of stress across the life course. Early trauma may influence the subsequent experience of pain, and the way that a child responds to chronic stress may, in part, determine future pain experience through the early setting or programming of hormonal, neural and behavioural stress response systems which may trigger and determine subsequent psychological and physical responses to pain. In other words, the body-self neuromatrix, which is a product of both sensory and psychological activation and determines an individual's experience of pain, operates in a co-dependent manner with the psychobiological stress response systems of the body. If this sounds familiar, and the theory of allostasis and notion of allostatic load come to mind as useful concepts in explaining the parallel ideas and interacting relationships between pain and stress, then you have been paying attention (if not, go back and read Chapter 2 before proceeding).

THE PAIN EXPERIENCE IN CHILDREN AND ANALGESIC MANAGEMENT OF PAIN

PAIN IN CHILDREN

The theories and models outlined above were developed based on pain in adults rather than pain experienced by children. But what is known specifically about the pain experience of children and how do these theories hold up when examining paediatric pain? A number of different versions of the biopsychosocial model of pain have been applied in order to understand the experience of acute and chronic pain across the different ages of childhood and into adolescence. A number of different methodologies have been used to assess the experience of pain in children and how children cope with pain. Methods of assessment of pain from illness, injury, or surgery include interviews (e.g., the Pain Experience Interview; McGrath et al., 2000); observation (direct or indirect via video, e.g., Vervoort et al., 2009); and questionnaires and pain-rating charts/visual analogue scales – for example, the Pain Experience Questionnaire (PEQ; Hermann et al., 2008); the Bath Adolescent Pain Questionnaire (BAPQ; Eccleston et al., 2005), the Chronic Pain Acceptance Questionnaire for Adolescents (CPAQ-A; McCracken et al., 2010), and the Fear of Pain Questionnaire for Children (FOPQ-C; Simons et al., 2011) – with children, their parents, and/or medical staff.

Various methods of induction of pain in the laboratory have used heat stimulation or cold-pressor tasks to assess responses to pain, tolerance and coping responses in healthy and clinical populations. In the studies referred to throughout this chapter, you will see a range of assessment methods included. Questionnaire assessment is the most frequently used, particularly for older children and adolescents, but, of course, for younger children, particularly preverbal, if assessment is direct rather than via parents and medical staff, then observation and interview are necessary. Excellent reviews of pain assessment and coping in children can be found in Gaffney et al. (2003), Eccleston et al. (2006), Hermann et al. (2007) and Huguet et al. (2010). For a more general discussion of biopsychosocial methodologies in child health research, refer back to Chapter 3.

An excellent example that articulates the pain experience of younger children is provided in an innovative qualitative study by Woodgate and Kristjanson (1996), who assessed the experience of acute pain in 11 children aged 2.5–6.5 years, hospitalized for abdominal, chest, plastic or reconstructive surgery. They used a variety of assessment methods, including extensive observation and interview (with children, parents and staff), to understand the pain experience in children. Whilst the language the children used to describe their pain reflected differences in age (e.g., older children using terms such as 'stabbing, jumping in and out', compared to simpler words such as 'owie' in the younger children), they note that there was a commonality to their pain experience, and it was the experience of pain itself which was the overriding factor in shaping their experience of hospitalization (Woodgate and Kristjanson, 1996). On the basis of these findings, Woodgate and Kristjanson put forward a model of acute pain experience in young children known as 'Getting better from my hurts', which identifies influences on their pain experience and the consequences of this experience, as shown in Figure 9.4. Pain described by the children was categorized as either pain that the children were experiencing at the time or potential pain which had the 'threat of hurting' (1996: 238). The pain experience was influenced by aspects of the child themselves, how others take care of them (including parents and nurses), and aspects of the non-social environment termed 'things out there' which included both pleasant and unpleasant symbols. Three types of coping strategy were used to deal with the pain experience: (i) 'hiding away'; (ii) 'fighting it'; and (iii) 'making it good', descriptions and examples of which are given in Figure 9.4.

'Things out there' = pleasant or unpleasant symbols in the child's non-social environment that directly or indirectly influence their pain experience

- Examples of pleasant/good symbols: sight of favourite soft toy, feel of comforting blanket
- Examples of unpleasant symbols: sight of needles/surgical gloves, sound of removal of surgical drain

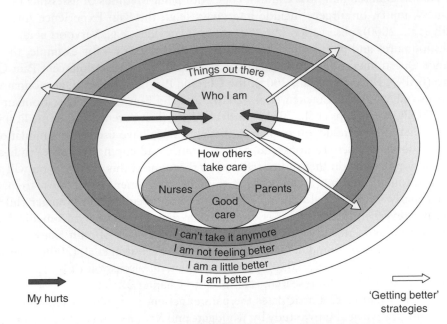

My hurts   'Getting better' strategies

'My hurts' = Central problem identified by the children. Process of getting better involves three conditions: (i) 'Who I am' (ii) 'How others take care' (iii) 'Things out there'	**'Getting better' strategies**	**Description and examples**
	1. 'Hiding away'	Withdrawing and distancing: not answering questions, avoiding eye contact, being quiet
	2. 'Fighting it'	Resistance to or attack on pain: tensing, pulling away, hitting, slapping or grabbing pain source, grimacing, crying, being angry
	3. 'Making it good'	Protection and comfort: guarded body movements, rubbing, patting, asking for help, distraction, fixed or serious facial expressions

FIGURE 9.4 'Getting better from my hurts': the young child's pain experience

Source: Woodgate and Kristjanson (1996: 238).

These authors emphasize the importance of the 'subtleness' (p. 240) of the pain responses observed in young children. The strategies of 'hiding away' (p. 238) and 'making it good' (p. 238), observed after a painful treatment, were expressed in quiet or serious behaviours, in contrast to the more noisy and overt pain responses associated with 'fighting it' (p. 239) in anticipation of, or during, a procedure. The emotions of 'fear, anxiety, anger, and sadness' (p. 240) were all observed as part of the pain experience and negatively influenced the children's pain (Woodgate and Kristjanson, 1996). This model of acute pain experience in young children shows the importance of the caregiver environment; in this case, the medical and nursing care, as well as that of the parents.

As this study by Woodgate and Kristjanson (1996) highlights, the distinguishing psychosocial characteristic associated with the pain experience for children is inevitably this caretaking role, whether provided by parents, family, those delivering care in the hospital setting or the school environment. These are the contextual social situations under the spotlight when considering the experience of pain throughout childhood including adolescence. Home, school and, when necessary, hospital are the environments which make up a child's world, and the actions of parents, teachers and peers, nurses and medical staff within them are vital to the outcome in a child's experience of acute and chronic pain. We return to this important theme later in the chapter.

Although the study mentioned above looked at young children, from toddler age up to school age, you may be wondering at what age infants start to feel pain. Before considering how the complex psychosocial interactions of the social context develop and play out in childhood and adolescence, we first need to go back a little further and consider how pain is experienced in infancy, from the developmental stage of the neonate ('neonate' is defined as from birth to 4 weeks old and is synonymous with the lay term 'newborn'; for more on this and related terms, see Chapter 4). Contrary to beliefs which existed prior to the 1970s, and continue to this day, that infants do not experience pain at least up until a month old, there is considerable evidence that young infants and children feel pain and respond to it and they also remember pain experienced (Schechter et al., 2003). In fact, Schechter et al. (2003: 13) point out that 'all the nerve pathways essential for the transmission and perception of pain are present and functioning by 24 weeks of gestation.' Take note that this is by 24 weeks 'of gestation', not 24 weeks after birth. So to answer the question about when children feel pain, there is evidence that, as neonates, children can certainly feel pain. In the context of the discussion above about setting the pattern of pain response, particularly in light of Melzack's (1999a) neuromatrix theory of pain, our interest here is in how the pain response develops throughout childhood and the psychosocial context in which the pain experience is shaped. In animal research, the effect of newborns not receiving analgesic pain medication has been found to lead to a 'rewiring' of sensory pain receptors in the spinal cord and to an increase in pain perception when they encounter future pain stimuli (Schechter et al., 2003). Similarly, they report that in newborn human infants who are not given pain relief during circumcision, a greater pain response has been seen to subsequent pain experiences such as immunization (Schechter et al., 2003). They argue that early experience of pain sensitizes the stress response system, leading to high levels of stress hormones which not only have psychological sequelae of distress and anxiety but also have deleterious physical effects (e.g., increases in heart rate, blood pressure and immuno-suppression) likely to compromise postoperative recovery. In other words, the pain experience is applicable to children of all ages, and applies as much to neonates as to adolescents, although it may be expressed in different ways. Common consensus is that children are particularly vulnerable to the consequences of pain if under-treated (Schechter et al., 2003).

PHARMACOLOGICAL PAIN MANAGEMENT: ANALGESICS AND ANAESTHESIA

Since we now know that neonates can feel pain right from the day they are born, the management of the pain experience is essential at least from birth onwards. Later on, we consider psychosocial interventions in pain management, but first we need to consider pharmacological pain management in children. As Schechter et al. (2003: 14) emphasize, 'for humanitarian, physiologic, and psychologic reasons, pain control should be considered an integral part of the compassionate medical care of children.' Many of the concepts that we have looked at so far in previous chapters of this book, such as hospitalization, treatments for leukaemia, and research ethics, have repeatedly pointed to the era of the 1960s or thereabouts as a turning point for the development of theories and improvement in treatment for children. In line with this, the 1970s are seen as the turning point for pain management in children. However, the documented lack of pain treatment and management in children, particularly with regard to the use of analgesic pain medication and anaesthesia, provides a chilling read, some aspects of which continued well into the 1980s.

Schechter et al. (2003) describe three categories of pain: (i) that of neonatal pain; (ii) postoperative pain; and (iii) pain associated with chronic disease. They document common cases in the 1980s of neonates undergoing lumbar punctures or having a chest tube inserted with minimal anaesthesia or children receiving minimal analgesia following cardiac surgery, an appendectomy, or a fractured femur (Schechter et al., 2003). They also report that, in the mid-1980s, children were not routinely sedated for aspiration of bone marrow or biopsies. Schechter et al. (2003) conclude that the most significant improvements in pain management have been postoperatively, during the hospital stay, especially for children of school age. However, there has been less of an improvement for postoperative pain management in younger children (particularly preverbal) and in children receiving day-case surgery (e.g., Gillies et al., 2001). Schechter et al (2003) point to neonatal and infant pain as being less well managed in comparison with management of pain experienced in older children, partly due to the false historical belief that neonates did not experience pain. In the context of chronic disease during childhood (e.g., sickle cell disease, HIV/AIDS, or cancer), despite developments, pain management is viewed as 'less adequate' compared to that of postoperative pain (p. 6). Although significant advances have been made, particularly for procedural pain in cancer, disease-related pain management across a variety of conditions is still described as problematic (Schechter et al., 2003). For example, work by Van Cleve et al. (2004) reported a lack of attention to pain in children with cancer who were largely cared for at home during the first year following diagnosis. A review published in this area 6 years later (Shepherd et al., 2010) still called for greater acknowledgement of the pain experienced in paediatric cancer patients in order to enable appropriate nursing care. Thus, the under-treatment of pain is still a substantial issue in pain management for children, despite an increase in knowledge about children's experience of pain. There are many reasons for this, which involve the concerns and sometimes misunderstandings of both parents and medical staff. This key issue in the management of paediatric pain is addressed by Friedrichsdorf and Kang (2007) in their review of how pain is managed in children with life-limiting conditions. They point out that, despite concern and a desire to relieve suffering, an aggressive approach to treating pain is often met with 'reluctance' by parents and medical staff. Friedrichsdorf and Kang (2007) summarize the 'myths and obstacles' reported in the literature regarding the use of opioids for managing pain in children as shown in Table 9.1. These myths and obstacles particularly highlight parental fear and practitioner education as important targets for addressing this issue.

So we know that the pain experience is a complex interaction between biological and psychosocial factors. We also know that, from a sensory perspective, children are just as capable of feeling pain as adults. I have outlined the importance of managing pain in children and the significance of treating pain in children on a number of levels. These levels include a minimizing of pain for purposes of reducing suffering in the short term, but also in order to reduce any future impact that the early pain experience may have. In terms of establishing the self-neuromatrix pattern, inadequate treatment of pain in early childhood may increase the experience of pain in later childhood or adolescence and lay the early foundations for chronic pain in adulthood. As Schechter et al. (2003) point out, although chronic and recurrent pain in children does not carry with it the economic burden of work absenteeism that is seen in adult pain conditions, pain and disability in children results in school absenteeism which may lead to social problems and future economic limitations, as well as the likelihood of adult pain, disability and dysfunction.

THE PREVALENCE OF PAIN AND DISABILITY IN CHILDREN

So how much of a problem are pain and pain-related disability in childhood? The prevalence of pain in children is difficult to assess, and pain of all types is often under-reported or under-recorded. Van Dijk and colleagues (2006) point to the fact that, whilst chronic pain prevalence is well documented in adults, we know a lot less about the incidence,

TABLE 9.1 Myths and obstacles associated with reluctance to use opioids for paediatric pain control

Parental concerns	Health-care practitioner concerns
• Fear of giving up	• Lack of sufficient education regarding managing pain
• Misconceptions of opioids as 'too strong for children'	• Misconceptions about frequency and severity of side-effects, such as respiratory depression
• Fear of side-effects	• Worries that opioids will shorten life expectancy
• Worry that their child will become 'addicted' to pain medications	• Concerns that escalating opioid doses will increase the likelihood of tolerance, and thus make pain control more difficult as the disease progresses
• Cultural or religious beliefs	

Source: Friedrichsdorf and Kang (2007).

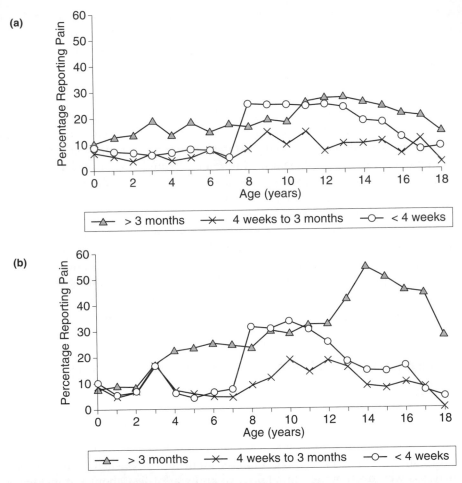

FIGURE 9.5   Age-specific prevalence rates of pain in (a) boys and (b) girls (0–18 years) shown separately. Lines represent pain of different duration. Data were based on one pain report per child

Source: Perquin et al. (2000: 55, fig. 1).

prevalence and pain experiences across various types of pain in children (for descriptions of prevalence and incidence, see Chapter 7). A large epidemiological study in The Netherlands of over 5,000 children aged 0–18 years reported pain in the past 3 months in over half the sample (54 per cent) and chronic or recurrent pain (most commonly limb pain, headache, abdominal pain or back pain) in over 25 per cent of participants (Perquin et al., 2000). As shown in Figure 9.5, prevalence was influenced by age and sex: for both girls and boys, the prevalence of chronic and recurrent pain increased with age; for girls, there was a leap in chronic/recurrent pain between the ages of 12 and 14 years, attributed to the onset of puberty and menstruation; and chronic/recurrent pain was significantly higher overall in girls than in boys (Perquin et al., 2000).

Data from another European study, this time using a sample of over 700 German children who were aged 10–18 years, show a similar increase in pain with age and similar pain locations (Roth-Isigkeit et al., 2004). In this study, pain in the past 3 months was reported by 85.3 per cent of the sample, chronic pain lasting more than 3 months was reported by almost half (45.5 per cent) of the sample, and recurrent pain in one-third of the sample (33.7 per cent). There were no sex differences found for pain duration or frequency in this study (Roth-Isigkeit et al., 2004). These pain figures are higher than for the Dutch sample, but bear in mind that the German sample consisted of older children and both found an increase of pain prevalence with age. Similar results have been found for acute pain in a Canadian study of the prevalence of acute, recurrent and chronic pain in a sample of 495 school children aged 9–13 years (van Dijk et al., 2006). These researchers report 96 per cent of children as having experienced acute pain in the past month, 57 per cent reporting recurrent pain and only 6 per cent reporting either currently having or having previously had a chronic illness. The most frequent acute pain was from headache (reported by 78 per cent of the sample). In addition to this period prevalence, a sex difference was found with significantly higher lifetime prevalence for acute pain (from accident/injury, stitches and bee stings) in boys compared to girls (van Dijk et al., 2006).

Finally, a recent German study looked specifically at children ($n = 2,249$) who fell into the category of severe impairment from chronic pain due to tension headache, migraine, functional abdominal pain or musculoskeletal pain and often with more than one type of pain (Zernikow et al., 2012). Almost a quarter of the German sample also had a diagnosis of clinical depression and almost one-fifth a diagnosis of clinical anxiety. Sex differences

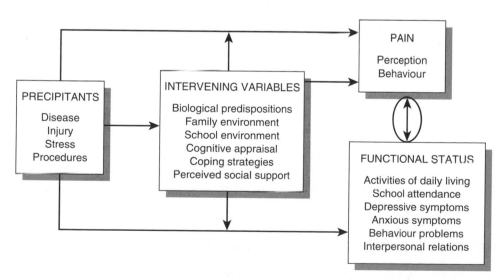

FIGURE 9.6 A hypothesized multidimensional biobehavioural model of paediatric pain

Source: Vetter (2012: 148, fig. 11.1); adapted from Varni et al. (1996); originally published in Varni et al. (1989). Reproduced with the kind permission of Springer Science+Business Media B.V.

were also observed, with girls over 13 years being more likely than boys to attend specialist pain centres (i.e., tertiary care services; Zernikow et al., 2012). These prevalence rates are variable, partly due to differences in methodology and definitions used between studies, particularly for reported chronic pain, and whilst sex differences exist, these are ambiguous at least until the age of puberty. Further data from Roth-Isigkeit and colleagues (2005) indicate that the extent of chronic pain experienced is, for some children and adolescents, sufficient to restrict activities of daily living related to varying levels of social and physical disability. Taken together, the evidence suggests that pain and pain-related restrictions or disability are significant problems for children and adolescents.

ROLE OF THE FAMILY, SCHOOL AND HOSPITAL IN PAEDIATRIC PAIN

Using the biopsychosocial approach to pain experience and management, we have established that pharmacological treatments are important in diminishing the sensory feedforward aspect of pain perception. Just as analgesic treatments have revolutionized pain treatment in the past 50 years, so too have the influence and acceptance of psychosocial aspects of pain in conjunction with these treatments. As flagged up earlier in this chapter, the biopsychosocial models of pain in children have emphasized the role of the family and school environment in influencing acute and chronic pain experiences. The biobehavioural model of paediatric pain first proposed by Varni and co-workers (1989) can be applied across acute pain, such as that from an injury or medical procedure, or chronic pain such as juvenile arthritis or sickle cell disease, and also includes stress as a precipitant of pain (Varni et al., 1996). The version of Varni et al.'s model shown in Figure 9.6 is from Vetter (2012), who adapted it to include important findings relating to the influence of the 'school environment' in chronic pain, for which evidence has accumulated and positioned the school environment, particularly in older children and adolescents, as key in relation to pain experience in chronic illness.

This model illustrates the interplay between precipitants such as stress, intervening variables, such as family and school environment, and functional status, including mood, behaviour and relationships, and pain. Note the bidirectional communication between pain and functional status in the adapted version of Varni et al.'s model shown in Figure 9.6. It is worth noting in relation to functional status or disability and school attendance, that a direct relationship between these variables and pain intensity is not always evident, implying that disability is a 'complex construct' involving the interplay of a number of psychosocial factors, particularly that of anxiety (Gauntlett-Gilbert and Eccleston, 2007; Cohen et al., 2010).

SPECIFIC CONSIDERATIONS IN ADOLESCENT PAIN

Given the prevalence of pain reported above and our focus in this section on the family and school environment, one important topic, which is beginning to receive increasing attention in pain research, is the influence of the adolescent peer environment on pain

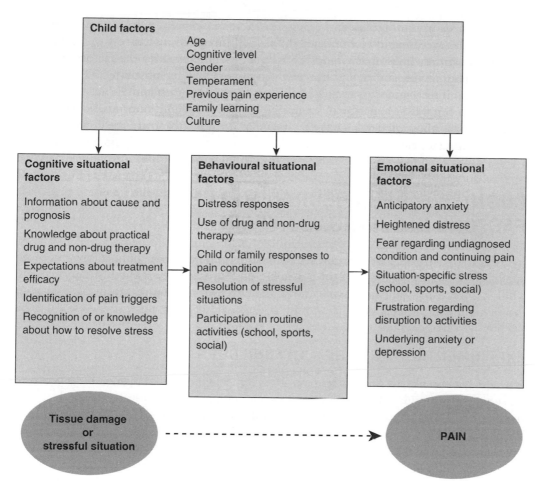

FIGURE 9.7   Situational and child factors that modify pain and disability

Source: Adapted in format from McGrath, P.A., and Hillier, L.M. (2003).

experience. In adolescence, the influence of peers or 'peer pressure' takes over to vary-ing degrees from the parental influence seen in younger children. The role of autonomy in adolescence was discussed particularly in Chapter 7, when I considered the mismatch between the characteristics of diabetes management. In relation to pain, the need for autonomy in adolescence means that parental advice is often rejected in favour of peer advice in managing pain, whether that is in relation to the expression of pain, pain behaviours or pain medication. Depending on the degree of pain, whether acute and requiring over-the-counter (OTC) medicine, or chronic and part of ongoing pain man-agement, this switch from family/parental locus of control to peer influence is vital in managing pain appropriately. For example, Hatchette and colleagues (2008) found that sex differences in how adolescents (aged 12–15 years) express pain to their peers and peer attitudes were found to influence the perception of ease of access to, and use of, OTC medications. In using the biopsychosocial model to identify the factors that contribute to pain and disability, and hence which factors may be most effective targets for psychosocial interventions to reduce pain in children, McGrath and Hillier (2003) very usefully conceptualize situational (cognitive, behavioural and emotional) factors and child factors as illustrated in Figure 9.7. Taken as a whole, these are the contextual factors that influence the pain experience.

COGNITIVE, BEHAVIOURAL AND EMOTIONAL FACTORS IN COPING WITH PAIN

In order to explore the vast literature that has developed in support of the biopsychosocial approach to managing pain, I now consider some of these contextual, situational and child factors, using the pain classifications of acute, chronic and recurrent pain given at the beginning of the chapter.

EXPERIMENTAL PAIN IN HEALTHY CHILDREN

A prequel, if you like, to considering pain states is the application of pain in the experimental setting with healthy individuals. A significant amount of pain research is conducted in this way in adults, although for obvious ethical and moral reasons less so with children. Work that has been done, particularly in the US and Canada, gives a useful baseline understanding of pain in the otherwise healthy context. For example, Lu and colleagues (2007) used a series of tasks to induce pressure, thermal heat, and cold (using the cold pressor test) in a sample of children and adolescents aged 8–18 years and assessed how they coped with the pain. The cold pressor test is a standard laboratory pain endurance (tolerance) and intensity test which involves participants submerging their forearm in a bucket of icy water for as many seconds or minutes as possible. Based on the pain intensity that the participants were able to endure, Lu et al. (2007) found the coping strategies of positive self-statements and behavioural distraction to be associated with 'pain resistance' as lower pain intensity was reported when using these techniques. Strategies of seeking emotional support and internalizing/catastrophizing were labelled as 'pain-prone' since the use of these was associated with a lower pain tolerance and greater reporting of pain intensity (Lu et al., 2007). In a similar study using just the cold pressor test, in a slightly younger sample of 7–14-year-olds, Piira and colleagues (2006) used visual images described in word form as attentional strategies. These strategies composed either external distraction (e.g., scene of playing ball in a park) or internal sensory-focusing (e.g., relating to water temperature or feeling cold). The control group received no visual images at all. Whilst pain tolerance was greatest for both intervention groups compared to the control group, an age difference emerged in which the youngest children (7–9 years) performed best in the external distraction condition, whereas the older children (10–14 years) performed just as well using either intervention (Piira et al., 2006). This demonstrates the importance of age in selecting the most effective type of distraction intervention.

ACUTE PAIN IN CHILDREN

Research examining acute pain in children has focused on three main areas: (i) routine medical vaccinations, injury and unplanned procedures, including emergency department admissions; (ii) dental anxiety and orthodontic pain; and (iii) the largest of these areas, postoperative pain. The use of secondary control coping has been found to be particularly beneficial in this context, with children using these coping strategies reporting less pain compared to those who used primary control coping strategies or relinquished control coping (Langer et al., 2005). An interesting study by Crandall and colleagues (2007) of adolescents aged 11–17 years, who had received an acute blunt traumatic injury (associated in the majority with injury following accidents), describes the 'struggle for internal control' that these adolescents experienced in dealing with their pain, reported in interview 1–11 days after the accident. Internal control is defined by the authors as 'behavioural and cognitive actions used to control and endure their pain' (2007: 229) and characterized by a passive, inward focus (e.g., staying still, not crying or screaming) which contrasts with 'loss of control' (p. 229) in which their distress was outward and overt (e.g., distress, resisting medical intervention, crying, screaming). They found that adolescents used internal control in order to 'maintain independence and self-control over their pain' (p. 233) and point out that the use of such behaviours is consistent with the autonomy of adolescence, but may mask the pain being experienced by these patients. They also point to the vital importance of the presence of both family and peers for support in managing their pain. Crandall et al.'s (2007) conceptual model of internal control is shown in Figure 9.8.

Studies of acute pain from dental and orthodontic treatment have also reported the common use of cognitive coping strategies, both internal coping strategies (e.g., 'I tell myself it will be over soon') and external coping strategies (e.g., 'I like it when the nurse holds my hand'), with internal strategies being the most frequently used in pre-adolescent children (Versloot et al., 2004; Van Meurs et al., 2005). It is the younger adolescent children (11–13 years) compared to older adolescents (age 14–17 years) who appear to experience more pain during orthodontic treatment (Brown and Moerenhout, 1991). In postoperative pain, Crandall and colleagues (2009) point to the importance of ameliorating anxiety preoperatively to reduce pain after surgery. They report evidence of significant relationships between prior anxiety and postoperative pain in their sample of children aged 7–13 years undergoing tonsillectomy. Amongst other factors, they stress the importance of previous surgical experience as an influencing factor in postoperative pain. In adolescents, evidence for links between preoperative expectations of pain and anxiety and postoperative pain experienced has also been found (Logan and Rose, 2005).

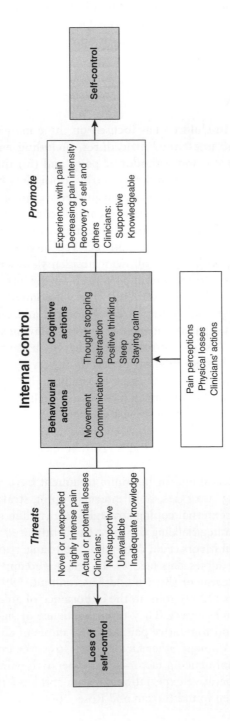

FIGURE 9.8 Conceptual model of 'internal control' of pain experiences in adolescents following acute blunt traumatic injury

Source: Crandall et al. (2007).

CHRONIC PAIN IN CHILDREN

Two of the most prevalent and well-researched chronic pain conditions in children are those of (i) juvenile chronic arthritis (JCA) and (ii) sickle cell disease (SCD).

Chronic pain in juvenile chronic arthritis

Juvenile chronic arthritis (JCA) is characterized by pain and stiffness in the joints (often in more than one part of the body at a time) which is 'unpredictable' and fluctuates with flare-ups and periods of remission, although for a subgroup the pain may be unremitting (Schanberg et al., 1997). Pain is seen as controlling the lives of children with JCA whose social life and future goals may become limited (Sallfors et al., 2002). The lived experience of children and adolescents with JCA has been described as 'oscillating between hope and despair', characterized by a 'disturbed order', 'dependency', 'ambivalence', and 'uncertainty' (Sallfors et al., 2002: 498). The use of coping strategies akin to secondary control coping strategies, relating to 'pain control and rational thinking' (e.g., reinterpreting pain sensations), has been linked to a lower intensity of pain and the experience of pain in fewer parts of the body in a sample of 56, 6–20-year-olds (mean age 12.4 years) with JCA (Schanberg et al., 1997: 183). More recently, Thastum and colleagues (2005) reported associations between level of pain in juvenile arthritis and pain-related health beliefs, particularly those beliefs relating to disability and harm about their pain problem. Thastum et al. (2005) also found associations between level of pain and the coping subscale of catastrophizing. The concept of catastrophization is an exaggerated, negative cognitive-affective state characterized by 'magnification, rumination and helplessness', frequently applied in the adult pain literature (Sullivan et al., 2001: 53; Buenaver et al., 2007).

In other chronic and recurrent arthritic pain conditions in children, compared to healthy controls (9–15 years), the greater use of pain catastrophizing, coupled with less expression and interpersonal communication of their pain experience, has also been reported (Vervoort et al., 2008). In a later study of children aged 7–15 years with juvenile arthritis, Thastum and Herlin (2011) found further evidence of dysfunctional health beliefs predicting greater pain over a longitudinal period of 2 years, indicating both the stability and course of pain belief in influencing pain outcome over time. Age and gender effects have also been seen in older adolescents (aged 16 plus) with JCA, boys reporting a greater ability to control and reduce their pain than girls (Sallfors et al., 2003). Similarly, perceptions of self-worth have also been linked to pain experience in adolescents aged 13–18 years with musculoskeletal pain (Guite et al., 2007).

Chronic pain in sickle cell disease

Sickle cell disease (SCD) is an inherited disorder of the haemoglobin, causing the red blood cells to develop abnormally (resembling 'sickles') and restricting the amount of oxygen they can carry and transport to the lungs (NHS, 2012). The sickle red blood cells cause a thickening of the blood and result in blockages in the blood vessels and a vaso-occlusive crisis (sickle cell crisis) which lasts on average between 5 and 7 days, but can be as short as a few minutes or as long as several months, causing episodes of intense pain (Barakat et al., 2007; Hollins et al., 2012; NHS, 2012). Complications include chronic anaemia, stroke, acute chest syndrome, vulnerability to infection, pulmonary hypertension and delayed puberty and small stature (Barakat et al., 2007; NHS, 2012). The pain caused by SCD can have a significant and daily impact on everyday functioning and social relationships, particularly for adolescents, and prevalence is greatest in those of African descent (Hollins et al., 2012).

Earlier work in children and adolescents with SCD focused on the negative aspects of cognitive, emotional and behavioural factors, such as stress, negative mood, negative thinking, and passive adherence (e.g., Gil et al., 1993, 2003). Barakat et al. (2007) found evidence for negative thinking to act as a mediator of pain intensity on depression and of the interference of pain with daily activities on the outcome of anxiety. More recent work has focused on the positive factors associated with resilience and adjustment in SCD, such as better quality of life, levels of hope, adaptive behaviour, and optimism (e.g., Pence et al., 2007; Ziadni et al., 2011). In particular, Pence et al. (2007) found that more optimistic adolescents (13–17 years) were better able to control their pain severity through more accurate medication use.

Demographic factors of age, sex and socioeconomic status have also been linked to pain in SCD. For example, whilst coping patterns have been found to stay relatively consistent in younger children (7–12 years) over a period of several months, for adolescents (13–18 years) these coping factors were more variable, which highlights both the opportunity for intervention and the instability of pain coping in older children (Gil et al., 1993). Barakat et al. (2007) report lower socioeconomic status, as defined by family income, to be linked to greater pain. This aspect of change across time for children with SCD is important. Hollins et al. (2012) point out that, whilst pain in SCD is episodic in childhood, it often becomes increasingly chronic throughout adolescence, and pain responses may begin to show the characteristic patterns of chronic pain which are seen in later adulthood. Evidence also points to the toll that having a child with SCD can take on parents, and the importance of maternal adjustment (Thompson et al., 1994), as well as to the reciprocal nature of relationships between the coping responses of the child and family functioning (Mitchell et al., 2007).

Chronic pain in other conditions

Other studies of chronic pain have considered not one specific condition but a variety of conditions, particularly when a specific condition, other than chronic pain itself, is not possible to diagnose. In adolescents (aged 12–17 years) with chronic pain conditions, including migraine, neuropathic pain, musculoskeletal pain, abdominal pain and diffuse pain, a pain-coping profile of avoidant coping (typical of isolation and social withdrawal) or dependent coping (such as catastrophizing) has been associated with greater somatic symptoms, anxiety, depression and disability, indicating that they were less able to cope with their pain (Claar et al., 2008). Similarly, Martin and colleagues (2007) found that children with chronic abdominal, headache, neuropathic or musculoskeletal pain who had higher levels of anxiety sensitivity (fear of anxiety-related sensations such as increased heart rate) were also more afraid of pain and, consequently, this linked to a higher level of pain disability.

Both age and sex differences in coping responses in chronic pain appear to emerge in children, with 8–12-year-olds showing differences in preference for the use of social support (girls' preference) over behavioural distraction (boys' preference), and adolescents (aged 13–18 years) showing greater use of positive self-talk than children (Lynch et al., 2007). Sex differences have also been found in how adolescents remember their experience of pain. An innovative study by Hechler et al. (2009) asked adolescents (aged 12–18 years) to report not just their current level of pain during an interview, but also to recall their memory of pain intensity in the previous time periods of 24 hours, 7 days, and 4 weeks. Adolescent girls were found to report higher pain intensity than boys within the time frame of 7 days and also 4 weeks, despite having similar medical diagnoses and being similar on other diagnostic criteria. The authors suggest that this may be due to expectations in gender role and point to the importance of pain memory in designing intervention programmes as remembered pain may influence future pain (Hechler et al., 2009).

RECURRENT PAIN

The most common form of recurrent pain in children is that of abdominal pain with prevalence as high as 25 per cent in 9–12-year-olds (see Dufton et al., 2011), representing a significant childhood problem with the potential for setting patterns of chronic pain in later life. These children have high rates of functional disability and a significantly reduced social life (Dufton et al., 2011), putting them at a disadvantage in the transition to adolescence. Using an experimental paradigm which combined elements of stress testing and the cold pressor task for pain tolerance and intensity, Dufton et al. (2011) compared the performance of children with recurrent abdominal pain or clinical anxiety and healthy control children without pain. They report greater reactivity as measured by increases in heart rate to the stress and pain testing in the sample with abdominal pain or anxiety (Dufton et al., 2011). In relation to coping, secondary control coping (in the form of acceptance, distraction, or positive thinking) has also been shown to reduce pain more effectively than involuntary actions or disengagement coping (such as avoidance in the form of escape or denial in the form of inaction) in children with recurrent abdominal pain (Thomsen et al., 2002) and this benefit of secondary control coping was also confirmed in the Dufton et al. (2011) study.

THE ROLE OF PARENTS IN THE PAIN EXPERIENCE

The dual effect between pain experience in a child and the impact on the parent(s) is important both for the health of the parent and for the reciprocal impact that the parental response has on the child's pain experience and level of disability. I have already hinted at this in considering various types of pain conditions above, but there is a surprisingly small amount of literature reported in this area, particularly for the parental effect on the child, compared to other aspects of the biopsychosocial pain experience and also compared to the amount of research on the parental effects and influence in chronic conditions more generally. Yet there is an emerging interest in this area. For an excellent brief review, see Palermo and Eccleston (2009) who highlight the importance of considering the parent in child and adolescent chronic pain. The way in which these interconnected relationships between parent and adolescent functioning operate is generating increasing interest. One model proposed by Vowles and colleagues (2010) includes both adolescent and caregiver psychosocial responses and pain management behaviours of the caregiver in relation to adolescent pain functioning, and on catastrophizing responses in both the adolescent and their parents.

The important influence of parental catastrophizing about their child's pain experience has also been demonstrated in healthy children and adolescents in a laboratory setting (Caes et al., 2011). Both maternal and paternal catastrophizing have been found to influence how the parent interacts with the child and also the level of pain reported, although sex differences between parents have also been noted. In particular, mothers appear to exhibit a greater degree of catastrophizing compared to fathers, and this difference was reflected in greater rumination rather than any differences in the components of magnification (exaggeration of the pain experience) and helplessness (Hechler et al., 2011).

THE ROLE OF EARLY LIFE PAIN EXPERIENCE ON SUBSEQUENT PAIN

Some of the most striking research to emerge in the area of pain in children, certainly for the lifespan perspective taken in this book, is that of the effect of early exposure to painful stimuli on subsequent pain experiences. To use the word 'striking' is perhaps an underestimation of the interest and excitement that this research topic ignites: this is a flag-waving, stand-on-your-chair level of interest; this really is important work, as not only does it relate to pain but it links to other key areas of interest in child health psychology, such as early life stress and adaptation. Whilst significant research has previously examined this phenomenon in animals, the application to human pain research is only just emerging. Recent work includes children who experienced pain early in life, either as hospitalized newborns (Hermann et al., 2006) or from burn injuries incurred between 6 and 24 months of age (Wollgarten-Hadamek et al., 2009). In these two studies, children were followed up at ages 9–14 years and 9–16 years respectively, and participated in standard experimental laboratory pain tasks, including thermal and mechanical stimulation techniques (Hermann et al., 2006; Wollgarten-Hadamek, et al., 2009).

In both studies, these school-age children, several years after the experience of early pain, showed elevated heat-pain thresholds and greater perceptual sensitization to thermal stimulation compared to controls. Hermann et al. (2006) report this as evidence of 'altered responsivity' to pain stimulation, with enhanced sensitization involving central pain pathways and elevation of pain thresholds associated with activation of the limbic system in pain feedback pathways. They theorize that this increased threshold 'masks' underlying sensitivity until sufficient pain input occurs, which explains why the children showed a higher pain threshold under low levels of stimulation, but when this became more intense the enhanced sensitization became evident (Hermann et al., 2006). A later study by Hermann's group examined the psychosocial context of this increased threshold/sensitivity in the 9–14-year-old children with neonatal intensive care unit (NICU) experience and found more catastrophizing in this group compared to controls. The mothers of the NICU children with more severe experiences exhibited more solicitous caretaking behaviour (i.e., showing special care and interest) in relation to their child's pain (Hohmeister et al., 2009). The mere presence of the mother was linked to an increase in heat-pain threshold in the child and less habituation to tonic heat. The authors highlight the dyadic result of neonatal pain experience on child cognition and the reinforcing effect of maternal behaviour. This simultaneous sensitization and inhibition is reminiscent of the PTSD models of stress associated with the third type of allostatic load discussed in Chapter 5.

PSYCHOSOCIAL INTERVENTIONS IN ACUTE AND CHRONIC PAIN

To summarize the evidence presented so far in this chapter, we know from at least as early as Melzack and Wall's (1965) proposed 'gate control theory' that psychosocial factors can influence an individual's experience of pain. This is just as true in children, for whom the situational context of the family and school has a key role within the biopsychosocial model. From pain in neonates through to adolescents, situational cognitive, behavioural and emotional factors, as well as child factors including demographics of age, sex, and previous pain experience, all make up the context of pain, which together with the sensory input determine the pain experience.

The group of coping responses that outperform all other coping responses are those of secondary control coping, and the type of coping associated with the most harmful or pain-perpetuating scenarios is that of catastrophizing, whether in the child or parent. Child factors relating to developmental stage of understanding and characteristic differences across age groups in dealing with pain, in particular the characteristic features of autonomy and control in adolescence, all have a major influence on the pain experience. Consequently, these biopsychosocial factors offer the potential for psychosocial intervention in the management of pain, alongside pharmacological treatment. We complete this chapter with a brief coverage of psychosocial interventions.

Psychosocial interventions to relieve pain, or alter the pain experience in children, have focused on acute pain (associated with medical procedures, vaccination and treatment in paediatric intensive care), chronic or recurrent pain (including recurrent headache and musculoskeletal pain) and pain in life-limiting conditions, each with their different characteristics and pain profiles. Non-pharmacological psychosocial intervention in the form of distraction and comfort through maternal touch has been found to help relieve acute pain in neonates and infants during vaccinations and medical procedures, either at well-baby clinics or in the hospital environment (see Johnston et al., 2012). A number of studies have reported skin-to-skin contact between mothers and newborns to reduce physiological pain arousal and provide comfort during painful procedures in the neonatal intensive care unit (NICU), although similar techniques using 'touch and talk' therapy in infants and toddlers in the paediatric intensive care unit (PICU) have found effects for comfort immediately after treatment rather than during treatment (Johnston et al., 2012). Johnston et al. (2012) note that more intense psychological intervention is necessary to reduce stress during the procedure, but that maternal comfort is sufficient after the procedure to facilitate adaptation and recovery from the procedure. There is enormous scope for future work in these younger age groups with limited or preverbal skills.

More work has been conducted with children of preschool age and above. In an excellent review and recommendation document by Duff and colleagues (2012), the use of a range of cognitive behavioural therapy (CBT) techniques, including 'progressive muscle relaxation training, guided imagery, distraction, modelling, graded exposure and reinforcement scheduling' (2012: 1) are highlighted as effective in reducing distress associated with painful medical procedures in children and young people, with distraction and general CBT being the most effective. Duff et al. (2012) emphasize that, despite this evidence base, demonstrating the efficacy and effectiveness of such interventions, they are not taken up routinely in clinical care, and cite clear guidelines provided by the British Psychological Society for dealing with invasive or distressing procedures in children, across age groups from infants and toddlers up to older children and adolescents (Gaskell, 2010). These refer to techniques for use prior to the procedure, and include aspects referred to in the models described in this chapter and previous chapters on acute and chronic illness, such as the environment, providing information, involving parents, and giving 'appropriate' control, as well as providing pharmacological intervention. Coping strategies (touch, music and singing, breathing techniques, and relaxation) and ways to deal with distress during procedures are also provided in these guidelines (Gaskell, 2010).

There is a wealth of research on psychosocial interventions in children and adolescents with chronic or recurrent pain conditions, including randomized controlled trials, which are held up as the gold standard in research design. In these studies, focusing particularly on headache, abdominal pain and musculoskeletal pain (e.g., fibromyalgia), or combinations of pain types (e.g., sickle cell disease), behavioural relaxation and CBT-based coping skills in children have been found to be effective for reducing pain across all three categories of condition, but to be particularly effective for reducing headache pain, including migraine (Eccleston et al., 2009; Sieberg et al., 2012). Palermo et al. (2010) also include biofeedback as an effective technique for pain reduction in these chronic pain groups. Used alongside relaxation, biofeedback enables the individual to receive information about their muscle tension through various means and this feedback provides useful guidance on how to relax further (see Morrison and Bennett, 2012). It is interesting that effective coping skills referred to in these interventions include the involvement of parents, trained to use operant strategies that reinforce their child's positive coping responses using reward systems (Eccleston et al., 2009; Palermo et al., 2009). Eccleston et al. (2009) point out that the effects of intervention on outcomes of mood and disability were more difficult to detect.

As mentioned above, one of the key distinguishing features between acute and chronic conditions is the dimension of time and, in interventions in chronic illness, the longer-term outcome beyond 3–6 months in relation to pain experience, functional status and disability is important and in need of further research. In line with our discussion of prior pain experience above, a further review specifically of childhood musculoskeletal pain, such as chronic regional pain syndrome (CRPS), by Clinch and Eccleston (2009) also stresses the importance of early intervention. Treatment time associated with administering such CBT-type interventions has been reported as averaging approximately 6 hours (Eccleston et al., 2009), which appears highly cost-effective given the advantages in pain reduction. Recent developments have also extended CBT approaches for managing chronic pain in children and adolescents to successful computerized versions and online web-based applications (Palermo et al., 2009; Velleman et al., 2010).

The intervention findings described above for chronic illness did not include cancer pain or pain in life-limiting conditions. To conclude this last section on interventions in pain, we consider the management of pain in life-limiting conditions. Friedrichsdorf and Kang (2007) provide a detailed list of CBT approaches, as well as complementary therapies, for use within this specific category of paediatric pain, as shown in Table 9.2, with clearly defined recommendations across each age group from infant to adolescent. These approaches are in line with the procedural BPS guidelines referred to above (Gaskell, 2010) and with the broader themes of coping discussed throughout this and previous chapters, the underlying aim of which is to restore physiological balance via reduction in pain and stress in order to reduce psychological distress and improve physical outcome.

In conclusion, psychosocial interventions to reduce pain have been shown to be effective across a range of acute, chronic, recurrent and life-limiting conditions, although to varying degrees. There is enormous potential for the development of a range and combination of cognitive behavioural therapy techniques tailored to specific conditions, and a need to assess systematically and scientifically both their efficacy under experimental conditions and their effectiveness in clinical practice. Helping children and adolescents draw on, develop, maintain and adapt effective coping mechanisms, within the context of family support, are at the heart of pain management and intervention. Pain is a complex, multidimensional phenomenon, and psychosocial interventions to reduce the sensory experience of pain provide a further example of the power of psychosocial factors to influence physical outcomes. In children, the impact and importance of these outcomes may be experienced not just during childhood but across the life course.

TABLE 9.2 Non-pharmacological approaches to paediatric pain management

Age	Pain behaviours	Cognitive-behavioural approaches	Complementary therapies
Infants	Avoiding eye contact Grimacing Difficulty sucking High-pitched crying Quivering chin Difficulty calming Wanting to be still Hiccupping Changes in breathing pattern	Use pacifier ('dummy') Swaddling Touch Distraction Music	Massage Sucrose solution Aromatherapy
Toddlers	Difficulty sleeping Loss of interest in play Increase in crying, irritability or restlessness Reduction in eating or drinking	Story-telling Blowing bubbles Toys Distraction Art and music therapy	Massage Warm/cool compress Aromatherapy
Preschool	Difficulty sleeping Loss of interest in play Quiet or curled Need to be held Says something hurts Reduction in eating or drinking	Distraction (cartoons) Offer favourite toy/object to hold Art and music therapy	Massage Reiki Emotive imagery Warm/cool compress Aromatherapy
School-age	Difficulty sleeping Moaning/crying Holding or protecting area of discomfort Loss of interest in play Decrease in activity level Complaining of pain Reduction in eating or drinking	Create a safe environment Dim lights, decrease noise, calm manner Power of suggestion Counting Art and music therapy Breathing techniques Visualization/guided imagery	Massage Reiki Progressive muscle relaxation Warm/cool compress Hypnosis (> 10 yrs) Acupuncture (>10 yrs) Aromatherapy Yoga/meditation/reflexology
Adolescent	Increasingly quiet Loss of interest in friends and family Decrease in activity level Increase in anger or irritability Changes in eating habits	Create a safe environment Dim lights, decrease noise, calm manner Distraction TV, video game, read a book, music Art and music therapy Breathing techniques Visualization/guided imagery	Massage Reiki Warm/cool compress Hypnosis Acupuncture Aromatherapy Yoga/meditation/reflexology

Source: Adapted from Friedrichsdorf and Kang (2007).

CHAPTER SUMMARY

In this chapter, we have examined the theories of pain experience, how children of different ages cope with pain, and the importance of the social context and role of the family in coping with pain. The experience of pain in neonates through to adolescents has emphasized the need for treating pain through a combination of pharmacological and psychosocial intervention. A range of acute, chronic, and recurrent pain experiences has been addressed, including surgical or postoperative pain, dental/orthodontic pain, pain following acute accidents, and pain associated with chronic illness, highlighting juvenile chronic arthritis and sickle cell disease. Changes in coping responses over time, with age and experience, have been addressed, and the response of catastrophizing has been contrasted with the more adaptive strategy of secondary control coping. I have also highlighted sex differences in pain and the impact of pain responses on level of disability.

This chapter links particularly well with the previous three chapters on acute and chronic illness and palliative care. As with these previous topics, the topic of pain experience and intervention underscores the life-course theme which runs throughout this book. Not only is the treatment of pain important for the child and their family during the pain experience, whether acute or chronic in nature, but how pain is dealt with in childhood has implications for lifelong psychophysiological responses to painful stimuli. This is another beautiful example not only of the biopsychosocial model in action, but also of its implications for the life-course trajectory in health and illness. In Chapter 10, I move on to consider the experience of illness not in the child themselves, but their experience of illness in a parent.

KEY CONCEPTS AND ISSUES

- Pain prevalence and intensity
- Acute, chronic, and recurrent pain
- The context of pain
- Catastrophizing versus secondary control coping
- Gate control theory, the body-self neuromatrix, and the neurosignature
- Pain stress
- The social context of pain
- Pain assessment
- Cold pressor test
- The under-treatment of pain in children
- Disability
- Pain resistance
- Internal control
- Anxiety sensitivity
- Role of parents, family, and school
- Cognitive behavioural therapy techniques and interventions in pain

FURTHER READING

For a very readable version of the original 'gate control theory' of pain and associated concepts (first published in 1982, following the advent of Melzack and Wall's (1965) revolutionary theory):

Melzack, R. and Wall, P.D. (2008) *The Challenge of Pain* (updated 2nd edn). London: Penguin Books.

One of the original papers on the neuro-matrix:

Melzack, R. (1999) Pain: an overview. *Acta Anaesthe-siologica Scandinavica*, 43(9): 880–4.

For one of the clearest accounts of the 'gate control theory' of pain with a modern-day clinical application, see:

Morrison, V. and Bennett, P. (2012) *An Introduction to Health Psychology*, 3rd edn. Harlow, Essex: Pearson Education.

One of the absolute best texts on child pain, including separate chapters on specific pain problems (sickle cell disease, cancer pain, headaches in children and adolescents, and pain and stress in the NICU), this is a must read, although be aware that the cost of the hardcover version would empty most student loan budgets (electronic library copies are available):

Schechter, N.L., Berde, C.B. and Yaster, M. (eds) (2003) *Pain in Infants, Children and Adolescents*. Philadelphia: Lippincott Williams & Wilkins.

An excellent text for everything you could want to know about pain, including in-depth coverage of pain pathways, mechanisms and processes with a lifespan perspective:

Holdcroft, A. and Jaggar, S. (eds) (2005) *Core Topics in Pain*. Cambridge: Cambridge University Press.

Practical, usable clinical guidelines from the British Psychological Society for age-relevant psychosocial interventions during acute medical procedures in children and adolescents:

Gaskell, S. (2010) Evidence-based guidelines for the management of invasive and/or distressing procedures with children. Position paper. Leicester: British Psychological Society (BPS).

USEFUL WEBSITES

The British Pain Society: www.britishpainsociety.org

The International Association for the Study of Pain: www.iasp-pain.org

THE EXPERIENCE OF PARENTAL ILLNESS AND DEATH

10

Covered in this chapter

- The child as carer
- Coping and adjustment: the impact of caregiving on the young carer
- Interventions to lessen the negative impacts on young carers
- Dealing with issues of death and dying
- Bereavement services for children

In this chapter, I stay focused on the experience of the child, and the effects of psychosocial factors on the child's health and well-being, but with a difference. Cast an eye back over the previous chapters: in Part I, we examined the influence of parental stress during pregnancy and the physical health outcomes of stress during childhood, including the experience of childcare, in otherwise healthy children; in Part II, we then focused on the experience of acute and chronic illness and pain during childhood, in which parents and family played an influential role in the child's care and were key components in the coping process. Whilst protecting a child from stress and trauma, helping them to cope, and comforting them during illness may seem a natural response which is part of parental caregiving, we also considered the incongruous experience of life-threatening and life-limiting illness in a child. Childhood death, or its threat, flies in the face of accepted cradle-to-grave expectations about the natural order of life. In a similar vein, before concluding Part II, there are two further and connected pockets of research that cannot be neglected. Both of these areas reflect the experience of life turning its tables on the common understanding of how things should be. These are (i) the experience of the child growing up with a parent or close family member who is unwell and/or disabled; and (ii) the experience of the child whose parent or sibling dies. Notice the reference here to siblings and close family members, as many of the points covered are relevant not only to parental illness or death; nevertheless, the emphasis here is on the parent, as reflected in the literature.

THE CHILD AS CARER

The first of these important topics is that of the young carer: that is, when children have caregiving responsibilities for a parent or close family member with physical illness and/or disability or with mental illness. In this scenario, rather than the parent caring for the child, we have a further cradle-to-grave paradox or incongruity: the child as caregiver, caring for an adult parent or helping to care for a sibling. This subject was largely overlooked for many years, but interest has gained significant momentum in the past couple of decades. Recent media interest has also helped bring this cause into the public domain, with well-known celebrities speaking with young carers in TV documentary programmes and supporting young carer campaigns.

Based on figures from the 2001 UK census, the number of young carers has been estimated at over 175,000 (ONS report, in McAndrew et al., 2012), but an investigation by the BBC in 2010 put this figure much higher; in fact, 'four times' as high, at 700,000 young carers in the UK (see http://www.bbc.co.uk/pressoffice/pressreleases/stories/2010/11_november/16/carers.shtml). This provides further evidence of young carers being an 'invisible', 'covert' or 'hidden' group, since there are more children providing care than are known about by social services (Jenkins and Wingate, 1994; Banks et al., 2002; Becker, 2007).

DEFINITION OF THE YOUNG CARER AND CAREGIVING RESPONSIBILITIES

So what is meant by 'young carers'? How much caring defines a young carer and what types of activities are classified as caregiving by a young carer? Whilst helping out with chores in the home and developing a caring attitude is one that most parents would encourage, what defines a young carer is taking on a substantial amount of caring activities on a regular basis which are associated with responsibilities beyond those usually given to children. Young carers were officially included in UK legislation under the Carers Act in 1995 and have since been more fully defined as:

> children and young persons under 18 who provide or intend to provide care, assistance or support to another family member. They carry out, often on a regular basis, significant or substantial caring tasks and assume a level of responsibility that would usually be associated with an adult. (Becker, 2007: 26)

The age at which children under 18 begin this caring role is frequently as young as 8–10 years (ONS report, in McAndrew et al., 2012), and care may be to a parent, sibling, grandparent or other relative (Dearden and Becker, 2004), although the focus in this chapter will be on caring for a parent.

It is worth noting that there are various definitions of young carers, and some include terms which distinguish between primary (i.e., main carer) or secondary carers (i.e., assisting the main carer; Pakenham et al., 2007). There are also differences in the terms used between countries, with 'young carer' being the preferred term in the UK, 'caregiver' in the US, and terms such as 'youth carer' sometimes used in the Australian research literature (Becker, 2007; Ireland and Pakenham, 2010b). It is also important to remember that having a parent with a physical or mental condition or disability does not automatically mean that the child will be defined as a young carer. As Lackey and Gates (2001: 327) rhetorically ask, 'Where is the line between normal expectations of family life and inclusion of youngsters in caregiving?', and with respect to young carers, 'How much is too much?'

Whilst there has been some considerable advancement in young carer research and practice in the past decade, these are still relevant questions to keep in mind. As Becker (2007) points out, whilst over one-fifth of children in the UK live with a parent who is unwell or disabled, many of these will not meet the definition of carer. Yet children growing up in families with a parent who has a chronic illness will undoubtedly have a different perspective on caring and understanding of illness from children raised in families for whom illness is an occasional inconvenience rather than a way of life, even if they do not perceive themselves as carers or are not required to engage in easily quantifiable caregiving tasks. Aside from caregiving, the concept of adjustment in children whose parent has a chronic illness has been investigated across a number of different chronic physical conditions, including rheumatoid arthritis (Turner-Cobb et al., 1998) and multiple sclerosis (for review, see Bogosian et al., 2010). The concept of caregiving is inherent in adjustment to parental chronic illness, and the experience and outcomes for the young carer provide a spotlight on adjustment in chronic illness and disability. Hence, the degree of variability within this role of young carer may vary from relatively low to high levels of caregiving and responsibility, as shown in the continuum of care by Becker (2007) in Table 10.1.

One demographic of the young carer population which most clearly stands out is the prevalence of single-parent families, reported as the situation for over half (56 per cent) of all young carers (Dearden and Becker, 2004). There are obvious practical reasons why the prevalence of young carers is higher in this group, responsibility falling on the child in the absence of partner support within the immediate family. Equally, the emotional and financial struggle that accompanies caregiving under these circumstances highlights this subgroup of young carers in terms of risk or vulnerability. As you will see below, social isolation is a potential negative outcome of caregiving, and the provision of social support a key factor in improving the situation of young carers.

WHAT TYPES OF TASK CONSTITUTE CAREGIVING?

The third national survey of young carers in the UK, conducted by Dearden and Becker in 2003 (Dearden and Becker, 2004; previous surveys in 1995 and 1997), draws from 87 young carer projects to include a total sample size of 6,178 young carers. Caregiving tasks provided by young carers were listed as falling into six categories, although young carers often performed tasks under several of these groupings. The six categories are described in

TABLE 10.1   A continuum of children's caregiving

'Light end' (low levels of caregiving and responsibility)	→→→ →→→ 'Heavy end'		'Very heavy end' (high levels of caregiving and responsibility)
'Routine' levels and types of caregiving including some help with instrumental activities of daily living	→→→ Caregiving tasks and responsibilities increase in amount, regularity, complexity, time involved, intimacy and duration		'Substantial, regular and significant' caregiving including considerable help with instrumental activities of daily living
Household tasks and caregiving tasks can be considered age and culturally appropriate for the child's age			Household tasks and caregiving tasks can be considered age and culturally inappropriate for the child's age
Most children			Few children
	Young carers providing 0–19 hours of care per week	Young carers providing 20–49 hours of care per week	Young carers providing 50+ hours of care per week
	Many 'hidden' young carers (unknown to service providers)		

Source: Becker (2007).

Table 10.2, along with the percentages of carers carrying out those tasks. As you can see from Table 10.2, for young carers the greatest percentage of caring is emotional support and domestic tasks. Table 10.2 also shows sex differences in tasks performed, with the greatest gender bias towards girls carrying out domestic and intimate tasks, although this sex difference is not apparent in all studies (Ireland and Pakenham, 2010b). Earlier work in this area described personal care tasks as presenting the most difficulties, and household tasks as being the most time-consuming for young carers (Lackey and Gates, 2001). Various scales have been developed to assess the extent of caregiving tasks performed by the young carer, such as the Multidimensional Assessment of Caring Activities (MACA-YC42; YC18), used across ages 6.5–22 years (Joseph, Becker, and Becker, 2009; Joseph, Becker, Becker, and Regel, 2009) and developed in the UK, and the Youth Activities of Caregiving Scale (YACS) for use with ages 10–24 years (Ireland and Pakenham, 2010a), developed in Australia. As might be expected, the degree of caregiving tasks tends to increase with age, reflecting an increased ability to perform the tasks adequately, and a greater number of care tasks were undertaken by children in single-parent families (Ireland and Pakenham, 2010a, b).

The type of illness or disability of the care recipient for whom young carers perform these caring tasks is predominantly for a physical or mental health condition, although learning difficulties and sensory impairments were also included in the Dearden and

TABLE 10.2   Percentage of young carers providing different caring tasks across six different categories, by gender

Caring tasks	Overall	Girls	Boys
Domestic tasks or household chores, e.g., cooking, cleaning, washing, ironing	68% (3,493)	65%	75%
General care or nursing tasks, e.g., giving medication, changing dressings, assisting with mobility	48% (2,443)	44%	45%
Emotional support, e.g., observing the carer recipient's emotional state, providing supervision or trying to cheer them up when they are depressed	82% (4,197)	13%	22%
Intimate care, e.g., washing, dressing, assisting with toileting	18% (913)	77%	78%
Child care, e.g., helping to care for younger siblings in addition to other caring tasks	11% (574)	8%	12%
Other, e.g., household or other administration, bill paying, translating for non-English-speaking relatives, accompanying to hospital	7% (337)		

Note: *n* = 5,116, missing cases 1,062. Figures do not add up to 100% since most carers are performing several caring tasks (up to four caring tasks per child recorded in report).

Source: Adapted from Dearden and Becker (2004: 7–8), using tables 5 and 7.

Becker (2004) report. Table 10.3 gives the breakdown of type of condition by relationship of care recipient to the young carer, and makes for interesting reading. It highlights the impact of having a sibling with a physical illness, as discussed in Chapters 6–8, as well as the high proportion of children with caring responsibilities for siblings with learning difficulties and parents with mental health needs.

TABLE 10.3   The nature of illness/disability of people with care needs

	Physical health	Mental health	Learning difficulty	Sensory impairment
Mother	57% (2,056)	50% (1,799)	7% (239)	4% (153)
Father	65% (625)	43% (414)	7% (72)	8% (81)
Sibling	49% (1,048)	10% (222)	63% (2,029)	3% (61)
Grandparent	88% (174)	19% (37)	5% (14)	6% (19)

Note: Figures will not add up to 100% since many people had more than one recorded condition.

Source: Dearden and Becker (2004: 7, table 4).

THE GLOBAL VIEW ON YOUNG CARERS

Caregiving by children under 18 years of age has been referred to as a 'global phenomenon' (McAndrew et al., 2012). Becker (2007) provides a useful global comparison of

TABLE 10.4   A global typology of levels of awareness and response characteristics to young carers

Level	Characteristics	Country/Region example
Advanced	• Widespread awareness and recognition of young carers among public, policy makers and professionals • Extensive and reliable research base • Specific legal rights (national) • Extensive codes and guidance for welfare professionals and national and local strategies • Multiple dedicated services and interventions nationwide	UK
Intermediate	• Some awareness and recognition of young carers among public, policy makers and professionals • Small research base • Partial rights in some regions • Small but developing body of professional guidance • Some dedicated services and interventions nationwide	Australia
Preliminary	• Little public or specialist awareness and recognition of young carers • Limited research base • No specific legal rights • Few, if any, dedicated services or interventions at national or local levels	USA
Emerging	• Embryonic awareness of young carers as a distinct social group within the 'vulnerable children' population	Sub-Saharan Africa

Source: Becker (2007: 42).

research conducted and policy developed on young carers, in which the UK is cited as the most well-developed country in respect of 'awareness' and 'recognition' of young carers as reflected in policy, practice and the provision of services. In Becker's (2007) classification, the UK is termed 'advanced' in its level of young carer awareness and response characteristics, with Australia as 'intermediate', the USA as 'preliminary' and sub-Saharan Africa as 'below preliminary' but 'emerging' as shown in Table 10.4. Whatever the running order, it is clear that the provision by children of day-to-day care for close relatives within the home is indeed a global issue. Although services for supporting young carers have improved considerably over the past 20 years, the issue of young carers, as with adult caregiving roles, is unlikely to diminish due to the trend for a reduction in acute care and an increase in caretaking within the home.

The Children's Society in the UK has developed six key principles for working with young carers and their families (for details, see Frank and McLarnon, 2008: 43–75) based on the central premise that:

> A young carer becomes vulnerable when the level of care-giving and responsibility to the person in need of care becomes excessive or inappropriate for that child, risking impacting on his or her own emotional or physical well-being or educational achievement and life chances. (Frank and McLarnon, 2008: 1)

The focus on working with the family as a unit, coordinating child and adult services, is central to the key principles proposed (for full details, see Frank and McLarnon, 2008). The importance of providing 'support for the whole family' is endorsed by policy and practice as documented by the UK Department for Education (Ronicle and Kendall, 2011).

Given the increased awareness of young caregiving roles, coupled with an understanding of the importance of young carers as a growing issue, this begs two questions. First, what impact does caregiving have on the health of the young carer; and, second, how can health psychology theory contribute to lessening any negative impacts and improving the future health of the young carer? As Pakenham et al. (2007) point out, much of the research on young carers has been qualitative and descriptive in nature. This seems entirely appropriate for a relatively new research area, and given the sensitive content and approach needed in getting access to, and gaining accurate information from, young carers. Quantitative empirical studies are now emerging, however, along with quantitative assessments of caregiving tasks as described above and of the experience of caregiving. In understanding the impact of caregiving on the young carer, we draw on a variety of research designs and methodologies, including qualitative and quantitative studies and cross-sectional, longitudinal, retrospective and prospective designs.

COPING AND ADJUSTMENT: THE IMPACT OF CAREGIVING ON THE YOUNG CARER

Thinking beyond the number, type or intensity of caregiving tasks performed by the young carer, there is the impact these tasks may have and the outcome on their psychological and physical health. Implicit in the description of young carers given so far is the concern that the experience of caregiving by children may impact on the normal healthy developmental process of childhood. There is a strong sense that being a young carer may disadvantage the life chances of the child and infringe on the 'good childhood' that all children are entitled to enjoy (see Chapter 2 for a description of the findings from the Good Childhood Inquiry). Box 10.1 lists a range of restrictions and difficulties experienced by young carers, which have been reported across a number of psychosocial domains, including emotions and psychological health, social relationships and activities, educational difficulties, and family relationships and the family unit.

BOX 10.1

Restrictions and difficulties experienced by young carers

Emotions and psychological health: feelings of emotional distress; increased levels of anxiety and depression; being overwhelmed or burdened by responsibilities; reduced self-esteem.

Social relationships and activities: a sense of isolation; being less able to participate in leisure activities outside the home; impact on friendships and dating; stigma associated with their parent's illness or disability.

Educational difficulties: missing school and having restricted educational opportunities.

Family relationships: worry about their parent's health and own or others' expectations about caring, and impact on family life; need to keep caring 'secret' or 'silent' due to fear of interference in their family situation, whether from professional services (fear of separation from the parent/being put into care if disclosed) or from stigma associated with social evalua-tion or peer pressure.

Sources: Becker et al. (1998); Frank et al. (1999); Becker (2000); Lackey and Gates (2001); Pakenham, et al. (2007); Ireland and Pakenham (2010a, b); Ronicle and Kendall (2011).

Such difficulties may create vulnerabilities for psychological and physical health problems. Whether the caregiving by a young person for a parent or other relative is due to a mental or physical health condition or other disability, there is plenty of evidence to suggest that the psychological health of young carers may be compromised (McAndrew et al., 2012). This increased vulnerability is not just during childhood, but may extend into adulthood, as may the caregiving role itself. The situation of the young carer can exacerbate the trials and tribulations of the adolescent transition to adulthood which are documented through-out this book. Our focus here is on physical health outcome in the child, but this link with psychological health is important particularly because of the potential moderating effects of psychological state on physical illness.

So what research evidence exists which documents the physical health outcomes of young carers? The answer to this is, surprisingly, very little indeed, particularly if we look at the physiological outcomes relating to endocrine and immune markers: here the over-whelmingly significant finding is an extremely large gap in the literature. Early work that we conducted on adjustment in children of parents with rheumatoid arthritis included the stress biomarker of cortisol measured in saliva (Turner-Cobb et al., 1998). In this sample of 25 children whose parents had chronic rheumatoid arthritis, children experienced almost 50 per cent more hassles per week and had significantly smaller social networks, as well as a greater number of behavioural difficulties, compared to 53 healthy control chil-dren. Yet there was no difference between the salivary cortisol levels in the children of rheumatoid arthritis parents compared to controls, possibly indicating physiological adap-tation despite the greater psychosocial difficulties experienced (Turner-Cobb et al., 1998).

This study was couched in terms of adaptation rather than focusing on young carers as such, and caregiving was not assessed but was inherent in the physical disabilities reported in the rheumatoid arthritis parents. In general, research on adjustment in children living with parental or sibling illness has a much longer legacy than that of the young carer literature but, as with this study on rheumatoid arthritis families, a direct focus on young caregiving may have been overlooked. It is still rare, however, to see physiological markers or physical illness indicators incorporated in adjustment research of this type.

Remember that whilst research on young carers is gaining momentum, it is still a comparative newcomer in the literature. There is a component of research conducted by Frank et al. (1999), under the heading of 'health and well-being', which provides some self-report retrospective evidence of physical health in former young carers. Asked the question 'Do you feel that your own health has been affected in any way, either from stress or from the physical demands of caring?', approximately 28 per cent of participants felt their physical health had been affected by caregiving as a child (Frank et al., 1999: 14). Responses included the onset of hair loss, developing asthma or the exacerbation of an underlying epileptic condition attributed to the stress of being a young carer (Frank et al., 1999). Physical health effects also continued beyond the period of caregiving, into adulthood, and descriptive reports from this study include back problems (as a result of lifting), inability to gain weight (implying a metabolic influence), allergies and ulcers (Frank et al., 1999).

Descriptive survey-style research and qualitative findings have generated evidence for the development of much-needed policy and practice to support young carers. Yet there is a lack of research which has systematically and clinically explored physical health outcomes in young carers during childhood and into adulthood. Endocrine and immune outcomes do not lend themselves particularly well to descriptive analysis, although there are some exceptions (see Chapter 3). In addition to the excellent qualitative work that has been conducted, quantitatively assessed physical health outcomes, including physiological markers, are crucial in explicating the underlying theory behind physical health outcomes. Whilst physiological markers have been investigated in adult carer literature, particularly in older carers and to a much lesser extent in parental caregiving for children with developmental disabilities (Gallagher et al., 2009), they have yet to be explored in relation to the young carer literature.

Yet the vulnerability perspective of caregiving is not the whole story. Research in adult carers – for example, in those caring for a dying partner with AIDS (Folkman, 1997) – has highlighted positive aspects of caregiving in which benefit-finding and finding meaning in the situation have provided a contrasting perspective to the negative aspects of caregiving. Similarly, in young caregivers, the growing literature does not paint a solely negative picture, far from it. In addition to the serious vulnerabilities described, there are positive aspects to caregiving in childhood, which have been observed across a number of studies. Pakenham et al. (2007) cite early anecdotal reports in the 1980s and 1990s (e.g., Kornblum and Anderson, and Segal and Simkins) which point to characteristics of psychological resilience in young carers, such as an 'enhanced skill development, maturity, independence, self-efficacy, self-reliance, self-esteem, sensitivity and empathy for others and a fostered capacity to accept responsibility' (Pakenham et al., 2007: 90). The study referred to above on adjustment in children of rheumatoid arthritis parents (Turner-Cobb et al., 1998) could be interpreted in light of physiological resilience despite psychosocial adjustment difficulties: even though the children were experiencing significantly more daily stress than the control children, at a physiological level they had adapted to their situation.

Findings from two methodologically different studies are particularly relevant in demonstrating these positive characteristics of resiliency. US researchers Lackey and Gates (2001) conducted the first retrospective study to focus on positive aspects of caregiving in adults who were young carers as children, caring for close relatives with physical illness (63 per cent of whom were caring for a parent). Prior to this work, landmark research had been conducted for the Children's Society in the UK by Frank (1995; Frank et al., 1999) which used predominantly an interview and case-study approach, and the cohort included carers for adults with mental health problems and alcohol/drug misuse. Although not originally designed to assess young carers retrospectively, the researchers were approached by 'former young carers' (Frank, 1995: 53–5), and subsequent work concentrated specifically on this retrospective focus in an adult cohort of former young carers (Frank et al., 1999). Whilst retrospective studies are often criticized for their memory bias and lack of adequate recall, in the case of former young carers, looking back retrospectively has proved to be a very useful technique.

In the study by Lackey and Gates (2001), not only could the adult participants relate their own experiences as young carers, but they were also able to provide information about the effect of the experience in shaping their adult life and to offer insight into the provision of support for children as carers. Using content analysis of semi-structured interviews with 51 adults, Lackey and Gates (2001) found both positive and negative effects of the caregiving experience and outcomes in adult life. The demographics of the cohort of participants is interesting, with the age range of young carers at the time of caregiving being as young as 3 years, up to 19 years, and the adults at the time of data collection being aged 19–68 years. The duration of caregiving ranged from less than a year to over 25 years, showing the caregiving status continuing beyond that of young carer, well into adulthood. The adults being cared for by the young carer had a physical illness diagnosis including cancer, stroke, cardiovascular disease, multiple or amyotrophic lateral sclerosis, respiratory disease, diabetes or arthritis. Lackey and Gates (2001) report a dichotomy of positive and negative experiences in all domains from the adults describing their experience as a young carer, and also for the effects of having been a young carer on their current adult life (see Table 10.5). The adult participants in this study also offered retrospective advice to 'be honest' with the young carer, particularly about the adult's condition, to involve them in 'decision-making' and to 'allow them free time' (Lackey and Gates, 2001: 325).

Whilst there is limited theory as yet developed to explain the impact of young caregiving on health outcomes, a theoretical framework to support this work is beginning to emerge. By way of contrast with the qualitative study of Lackey and Gates (2001), Pakenham et al. (2007) examined positive and negative aspects of caregiving using a self-report questionnaire assessment and quantitative analysis of the young carer experience. This study is described in Box 10.2.

TABLE 10.5 Positive and negative experiences of young carers as children, and positive and negative outcomes as adults, reported retrospectively in sample of 51 adults who were previously young carers

As young carers	Positive experiences	Negative experiences

General	Liked …
	  Responsibility
	  Able to help/'be part of the family'
	  Felt 'appreciated', 'needed',
	   'important', 'useful'
	  Pride at learning new skills
	  Being around adults helped them
	   'grow up faster'
		Disliked …
		  Too much responsibility
		  Watching loved one suffer
		  Unpleasant sight/smells
		  Felt helpless

Family life	Closer, stronger	Changed dynamics Increased tension and stress Change in finances

School life	School provided a 'break' from caring
	Help and encouragement from adult
	  being cared for
		Less time for homework and
		  extracurricular activities
		Missing school and special events

Social life	Supportive friends who understood	Limited friendships Impact on dating: restricted or married early to escape caregiving situation
As adults	**Positive outcomes**	**Negative outcomes**

	Developed into more caring and
	  nurturing adult
	Understanding of chronic illnesses
	Caregiving influenced career choice
	Sense of having put life into perspective
		Unresolved anger and guilt
		Fear that they would have chronic/
		  terminal illness
		Unresolved grief over lost role that cared-
		  for parent was not able to perform
		Established need to over-care for others

Source: Lackey and Gates (2001).

BOX 10.2

Applying a theoretical framework to the positive and negative experiences of young carers

Source: K.I. Pakenham, J. Chiu, S. Bursnall and T. Cannon (2007) Relations between social support, appraisal and coping and both positive and negative outcomes in young carers. *Journal of Health Psychology*, 12(1): 89–102.

Rationale: The development of a theoretical framework linking the young carer experience with outcomes is important in advancing understanding and intervention in research and practice

(Continued)

(Continued)

with young carers. Whilst Lazarus and Folkman's (1984) stress and coping model (see Chapters 2 and 5) has been applied to the concept of adjustment in children who have a parent with an illness or disability, and in adult caregiving, the authors point to the fact that it has not yet been applied to the young carer scenario. They set out to examine components of the stress-coping model within the context of caregiving in young people and to focus on the positive aspects of stressful situations, some of which have not previously been examined in young carers. Note that, although the authors refer to stress appraisal, coping strategies and coping resources as 'mediational processes' in their rationale, this study does not specifically set out to address mediation in its hypothesis or in statistical analysis (Figure 10.1).

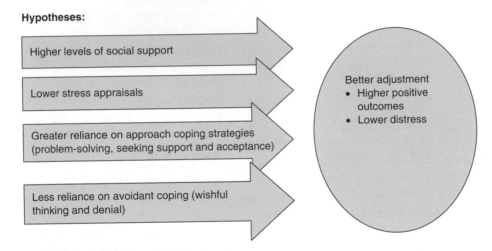

FIGURE 10.1 Hypotheses tested in study by Pakenham et al.
Source: Based on Pakenham et al. (2007).

Participants: One hundred young carers aged 10–25 years (72 per cent female; 81 per cent Australian; family size ranged from 2 to 13 people), caring for a parent or parents with a physical or mental illness or disability.

Design and methods: Cross-sectional design using self-report questionnaire assessment of (i) demographic variables; (ii) caregiving variables, including the family situation and context of the caring undertaken (degree of choice in caregiving situation), level of parental impairment, and unpredictability of the illness or disability; (iii) stress process variables of appraisal, social support, and coping strategies; and (iv) adjustment of the young carer: (a) negative outcomes of emotional distress (depression, anxiety, somatization) and (b) positive outcomes of positive affect, life satisfaction and benefit-finding.

Method of analysis: Correlation and four hierarchical regression models (run separately for each of the dependent outcome variables). Order of variable entry into regression: caregiving choice; social support; stress appraisal; and coping strategies.

Key findings: Demographic variables were not significantly related to the outcome measures in this study. Interestingly, 'choice in caring' was the only caregiving context variable to correlate significantly with the outcome variables. Significant bivariate correlations found positive outcomes to be associated with higher social support (number and satisfaction) and use of coping strategies of problem-solving, acceptance and seeking support. Greater distress was associated with poorer social support and use of coping strategies of wishful thinking and denial. In regression analyses, choice in caregiving was significantly associated with positive affect and inversely with distress. Reinforcing the correlations found, social support was consistently the strongest and most consistent predictor of positive outcomes (positive affect and satisfaction with life) and inversely related to the negative outcome of distress, but not linked to benefit finding. Surprisingly, stress appraisal was not associated with any of the outcome variables, but the coping strategy of wishful thinking was related to greater distress. The authors also report a trend for the coping response of acceptance being associated with benefit-finding and of the use of problem-solving being associated with positive affect, although these did not reach the 0.05 significance level.

Conclusions: Positive adjustment in young carers was predicted by greater choice in the caregiving context and the quality, and to a lesser extent the quantity, of available social support. Distress was predicted by poorer support satisfaction and greater use of wishful thinking as a coping strategy. There was also some tentative indication that the coping strategies of problem-solving and acceptance were linked to more positive affect and benefit-finding, respectively. In relation to benefit-finding, although this outcome variable was the least well predicted of all the outcome variables by the factors investigated in this study, the authors note that this measure captured the experience of benefit-finding for the entire age group, suggesting that even the youngest children (10 years old) experienced this positive outcome from care giving.

Implications: This study points to the potential benefits of interventions for young carers which specifically address the development of social support, cognitive stress appraisal and coping skills techniques. In addition to reducing distress, the 'enhancement' of positive outcomes in response to caregiving requires attention in young carer interventions.

Points to consider

- How do the coping responses identified as being associated with better outcomes in this study fit with the primary, secondary and disengagement coping categories highlighted in Chapter 6?
- How could these findings be incorporated into the type of psychosocial intervention suggested?
- How might these important theoretical constructs be developed in future research with young carers and what other variables or theoretical framework might contribute to research in this area?

TABLE 10.6   Positive and Negative Outcomes of Caring Questionnaire (PANOC-YC20)

Below are some things young carers like you have said about what it feels like to have to look after someone. Please read each statement and tick the box to show how often this is true for you. There are no right or wrong answers. We are just interested in what life is like for you because of caring.

1 Because of caring …	I feel I am doing something good
2 …	I feel that I am helping
3 …	I feel closer to my family
4 …	I feel good about myself
5 …	I have to do things that make me upset
6 …	I feel stressed
7 …	I feel like I am learning useful things
8 …	my parents are proud of the kind of person I am
9 …	I feel like running away
10 …	I feel very lonely
11 …	I feel like I can't cope
12 …	I can't stop thinking about what I have to do
13 …	I feel so sad I can hardly stand it
14 …	I don't think I matter
15 …	I like who I am
16 …	life doesn't seem worth living
17 …	I have trouble staying awake
18 …	I feel I am better able to cope with problems
19 …	I feel good about helping
20 …	I feel I am useful

Note: Items are rated on a 3-point scale: 0 ('never'); 1 ('some of the time'); 2 ('a lot of the time'), yielding two 10-item subscales: (i) positive outcomes, (ii) negative outcomes (both ranging in score from 0 to 20). Positive items are highlighted for the purposes of this chapter.

Source: Joseph, Becker, Becker and Regel (2009: 520, appendix 2).

A scale which specifically measures the positive and negative effects of young caregiving, the Positive and Negative Outcomes of Caring Questionnaire (PANOC-YC20), has been developed by Joseph and colleagues (Joseph, Becker, and Becker, 2009) in the UK as shown in Table 10.6. A score of less than 12 on the positive outcomes subscale and a score of greater than 8 on the negative outcomes subscale is considered cause for concern, requiring clinical intervention.

In interpreting the impact of caregiving tasks, Ireland and Pakenham (2010b) describe the positive and negative aspects of young caregiving in terms of the 'costs and benefits' involved. Ireland and Pakenham (2010a) describe an association between the positive outcome (benefit) of greater prosocial behaviour and the negative outcome (cost) of poorer health in young carers involved in a greater number of care tasks. Similarly, a greater emphasis on social or emotional care tasks simultaneously predicted poorer health and greater prosocial behaviour, although these researchers acknowledge that it may be those who are more prosocial to begin with who engage in greater amounts of caring. This theoretical interpretation of the young carer experience adds to the work described by Pakenham et al. (2007) and further highlights the need for development of mediation and moderation constructs. One example given as a possible driving force behind these relationships is that of parental attachment, which acts to influence adjustment processes and may play an important role in 'shaping' young carer outcomes (Ireland and Pakenham, 2010a: 729).

This notion of early experience shaping physical health outcomes into adulthood fits well with the life-course perspective taken throughout this book. As applied specifically to young carers in this chapter, the impact of this life experience can be seen as having a central role in contributing to allostatic load or accumulated lifetime stress. If you contrast with the adult caregiver literature, cutting-edge research highlights the impact of the caregiving role in older age being dependent on previous life-stress experience. In the case of young carers, we are looking through the opposite end of the kaleidoscope of accumulated lifetime stress, and considering the impact of subsequent life stress from the perspective of underlying allostatic load following the childhood experience of caregiving.

Most of the studies referred to so far have included a range of illness conditions, some including physical and mental health conditions and disability, others focusing on just physical illness. More recently, studies have started to explore the impact of specific characteristics of the caregiving context, such as choice in caregiving (Pakenham et al., 2007; see Box 10.2). Ireland and Packenham (2010b) have directly addressed differing characteristics between caring for a parent with a mental health condition and a parent with a physical condition using a cross-sectional study. In their sample of 81 young carers aged 10–25 years, they found gradual illness/disability onset, being male, isolation, lower perceived maturity, and less choice in caregiving to predict poorer adjustment (defined as having more emotional and behavioural difficulties, less prosocial behaviour, and poorer physical health as rated on a scale of 1–5). Those who had a parent with a physical illness/disability were found to 'worry' more about their parent compared to those whose parents had a mental illness, for whom 'caregiving discomfort' was higher (Ireland and Packenham, 2010b). Other contextual variables in want of further study include predictability of the condition, variability in symptoms, and age at illness onset.

A focus on characteristics, tasks and outcomes related to specific illness conditions is also emerging in the literature. In their Norwegian study, Syse and colleagues (2012) drew attention to the fact that there are increasing numbers of children who have parents diagnosed with cancer. Parental choice to delay child-bearing, coupled with increased technology to detect cancer, means that more parents are engaged in child-rearing at the time of diagnosis and treatment for cancer (Syse et al., 2012). They point out that 20 per cent of children whose parent is diagnosed with cancer will experience the death of the parent, but this leaves 80 per cent who live with cancer and its treatment in a parent. Whilst many cope well, some may suffer from emotional and behavioural problems and a smaller proportion experience more severe psychological difficulties or even trauma (Syse et al., 2012). Death of a parent is covered later in this chapter.

A recent longitudinal study of 88 families in which one of the parents had multiple sclerosis provides early evidence of caregiving characteristics specific to this population (Pakenham and Cox, 2012). These researchers utilized a number of questionnaires, including the YACS, to assess the type and amount of caregiving tasks performed by 130 young carers aged 10–20 years. They also used a range of outcome measures to assess behavioural, emotional and social functioning, somatization, positive affect and life satisfaction at two time points separated by 12 months. Given the longitudinal nature of this study, the effect of caregiving at time 1 on adjustment at time 2 was able to be investigated. Specific to the caregiving context of multiple sclerosis, poorer adjustment in the young carers was linked to greater amounts of instrumental care and social-emotional care, whereas better adjustment was seen in those who were involved in more personal-intimate care. This pattern is different from the poorer outcomes previously found for personal-intimate care in studies with more general, all-inclusive young carer populations. It is also of interest that in this study, increased amounts of caregiving summed across all categories were associated with greater somatization.

These findings by Pakenham and Cox (2012) advance the theoretical framework behind the effects of caregiving on adjustment and outcome in young carers. The authors describe their effects in terms of 'parentification' (Boszormenyi-Nagy and Spark, 1973) versus 'attachment' theory (Bowlby, 1969; see Chapter 2). 'Parentification' has been described as a situation in which 'children … are parent to their parents, and fulfil this role at the expense of their own developmentally appropriate needs and pursuits' and it 'entails a functional and/or emotional role reversal in which the child sacrifices his or her own needs for attention, comfort and guidance in order to accommodate and care for logistical and emotional needs of the parent' (Chase, 1999: 5). It has obvious applications to the experience of young carers and is an interesting and appropriate framework to consider within the context of the young carer. However, as seen above, the experience of the young carer is not by any means all negative, and there is no inevitable pathological result, particularly if appropriate support is in place. The term 'adaptive parentification' has also been used to describe parentification from a more positive, adaptive or functional perspective (Chase, in Pakenham and Cox, 2012). Packenham and Cox (2012) report their findings as consistent with both attachment theory and that of parentification theory. They argue that, in providing personal care tasks, attachment bonds are increased between the young carers and their parent with multiple sclerosis, increasing attachment and facilitating adaptation. When young carers are required to perform greater amounts of instrumental and social-emotional tasks, the experience of parentification is more likely since these tasks involve more 'adult-like interactions'; for example, speaking to health professionals on behalf of the parent or trying to keep the parent safe (Packenham and Cox, 2012: 342). This study provides much-needed longitudinal data and adds to the theory supporting research findings and practice in young carers. Yet there is much more research still to be conducted into the differential effects of early life caring in relation to specific physical health conditions.

INTERVENTIONS TO LESSEN THE NEGATIVE IMPACTS ON YOUNG CARERS

Based on these descriptions of young caregiving, key recurring psychosocial themes are those of social support, cognitive appraisal, coping, and resilience. Important theoretical factors are attachment versus parentification, and negative versus positive outcomes or resiliency, whilst a central concept includes the intergenerational dimension of time and longevity of effects from childhood through to adulthood. Findings from the study of Packenham et al. (2007), described in Box 10.2 above, demonstrate the value of increasing both the number of support contacts and the quality of support received, developing the coping responses of problem-solving, acceptance and seeking social support, whilst minimizing the coping strategies of wishful thinking and denial. If these are the key elements, then have they been applied and incorporated into young carer interventions and what are the outcomes? Before we can consider these questions, there are a few caveats which cannot be ignored. As noted above, the first caveat, which is an integral challenge to the provision of intervention and support to young carers, is that of identification of the young carer in the first instance. Moore and McArthur (2007) report four major barriers to the provision of support to young carers in Australia, identification being one of them, as given in Box 10.3.

BOX 10.3

Major barriers to providing support to young carers

Source: T. Moore and M. McArthur (2007) We're all in it together: supporting young carers and their families in Australia. *Health and Social Care in the Community*, 15(6): 561–8.

Population sample: 50 young carers (age range 9–24 years): 26 male; 24 female.

Methodology: interview

Barriers identified:

1 Reluctance within families to seek assistance for fear of child removal, negative intervention and increased scrutiny.
2 The families' lack of awareness of available services.
3 A lack of flexibility and responsiveness to the holistic needs of families.
4 A lack of service collaboration.

This study also highlights the fact that young carers themselves did not necessarily identify as being a young carer or, if they did identify as such, they did not want to acknowledge it for fear of bullying or harassment by peers at school. Moore and McArthur (2007) empha-size that the needs of each member of the family should be recognized within the context of joined-up service provision for family members. In terms of policy and practice, health psychology principles have also been used by service providers to assess young carers' needs more adequately, such as the 'theory of change' process approach used by Butler and Astbury (2005) in UK service provision. One application of this approach was to help examine and develop routes through which young carers are identified, with the end result of promoting identification within schools rather than primarily through social ser-vices (Butler and Astbury, 2005).

Our second caveat, which is central to the development of psychosocial support and intervention for young carers, is the perspective that simply providing support to the child independently of the adult services received by the parent is not only inadequate, but may be counterproductive. McAndrew et al. (2012: 13–14) caution that in some instances the provision of support may result in 'the unintentional impact of rewarding carers, and thus, reforcing their caring role'; particularly as this may increase time spent on caring tasks, there may be an unwanted effect of poorer adjustment and further educational and social-emotional repercussions. To avoid this, support to the whole family as a unit, taking account of the various characteristics of the illness and dynamics of the attachment rela-tionships involved, with continued support at an age-appropriate level, is recommended. Yet the need for support in young carers is substantial and should not be underestimated (Moore and McArthur, 2007). So it is that McAndrew et al. (2012: 14) describe this dilemma in the provision of support to young carers as a 'complex challenge'. They emphasize the need for interventions to 'enable and empower the whole family to make their own changes' (McAndrew et al., 2012: 14). So, rather than simply providing sup-port, the goal is to encourage mutual support within the family and also to develop sup-portive links outside the family, fostering the characteristics of resilience.

This notion of resilience, first noted in some of the children evacuated during the Second World War (Hicklin, in Glover, 2009), has emerged within several of the topics already considered in previous chapters. To describe this concept more fully, resilience is defined as 'having the capacity to resist or "bounce back" following adversity' and is composed of 'individual, family and community factors' (Glover, 2009: 5). It has been the cornerstone of research by the UK charity Barnardo's, which has developed interventions to improve well-being in children across a range of vulnerabilities based on key elements of resilience, such as in the ARCH (Achieving Resilience, Change, Hope) project (Glover, 2009). A national-level project dedicated to providing support for young carers is the Children's Society Include Programme (see www.youngcarer.com), managed by Jenny Frank (see ref-erence citations above). The Include Programme provides a range of information, training and support for young carers, their families and those providing services for them, and conducts a growing number of projects in this area. For example, one of the successful services provided by this programme, in collaboration with the YMCA youth charity, is the Young Carers Festival. This is an annual event that started in 2000 and 'provides the oppor-tunity for young carers from across the UK to get their voices heard about changes they want to see by taking part in participatory consultations to inform future work and to be communicated to government' (www.childrenssociety.org.uk). The Children's Society reports that these festivals, designed to be fun weekends for young carers, have grown in popularity since their inception and currently have about 1,800 attendees each year.

As can be seen from this review of young carer experiences, outcome and interventions, the identification of young carers and an understanding of the young carer role have led to a monumental change in service provision and support. However, whilst we have a good idea about the psychosocial theory informing the experience of young carers, there remains a significant amount of research to be conducted with respect to theory-driven, systematically tested interventions targeted to improve the lives of young carers.

DEALING WITH ISSUES OF DEATH AND DYING

Before leaving this topic of the experience of parental illness, one last aspect needs to be addressed. This is the experience of the child when faced with death or the possible threat of death in a parent or sibling due to illness. Children's understanding of death was covered in Chapter 8, and this understanding very much informs the experience of death and their response to it. There we considered some myths about childhood grief and bereavement and concluded that a sensitive, yet open and honest, approach is important in talking to children about issues of death and dying, in a way that the child can understand, and appropriately in line with their developmental level. There is general consensus that, below the age of about 9 years, children have difficulty understanding the concept of permanency (i.e., that someone has gone and will not be coming back) and, as such, a fuller understanding of death is usually only feasible for children from about 10 years upwards (e.g., Black, 1976). Yet children younger than this still have a considerable need to make sense of death and loss, and require age-appropriate communication and support. Misunderstandings can lead to later emotional difficulties if direct and honest communication, sensitive to their age and developmental level, is not provided. We are focusing here on parental death, but work in this area similarly includes death of a sibling in terms of the gravity of impact and effect that it may have.

The circumstances under which a parent dies, and the characteristics of the death, are also important components of the impact on the child. For example, the sudden death of a parent from a cardiovascular event, such as a heart attack, or from suicide both bring with them challenges different from the death of a parent who dies following a long battle with cancer. Yet, whatever the cause, the death of a parent has been described as 'an incomparable stress' (Rolls and Payne, 2003: 423) which has both immediate and longer-term, life-course effects on the child. Black in the 1970s was amongst the first wave of clinicians and researchers to draw attention to the increased impact of parental bereavement in childhood on psychiatric referral (e.g., Black, 1976). She also drew attention to the fact that a great majority of bereaved children in fact cope well with this major source of stress, and generated interest in the factors that positively influence the grieving process in children.

The impact of parental bereavement may show itself differently depending on the developmental stage of the child at the time of parental death and, furthermore, different effects may emerge throughout the stages of childhood, adolescence and into adulthood as that child develops. The effect of parental death on a child before the age when they can understand the concept of permanency may carry with it the potential for later effects as that child transitions through the stages of childhood and into adulthood. The objective life event of bereavement generates a subjective grief reaction which requires working through a complex array of emotions. The concept of 'mourning' is distinguished from 'bereavement' and 'grief' as 'the conscious and unconscious intrapsychic processes, together with the cultural, public or interpersonal efforts that are involved in attempts to cope with loss and grief' (Corr, in Stokes, 2004: 142).

Grief is a natural and normal response to death and is often referred to as a 'journey' (Stokes, 2004). Researchers have been documenting various components of the grieving process since the 1940s, highlighting important stages which an individual reaches in coming to terms with loss. Key theorists in this area include Linderman (1944), Bowlby (1961) and Kubler-Ross (1969), with theories based on the experience of a range of often conflicting emotions, including anger and denial, whilst detaching from the loss of the loved one, leading to an eventual readjustment and acceptance of the loss (for an excellent review and comparison of theories, see Kirwin and Hamrin, 2005). For children, this process is even more intimately bound up with the process of attachment (see Bowlby, 1969, 1980; and Chapter 2 for more on attachment theory). More recent theorists (e.g., Stroebe, 2008) view these stages as less fixed than first proposed, with periods of 'oscillation' between conflicting emotions, and greater emphasis is now placed upon the social, cultural and individual context, with the grieving process being seen as different for different individuals. Based on the theoretical framework proposed by Tonkin (1996), Stokes (2004) emphasizes that grief is not something to 'get over', but rather a process of adaptation whereby the individual learns

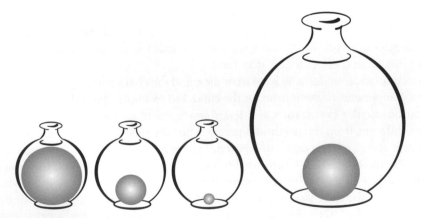

FIGURE 10.2   'Message in a bottle': Tonkin's (1996) ideas in the metaphor of a ball in a bottle
Source: Stokes (2004: 140); original source: Tonkin (1996).

how to live with the loss and to develop an adaptive coping style and increase their perception of hope and control over their life. Stokes (2004) symbolizes Tonkin's ideas in the metaphor given in Figure 10.2. This symbolizes that the pain experienced from grief does not simply diminish over time through a series of stages, as first suggested in original theories of grief. Instead, an individual can develop ways of coping with the grief, using techniques such as cognitive behaviour therapy to adapt to their new situation and to deal with their feelings of grief when they occur, and through development of supportive networks. Thinking back to the stress theories discussed in Chapters 2 and 5, if grief is the stressor then successful adaptation to grief is to increase the resources available to deal with or contain it.

Supportive intervention at an early stage is seen as essential in promoting adaptation and preventing the later development of pathological or unresolved grief. The first year following bereavement is generally viewed as an important time frame across all age groups including children. Yet, in the case of children, further support and explanation will need to be provided in different ways as the child develops and is able to take on board a more complex understanding of death and loss and the implications of these for their life. Anniversaries (e.g., birthdays or anniversary of the death) and important life events (e.g., starting school, getting married) may signify poignant reminders of the earlier loss, taking on different meanings and requiring additional support and adaptation. In their review of cross-sectional and longitudinal literature on parental loss and bereavement, Biank and Werner-Lin (2011: 271) describe this long-term process as 'growing up with grief', and point out that 'successful grieving is not measured in the termination of grief, but rather in the child's functional adaptation to prolonged grief' (2011: 275). They summarize the long-term trajectory of effects following the loss of a parent early in life, as impacting across the biopsychosocial domains of relational, social, emotional and physical development, throughout the life course, as described in Figure 10.3. Biank and Werner-Lin (2011) emphasize the importance of support and nurturing from the surviving parent in facilitating the child's adaptation to parental loss. Yet they point out that this presents its own difficulties as the surviving parent has their own grief to deal with and this is further compounded by other 'disruptions in family life' created by parental death (2011: 274). The outcomes in adulthood presented by Biank and Werner-Lin (2011) reflect both mental and physical health issues.

A handful of studies has directly assessed physiological stress reactivity to everyday stressful events (hassles) specifically in adolescent or adult populations who have experienced parental loss as children. For example, Luecken et al. (2009) assessed ambulatory blood pressure, self-reported stress, and perceived parental caring from the surviving parent during childhood via questionnaire, in a sample of 91 undergraduate students aged 18–29, of whom just under half had experienced parental bereavement before the age of 17 (with a period of at least 2 years prior to study entry). Interestingly, this study found a lower blood pressure for the parental loss group, despite a similar level of daily hassle stress. Just as in the findings reported above on adjustment to parental chronic illness during childhood (Turner-Cobb et al., 1998), this study indicates an altered underlying physiology which could imply a toughening, developed resistance, or 'stress inoculation', in

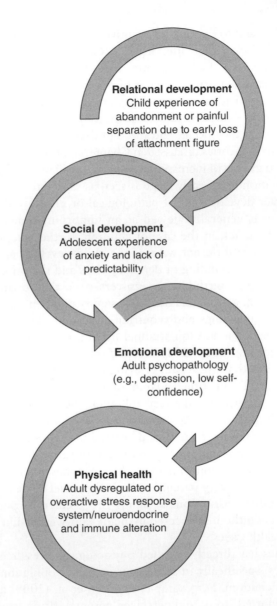

FIGURE 10.3   Long-term trajectory of grief showing impact across biopsychosocial domains of development
Source: Adapted from information in Biank and Werner-Lin (2011).

this parentally bereaved group of young adults. When exploring the outcomes of self-reported stress and emotional response (negative affect), Luecken et al. (2009) report stress sensitization with the parentally bereaved participants showing a greater negative response with the addition of poorer parental caring, but inoculation from the effects of stress when parental caring was high. Similarly, whilst several studies have reported dysregulation of cortisol in bereaved children or adults bereaved during childhood, the direction of effects varies, some reporting higher basal cortisol levels whilst others reporting lower basal levels or awakening responses (Hagan et al., 2011). Combining a longitudinal protocol with an experimental design, Hagan et al. (2011) measured salivary cortisol response in a sample of 55 parentally bereaved adolescents and young adults (aged 14–22 years). In this study, positive parenting was assessed by a combination of questionnaire and coded interview observations on two occasions, once at approximately 13 months after parental death (4–30 months prior to study entry) and 11 months later. Measures of recent negative life events and mental health were then assessed 7 years post-parental death, in addition to measuring cortisol before and after a 'conflict discussion task' between the participant and their caregiver. As shown in Figure 10.4, a combined effect of greater exposure to recent negative events and lower levels of past parenting was associated with a greater total cortisol output during the conflict task, indicating a greater reactivity in this sample of adolescents. In other words, it was under conditions of higher negative life event stress that the effect of less nurturing past parenting was observed. Importantly, those with high levels of parenting reacted less to personal conflict stress in the face of negative life events, highlighting once again the importance of positive parenting in moderating the effect of parental death on physical health.

The psychological stress experience of parental death fits well within the framework of stress concepts and theories outlined in this book, such as the mosaic patterning of life

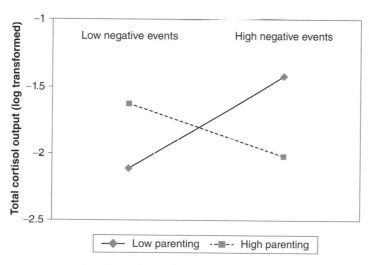

FIGURE 10.4   Interaction of parenting and life events on cortisol in a sample of bereaved adolescents

Source: Hagan et al. (2011: 236).

stress, allostasis and allostatic load. In fact, the study by Hagan et al. (2011) is a perfect example of the notion inherent throughout this book, that of early life stress having an impact on physical health not just during childhood but shaping adult physical health.

BEREAVEMENT SERVICES FOR CHILDREN

Whilst the initial impact of death and early stages during the first year are a crucial time for support and intervention to facilitate the process of grief, work outlined above shows the importance of continued follow-up of bereavement services throughout development. In the past couple of decades, there has been a significant growth in the provision of community bereavement services to children in the UK (Rolls and Payne, 2003). A leading charity behind this work in the UK is that of Winston's Wish, founded in 1992 by clinical psychologist Julie Stokes, which was set up to help children who are bereaved of a parent or sibling. Initially working with bereaved children locally in Gloucestershire, UK, the work of Winston's Wish has expanded nationwide and operates in collaboration with national organizations such as the Childhood Bereavement Network and social services. The incredible services provided by Winston's Wish include a range of support from written information to weekend residential camps for children aged 5–18 years, including both more immediate and continued support for bereaved children.

The goal of interventions to support the grieving process in children is to facilitate healthy adaptation, fostering the notion of resiliency which we discussed earlier in this chapter. A recent line of research in this area has started to investigate the concept of 'post-traumatic growth' in children who are parentally bereaved. Work by Wolchik and colleagues (2008) suggests that during the early stages of grief (in this study, assessed at 9 months post-bereavement), factors of cognitive appraisal, an individual's coping strategies, and ability to seek support (particularly the support of the surviving parent or guardian) can predict post-traumatic growth 6 years later as adolescents or young adults. In this prospective quantitative study, post-traumatic growth was observed in four areas: 'relating to others', 'new possibilities', 'personal strength' and 'appreciation of life' (Wolchik et al., 2008). In a similar vein, other research has specifically examined factors which were found to be useful in dealing with parental bereavement following the involvement in childhood bereavement services. For example, in a qualitative interview study, Brewer and Sparkes (2011) identified seven key themes: expressing emotion, physical activity, positive adult relationship(s), competence, friendships/social support, having fun/humour, and transcendence (i.e., a sense of gratitude, an appreciation of life and optimism for the future).

Longitudinal work is also beginning to emerge with respect to physiological outcome measures following bereavement intervention. In line with the key factors of parenting and life-stress exposure in determining physiological responses following bereavement described above (Luecken et al., 2009), later work reports a 12-week intervention for

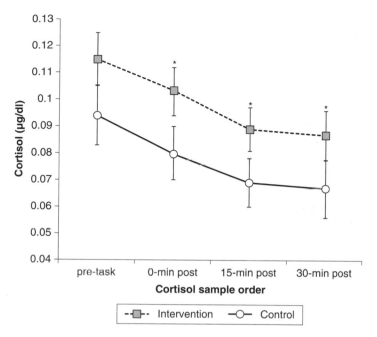

FIGURE 10.5 Cortisol levels before and after a conflict discussion task
Source: Luecken et al. (2010: 787).

parentally bereaved children (mean age 11.5 years) and their surviving parent/guardian (Luecken et al., 2010). The intervention was found to prevent an attenuated or dysregulated cortisol response as adolescents, 6 years later, compared to a control group of bereaved children who received only self-guided materials for use at home. Based on the earlier intervention of Sandler et al. (2003), the intervention for bereaved children involved the development of positive coping skills and adaptive beliefs relating to negative events, aimed to increase self-esteem/self-efficacy and to reduce inhibitions in grief expression; and for the parents/guardians, there was an emphasis on increasing positive parenting skills and reducing the child's exposure to stress (Luecken et al., 2010). They assessed physiological outcomes by measuring cortisol responses to a laboratory social stressor 6 years after the intervention. As shown in Figure 10.5, the intervention group had a greater stress response than the control group, indicating a suppressed response in the control group and a more normal response in the intervention group. Such work assessing the outcomes of bereavement services is still in the early stages but, taken together, these qualitative and quantitative, psychosocial and physiological outcome measures reveal not only the importance of early intervention, but also the long-term outcomes of such interventions across the full range of biopsychosocial effects.

Although they are very different in circumstances, there are several parallels between the experience of, and services offered to, young carers and children who are bereaved.

Both groups have experienced loss and, for some children, the caring role will ultimately lead to the experience of death of their parent. The development of coping skills and characteristics of resiliency are key elements in adaptation to the situation of the young carer and to parental bereavement. Both are associated with short-term and longer-term physiological responses and health outcomes, across development and into adulthood. Coping skills, the quality of parenting and exposure to future life stressors all influence these outcomes. Both young carers and children who experience the death of a parent require interventions with an emphasis on developing social networks and the quality of supportive relationships.

CHAPTER SUMMARY

In this chapter, I have considered the experience and effects of a child growing up with a parent or close family member who is unwell and/or disabled. I have looked at what defines a young carer and at both the positive and negative outcomes of caregiving at a young age. The second topic considered was that of the experience of the child when a parent dies and the biopsychosocial impact of bereavement. I also referred to the experience of death in a sibling or other close family member. Importantly, I examined the impact of caregiving and of parental death, not just during childhood but into adulthood, with reference to changes over time consistent with social and developmental maturity. Notions of resilience and stress inoculation apply to both the young caregiving experience and the experience of being parentally bereaved as a child. Different study designs were drawn upon to illustrate these relationships, including those which assessed outcomes and experiences during childhood and adolescence, but also those asking adults to reflect on their experience as children. Psychosocial support was highlighted as central to interventions in both caregiving and following bereavement in children and adolescents.

This chapter concludes Part II of the book. The final chapter takes a 'bird's-eye' view of health risk and resiliency, drawing together key concepts across both parts of the book, with a focus on health promotion and the future landscape of child health research and practice.

KEY CONCEPTS AND ISSUES

- Young carer/young caregiver/youth carer
- Positive and negative aspects of young caregiving (costs versus benefits)
- Resilience
- Parentification and adaptive parentification
- Parentally bereaved
- Bereavement, mourning and grief
- Grief as a process involving oscillation

- Stress inoculation and resistance
- Psychosocial support and intervention

FURTHER READING

YOUNG CARERS

A well-written and-designed document which summarizes recent UK survey findings, provides information on relevant legislation, and details the six key principles of practice for young carers, with poignant quotes:

Frank, J. and McLarnon, J. (2008) *Young Carers, Parents and their Families: Key Principles of Practice*. London: The Children's Society.

A useful document with excellent case studies of families in which young carers are the key context:

Ronicle, J. and Kendall, S. (2011) Improving support for young carers: family focused approaches. Department for Education, Research Report DFE-RR084. York Consulting LLP.

An insightful qualitative study of adults who were carers as children:

Lackey, N.R. and Gates, M.F. (2001) Adults' recollections of their experiences as young caregivers of family members with chronic physical illnesses. *Journal of Advanced Nursing*, 34(3): 320–8.

An excellent longitudinal quantitative study:

Pakenham, K.I. and Cox, S. (2012) The nature of caregiving in children of a parent with multiple sclerosis from multiple sources and the associations between caregiving activities and youth adjustment over time. *Psychology and Health*, 27(3): 324–46.

GRIEF AND BEREAVEMENT

I could wax lyrical about this book. If you read nothing else, read this. Not only an excellent book with insight for practitioners working with children who have been parentally bereaved, it is also beautifully written and presented, with a sensitive yet practical account of bereavement – non-technical but with academic references:

Stokes, J.A. (2004) *Then, Now and Always. Supporting Children through Grief: A Guide for Practitioners*. Cheltenham: Portfolio/Winston's Wish.

Potentially time-limited but a remarkable book nonetheless, this book uses stories mainly from the Harry Potter series as illustrations to help children who have been bereaved. Cross-referenced with Julie Stokes's book above, it provides a further example of using fictional characters and literature as a therapeutic tool in bereavement:

Markell, A. and Markell, M.A. (2008) *The Children who Lived: Using Harry Potter and Other Fictional Characters to Help Grieving Children and Adolescents*. New York: Routledge.

An excellent review based on a lifespan perspective, incorporating a case study:

Biank, N.M. and Werner-Lin, A. (2011) Growing up with grief: revisiting the death of a parent over the life course. *Omega: Journal of Death and Dying*, 63(3): 271–90.

An example of a longitudinal study combining an intervention and a laboratory-based social stressor task with cortisol response assessed:

Luecken, L.J., Hagan, M.J., Sandler, I.N., Tein, J.Y., Ayers, T.S. and Wolchik, S.A. (2010) Cortisol levels six years after participation in the Family Bereavement Program. *Psychoneuroendocrinology*, 35(5): 785–9.

USEFUL WEBSITES

YOUNG CARERS

Carers Trust (merger of former Princess Royal Trust for carers and Crossroads Care): www.carers.org

The Children's Society: www.childrenssociety.org.uk

The Children's Society Include Programme website (includes school resources): www.youngcarer.com

Macmillan cancer support: www.macmillan.org.uk/cancerinformation/ifsomeoneelsehascancer/youngcarers2010

Spurgeons: www.spurgeons.org/young-carers

GRIEF AND BEREAVEMENT

Childhood Bereavement Network: www.childhoodbereavementnetwork.org.uk

Winston's Wish: www.winstonswish.org.uk

SUMMARY AND THE WAY AHEAD

11

Covered in this chapter

- Summary of health risks and resiliency factors
- Promoting and maintaining health
- Psychological factors and issues in child health not mentioned
- The role of health psychology in future child health

In this final chapter, I bring together the underlying themes, issues and concepts that have recurred throughout this book. Some of these were obvious to me from the inception of the book, whilst others have suggested themselves, sometimes rather audaciously, during the process of carefully sifting through the research literature and various sources of information whilst compiling these chapters. The ten preceding chapters cover a range of psychological issues related to child health, from the effects of stress during pregnancy to issues of relevance to adult survivors of childhood cancer. Some of the topics covered might at first glance seem perhaps rather disparate. Whilst in many respects they are distinct areas, each with its own theories, models and paradigms, when taken as a whole, a clear picture emerges relating to psychological factors of risk and resilience in child health. These psychological factors underlie much of the current health promotion and intervention strategies, and pave the way for future developments in child health. In addition to summarizing these concepts and discussing a biopsychosocial strategy for promoting and maintaining health in children, this chapter also examines what the future holds. Taking these concepts, theories and models as a whole, it examines how psychological research and practice can help shape the future of child health and illness from a life-course perspective.

SUMMARY OF HEALTH RISKS AND RESILIENCY FACTORS

Some of the themes, issues and concepts covered in this book have caused me (metaphorically speaking) to stand on my soapbox, arms waving furiously. In some cases, this is because of a key recurring concept or unifying theme; in other cases, because of the under-studied nature of important areas of research, gaps in the literature, or the identification of parallel research areas which appear to pay very little regard to one another, despite making use of similar underlying concepts. I start with the key recurring concepts and themes, then move on to point out some of the inconsistencies and gaps identified in the literature.

KEY RECURRING CONCEPTS AND UNIFYING THEMES

The central concept around which this book has revolved is that of the biopsychosocial model, supporting the mind–body connection. This is, however, a rather broad model and needs further refinement for understanding child health psychology as applied here, in order to define the biological, psychological and social content relevant to the topics considered. It should be obvious by now that the overriding themes that dominate this book are those of the presence, severity and impact of early life adversity and the life-course perspective. The experience of early life adversity creates a *potential* health risk during childhood and throughout adult life. Potential, that is, since it is important to remember that this is not a given; instead, early life adversity in its various forms and levels of severity also offers opportunities for the development of resiliency. An example of this is given in Chapter 10, when discussing the psychosocial impact of young carers looking after a parent or close family member. The young carer literature contrasts the risk of 'parentification' (role reversal with child parenting the parent) with the potential for developing resiliency through increased maturity and coping ability. Furthermore, at a theoretical level, the lessons learned from the harmful effects of early life adversity on health outcome provide useful indicators from which to build intervention tools at the level of both recovery and prevention. Risks to health across the lifespan include stressful events, whether cataclysmic, repeated acute, or chronic enduring stress, and these are borne out in the recurrent themes of stress, threat and challenge throughout the book.

Early life adversity is another term for stressful events or conditions experienced early in life, often focused on the first 3 years of development but, as detailed in Chapter 4, it can include the prenatal experience or, more generally, stress during the wider childhood years (see Chapter 5). The transactional model of stress and coping outlined in Chapter 2 pervades all of the topics covered in subsequent chapters. There are various classifications or taxonomies of stress used throughout this book, but the overriding factors in terms of the impact of stress are severity, duration, controllability, predictability and the presence of social evaluative threat (a threat to the self, based on the social judgement of others; see Chapters 2 and 3 for a fuller description of social evaluative threat). The psychosocial impacts of socioeconomic inequality and child poverty are underpinned by this concept of social evaluative threat, and it is inherent in the conclusions of the Good Childhood Inquiry referred to in Chapter 2. In other words, the concept of stress pervades all the topics considered throughout this book, although in different forms and orders of magnitude. The ability of an event to activate the physiological stress response systems of the body, and the ability of psychosocial resources to enable a return of these physiological systems to pre-stress levels, known as adaptation, are of central importance. Stressful events have the potential not only to generate a stress response at the time the stress occurs, but also to alter the basal underlying levels and circadian rhythms, as well as to change the level or starting point at which subsequent stress reactivity occurs. This is so enormously important in children, due to their ongoing physiological, social and cognitive development, and has implications for lifelong health. Indeed, it was argued in Chapter 1 that an early stressful environment creates a 'biological embedding' (a laying down of biological 'wiring' which dictates future responses).

Across the topics explored in this book, the process of stress repeatedly emerges not as a simple dose-response effect (i.e., the more you experience, the greater the impact), but as a complex constellation or life stress 'mosaic' in which combinations of acute and chronic stress, experienced in double or multiple and often overlapping 'hits', serve to shape the physical health outcome. The underlying theory that accounts for these stress impacts across different topics is that of allostasis (adaptation through change) and the notion of allostatic load (accumulated lifetime stress). Early life adversity, then, offers a theoretical perspective from which to understand adult health as well as child health. It also serves to suggest psychosocial factors which might be targeted in order to lessen the impact of stress during childhood with the goal of improving lifelong health. These psychological factors which have arisen repeatedly throughout the book include those of social support versus isolation and loneliness, and adaptive versus maladaptive coping responses. An emphasis on adaptive secondary control coping (e.g., acceptance, distraction, cognitive restructuring, positive thinking) and, to a lesser extent, active primary control coping (e.g., problem-solving, emotional expression or modulation) has repeatedly emerged as more favourable than withdrawal techniques of disengagement coping (e.g., avoidance, denial, wishful thinking) or the emotional over-reaction of catastrophization (see Chapters 6, 7, and 9). The importance of coping responses and social support emerge at both the individual child level and at the level of the family, with parental (maternal and paternal) coping responses and social support (both provided to the parents and the support parents provide to the child) being central to child and family health.

The family context is a strong theme throughout the book and forms part of the social context or environment through which the impact of stress is experienced. Adaptation emerges as a top contender for unifying concepts, with failure to adapt presenting a high risk for poor health outcome, and the ability to adapt resulting in the development of resilience. The theory of allostasis rests on this notion of adaptation through change, and the ability to develop characteristics of resiliency could be seen as the ultimate test of the ability to adapt in the face of difficult or novel circumstances. Secondary control coping is characteristic of adaptive styles of coping and repeatedly emerges as the most useful set of coping strategies across a range of circumstances and health outcomes.

Individual differences, such as child temperament, also recur as important variables to influence the stress experience and health outcome. For example, this was seen particularly in relation to cortisol levels in healthy children transitioning to school, in which the combination of temperament and social environment influenced health outcome of the common cold (see Chapter 6). It is important to note that a particular temperament, such as the more introverted child or, alternatively, one with a more surgent or extroverted temperament, cannot necessarily be said to fair better, but it is the combination of temperament, peer interaction and environment that determines the outcome.

Likewise, lifestyle and health behaviours (e.g., diet, exercise, condom use, smoking, sleep, vaccination) are also important contenders for the top spot as contributors to health in children. Viewed from the elaborated biopsychosocial perspectives presented in Chapter 2, health behaviours act as moderators and mediators of psychosocial factors on physiological change and health outcome (i.e., psychosocial factors act in conjunction with or through health behaviours). That is, health behaviours, lifestyle and habit emerge as the 'bridging factors' between psychosocial concepts and health outcome. At one level, psychological techniques can be used to change health behaviours (e.g., to encourage healthy eating or to reduce the attractiveness of smoking) and in doing so avoid negative health outcomes (e.g., obesity or lung disease). On a slightly more complex level, encouraging good sleep hygiene, for example, may provide improved cognitive capacity to develop adaptive coping responses to deal with chronic stress situations. Health behaviours are relevant at various levels and applications to all child and adolescent populations considered in these chapters, but perhaps the most

TABLE 11.1   Key recurring concepts, unifying themes, theories and models in child health psychology

Recurring concepts	Unifying themes	Theories and models
• Stressful events (severity and duration), threat and challenge • Controllability and predictability • Reactivity • Basal endocrine levels and circadian rhythms • Adaptive versus maladaptive coping responses: secondary control coping, catastrophization • Individual differences: temperament, socioeconomic status (poverty) • Lifestyle, health behaviours and habit • Cognitive and social development	• Early life adversity • Life-course perspective • Resiliency • Adaptability • Survivorship • Social support versus isolation and loneliness • Parental/family context • Social context • Open communication	• Biopsychosocial model • Time-course perspective • Transactional model of stress and coping • Allostasis and allostatic load • Social cognition models • Attachment theory

striking illustration of their importance is seen in the impact on late effects in long-term adult survivors of childhood cancer (Chapter 6). Furthermore, social cognition models provide an excellent framework in delivering interventions to change health behaviours, as detailed below.

A further theme that runs through the book is that of communication, particularly that of openness in communication. The need for openness and honesty in communication repeatedly emerges, whether in communication between parents and children, or between health professionals and parents or children. Prominent examples are those of communication concerning illness diagnosis, prognosis, treatment side-effects and issues of death and dying (see Chapters 7, 8 and 10). Table 11.1 lists some of these common concepts and themes across different topics in child health psychology.

POPULATIONS, ILLNESS CONDITIONS AND RESEARCH METHODOLOGIES

A range of illness populations has been mentioned in discussing the various topics, from acute illness in otherwise healthy children to severe life-threatening conditions and chronic illnesses. Healthy populations have been referred to and highlighted as a useful group to observe in relation to the occurrence of acute illness, such as the common cold and flu, in order to build theory which can also be applied to chronic conditions. Acute infection was flagged as an important paradigm for examining the effects of stress on endocrine and immune changes and health outcome. The most prominent of the physical health conditions in the psychosocial literature relating to children include asthma, sickle cell disease, diabetes, acute lymphoblastic leukaemia, juvenile rheumatoid arthritis, obesity, and human immunodeficiency virus (HIV). Accidents were also considered, their incidence being particularly high in children, and in adolescents when viewed as accident-prone risk-takers.

From a methodological perspective, a broad range of methodologies has been considered, from both quantitative and qualitative approaches, including questionnaire assessment (including web-based surveys), interview, diary recording, the use of endocrine and immune biomarkers, laboratory stress-testing paradigms and MRI scanning. Emphasis has been on the use of appropriate methodologies for the research questions being addressed. In particular, the benefit of using mixed methods approaches to the same question has been highlighted. By far the most important approach to assessment of psychosocial factors on child health has been shown to be the longitudinal assessment of a range of process and outcome variables, using biopsychosocial markers of stress and other psychosocial assessment, physiological alteration and health outcome. A number of cohort studies has been examined, particularly in relation to childhood cancers. Throughout the topics addressed, a repeated call for research which examines the physical health effects of childhood stress across various stages of adulthood has been made. The practicalities and costs of such longitudinal work are naturally problematic, and meeting the requirements for scientific rigour presents a challenge. Yet an exciting body of research is emerging with respect to adult physical health outcomes, from various types of longitudinal studies, including those of large epidemiological cohorts. With the application of a range of methodologies and assessment techniques, much-needed further work in this area offers great potential for understanding the health implications of child and adolescent adversity.

Some age cut-offs have been identified, such as the 5-year-old age group (pre-adrenarche) being more vulnerable to certain pathogens against which T-helper 1 (Th1) immunity normally defends (e.g., common cold and flu viruses); before adrenarche, there is a greater balance towards Th2 immunity in children (see Chapter 2). In a similar vein, understanding of the concepts of stress and illness by children has re-emerged as an important topic of discussion concerning developmental stages of understanding versus a more fluid conception of the nature of illness. An early understanding of stress at 8 years and older has been identified, but even at 4 years old, children have reported being aware of the concept of stress.

MINDING THE GAPS AND IDENTIFYING PARALLEL UNIVERSES IN RESEARCH

In considering the distinct but related areas of child health psychology discussed here, most experts in each area would undoubtedly argue, quite rightly, that further research is needed. Exactly what that research comprises depends upon the perspective or clinical need of the researcher, and their own focus on the relative ingredients of biological, psychological and social factors they consider to be important. There are three areas that particularly stand out from my own perspective when reviewing these topics, and I raise these here as suggestions for future research.

The first is that of stress reactivity testing in children, using a social stress test. As highlighted in Chapter 5, further work is needed to establish an appropriately meaningful stress test for children under the age of approximately 11 years. This corresponds to the period of childhood when cortisol reactivity is thought to be relatively low (i.e., hypocortisol phase) or unresponsive. Not all studies using stress tests have found this, but there is considerable heterogeneity or variation in the content of the tests used and in the results. Understanding more about the underlying mechanisms in childhood reactivity to stress in healthy children of different ages is not only worthy of study for theoretical reasons but would enable a more reliable comparison when seeking to understand stress reactivity responses in children with acute or chronic conditions. Developing stress tests which incorporate reliable, consistent and meaningful social evaluative threat for children is a necessary challenge in being able to establish norms of reactivity accurately across different age groups. In a similar way, further detailed assessment of the cortisol awakening response (CAR) in both the pre/post-adrenarche and pre/post-pubescent age groups is needed before assessment of stress responsivity can be fully interpreted.

A second area that is striking when considering the chapters in this book is the lack of research in young carers, which includes physical health outcomes and, in particular, physiological assessments of endocrine and immune markers. This in part reflects the relatively new interest in this research area (see Chapter 10). A parallel research area is that of the physical health and physiological assessment of those who are carers for people at the other end of the lifespan, in old age, particularly for those with dementia or Alzheimer's disease. There have been some remarkable studies in adult carers of these older adults, but as yet there is virtually nothing in the literature which examines the biomarkers and physical health outcomes in young carers, either during childhood or in later life.

The third area of neglected research that deserves a mention is that linking pain (Chapter 9) and stress (Chapter 5). Whilst some links have been made and written about for decades, for much of the time these two areas operate within parallel research domains. What is particularly striking when considering these areas in relation to child health is the life-course trajectory. Early experiences of pain can prime or set the pain response system to respond to future pain experiences, just as early experiences of stress may prime or set the stress response system to respond to future stress experiences. Both also involve a re-experiencing or heightened sensitivity experience based on previous life stress or pain. Furthermore, the links between these two response systems, the overlapping physiological systems utilized by both, and the social context in which responses are exaggerated or attenuated may hold the key to relieving many stress- and pain-related conditions. Central to both are psychosocial experiences, adaptation, adjustment and the goal of normalizing response systems through psychosocial intervention. One application of this is to hospitalization, in which both stress and pain shape the experience, and past experience has been found to predict future responses to hospitalization.

PROMOTING AND MAINTAINING HEALTH

Intervention strategies for promoting and maintaining health have been included in each of the preceding chapters, across a range of acute and chronic conditions and in healthy children and adolescents. A variety of cognitive behavioural techniques and stress reduction techniques and interventions which develop adaptive coping responses and facilitate social support have been highlighted, relevant to the specific acute or chronic illness context. Cognitive behavioural therapies (CBT) and stress-reduction techniques have been particularly effective in relation to medical procedures, hospitalization, and pain control in children and adolescents. One specific type of relaxation technique, which has seen a significant increase in popularity over the past decade, is that of mindfulness-based stress reduction, and this technique has been applied to children and adolescents as illustrated in various chapters of Part II. Some adaptations of the original mindfulness meditation techniques now include specific CBT components. Such techniques tap into the characteristics of stress, aiming to induce relaxation by reversing these characteristics; for example, increasing control, reducing unpredictability and challenging social evaluative threat, thus calming the stress and pain responses. The early education of relaxation strategies to reduce examination stress in children has potential for longevity in the learning of useful skills which can be applied throughout schooling, as well as serving to keep stress responses to a minimum and retain a high threshold for stress responsivity to other life stressors. There is enormous potential in these psychosocial interventions, which can only be improved with increased theoretical knowledge of the underlying mechanisms as suggested above.

The other domain in which psychosocial interventions can challenge acute and chronic conditions in children and adolescents is via preventive measures. The need for early intervention is key to most powerfully effecting health outcomes in children, with potential to improve health into adulthood. Health psychology models that have been instrumental in promoting health in both healthy populations of children and in illness populations are the social cognition models referred to in Chapter 1, such as the 'health belief model' and the 'theory of planned behaviour'. Many health promotion interventions have successfully used such models to influence a range of health behaviours in children, adolescents and their parents. Examples include healthy eating and exercise campaigns to prevent obesity; condom use to prevent sexually transmitted diseases; smoking prevention and cessation; vaccination of children against measles, mumps and rubella (MMR) or human papillomavirus (HPV) which causes cervical cancer; and the promotion of sun safety to reduce the risk of skin cancer.

Beyond these types of intervention to prevent specific conditions, a broader but equally important health promotion involves increasing knowledge and changing accepted cultural norms about health and disease. As seen throughout many of the chapters in this book, a sense of fear and isolation is deleterious to adaptive coping with stress and illness, and this can have a subsequent effect not just on the experience of being ill but may further influence physical health via underlying physiological mechanisms activated by stress and related emotions. Health promotion techniques which attempt to develop a culture of understanding about illness, explain the experience of living with a chronic illness such as diabetes or a condition with a visible difference, talk about stress and how to recognize it, and prepare children in case they do encounter the need for medical procedures or hospitalization, can also make a significant contribution. There are examples of these throughout this book. Children understand more about health, illness and death than they may sometimes be given credit for. We see this in the studies presented on children's cognitive understanding of health and illness, in which children as young as 4 years had some understanding of stress and health. In studies of bereavement and children receiving palliative care, understanding of death was not always predicted by staging models. Instead, a gradual understanding appears to emerge, largely dictated by the child's ability to understand the concept of permanence. Around the age of 9 years is generally the distinguishing time point for understanding death, but, as with understanding health and illness, this varies according to factors including developmental maturity and life experience.

PSYCHOLOGICAL FACTORS AND ISSUES IN CHILD HEALTH NOT MENTIONED

The main focus in this book has been on the child rather than on the parent. For this reason, topics of interest to health psychologists, such as the effect on parents of caregiving for a child with physical illness or disability, whilst being mentioned, have not been focused on to any degree. This is an important topic and one of current interest in the literature (see, for example, Bella et al., 2011, on mothers of children with cerebral palsy; or Rempel et al., 2012, on parenting children with congenital heart disease), but the focus of the topic is on the parental experience and effects, rather than that of the child *per se*. Many of these issues would, however, be the subject of a different text with the focus on parenting, rather than the focus on the child, as is the perspective taken in this book.

There are also further pertinent issues, such as behavioural conditions (e.g., attention deficit hyperactivity disorder [ADHD]) and physical disabilities, which are mentioned in this book (see Chapters 6, 7 and 9), but not focused on to a large extent, or that of sudden infant death syndrome (SIDS) which was considered beyond the scope of the book. The unifying theories, models and approaches used throughout the book in tackling the various issues addressed are applicable to these topics. I have focused on current topics which are being placed at the forefront of government agendas and public interest in applying the theories and models outlined, but they can equally be applied to these other topics. Similarly, there are topics which are currently increasing in interest in related areas of psychology, including social psychology and mental health outcome, such as substance misuse, alcohol consumption, and binge drinking in adolescents. Whilst mention was made of these health behaviours, the outcomes are not currently the focus of this text, but this is not to deny their importance or relevance in child health psychology. The focus in this book is on the components and applications of biopsychosocial models which fit within a psychoneuroimmune perspective.

THE ROLE OF HEALTH PSYCHOLOGY IN FUTURE CHILD HEALTH

In the very first chapter of this book, I took an historical perspective with reference to health and medicine as far back as medieval times. In Chapter 6, I examined the experience of hospitalization for children before the 1960s; there were also references to historical practices in research methods and ethics in children in Chapter 3. In reading these accounts, what stands out is the significant and steady improvement in medical and research practice from about the late 1960s onwards. Viewed through the long lens of what medical historians and politicians might metaphorically refer to as a 'retrospectroscope', some of the health-related practices of the past seem rather outrageous to us now, and recent discoveries rather obvious once they are allowed to take their place in everyday practice. As explored in this book, health psychology has a considerable amount to offer in relation to child health and it has the necessary tools to shape that future.

It now remains to project forward and consider what child health might look like in future years with the input of health psychology. Yet predicting the future of health psychology research and practice as applied to children might feel slightly overwhelming, if not rather ominous. In true psychological style, perhaps I can turn this into a question and reflect it back to you as the reader. Having read the preceding chapters, or at least, I hope, some of them, and combining this with your own knowledge of child health psychology research and/or practice, what would you consider to be the key psychological concepts, methodologies and interventions for developing, promoting and maintaining health in children? It is worth thinking about where child health psychology is heading in the future, in terms of both realistic goals for the more immediate development of child health from a biopsychosocial perspective and what the longer-term view has in store. Box 11.1 presents an exercise in 'futurology', asking you to think about the future of child health, in particular how health psychology might influence health outcomes through research and practice.

BOX 11.1

Shaping the future of child health psychology

Think about where child health psychology is heading in the future.

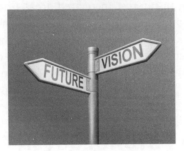

FIGURE 11.1   Future vision
Source: Shutterstock 66324592.

- How could the future of child health be shaped by health psychology theories and models?
- What do you consider to be the top three realistic goals for the development of child health from a biopsychosocial perspective?
- How could health promotion programmes be most effectively delivered to parents, children and adolescents?
- Which health behaviours would be most effective to target?
- What would be the most significant child health conditions that a psychologist would be needed to deal with?
- What might health-care delivery look like in 50 years' time? Consider the hospital environment, outpatient facilities and care for children at home.
- How would interventions be most effectively delivered?
- What type of technological advances might be needed for effective delivery of health care, health promotion and health interventions?
- What ethical restrictions and requirements might be necessary in this environment?

Futurology, or the 'science' of predicting the future, has been applied most readily to tech-nological advances and human–computer interaction. Also termed 'crystal ball gazing', given the element of guesswork and uncertainty inherent in attempting to predict the future, there is an attractive and useful aspect to pondering what life may look like in the years ahead, not least because it helps define goals and objectives towards reaching them. In a very aptly named article ('The psychology of futurology and the future of psychol-ogy'), Tetlock (1994) reviews work by Nickerson (1992) which takes this futurological approach to human factors and applies it to the potential role of psychologists in a future world. Tetlock points out that the extent of the role for psychologists depends on whether a 'pessimistic' or an 'optimistic' view of the future is taken. A greater role for psycholo-gists is speculated if there are more difficulties in society and the outlook less positive, but in an optimistic scenario, psychologists are speculated to be even more in demand. The education of children and the practice of preventive health care are two important areas outlined for psychologists (Nickerson in Tetlock, 1992). Whilst this review may have been undertaken 20 years ago and, granted, advances have been made since this time, the vision of future health has not changed greatly.

More recently, in his presidential address to the American Psychological Association (APA) in 2009, Bray (2010) set out his 'initiatives and recommendations for the future of psychology practice and science' (p. 355). Part of this directly refers to health education and promotion in children, with recommendations for 'cost effective treatment for use in school-based interventions for preventing and treating overweight and obesity in children and adolescents' (p. 364), as well as a range of cognitive, social and behavioural therapies for ADHD. Bray (2010) calls for the involvement of psychologists in developing public policy to avoid rigid regulations which might 'undermine' research in areas such as clinical governance and ethics (p. 365). He also cautions about the application of technology and the need to be mindful of human engineering and human factors in designing computer-ized systems which are intended to facilitate research and clinical practice but, if badly designed, may be counterproductive to research and even to health (Bray, 2010). The mantra repeated by Bray at the start and finish of his address, that 'the best way to predict the future is to create it' (pp. 355, 367) is both inspiring and challenging. Armed with this wealth of health psychology research knowledge and practice, there is plenty of scope for creating a very positive future in child health. Implementation of this knowledge is often more of a challenge than expected, not only at the individual and community level but also at a societal and political level.

This discussion has so far been focused on developed countries and child health expec-tations in the developed world. From a wider, worldwide perspective, it is worth remem-bering the child-related aspects of the Millennium Development Goals (MDGs) set by the World Health Organization, discussed in Chapter 1. These have the aim of being achieved not 50 years in the future, but by 2015, and take a worldwide perspective on child health in order to (i) 'eradicate poverty and hunger'; (ii) 'reduce child mortality'; (iii) 'improve maternal health'; and (iv) 'combat HIV/AIDS, malaria, and other diseases'. In the developed world, acceptance of psychological practices has become mainstream in many areas of health and medicine, and has been, perhaps, even more widely accepted in child health psychology where the need to relate at a psychosocial and emotional level is seen as greater than in adults. There have been many changes in the hospital environment (see Chapter 6) and in the delivery of care within and outside the hospital environment since the 1960s. Together with advances in medical treatment and technology, health outcome for children has seen monumental changes. New threats and risks to health emerge, however, and the health-care and prevention context is constantly changing, and psychological approaches and the delivery of psychosocial techniques need to change in response. As seen throughout the chapters in this book, these need to be tailored not just to children but to their parents, carers and family.

From the central biopsychosocial perspective of this book, with a focus on lifespan trajectories of health and illness, I would like to conclude with a mention of one further study which is a useful reminder of the importance of establishing early expectations of health and well-being in children. In their cohort analysis of over 20,000 adolescents enrolled in the US National Longitudinal Study of Adolescent Health, McDade et al. (2011) examined links between adolescent expectations for the future (chances of attending college and living to middle age) and engagement in health behaviours (physical activity, consumption of fast food and smoking). They found health behaviours to be strongly predicted by expectations for the future, independently of parental education, and conclude that perceived life chances are an important predictor of health behaviour factors which form an important link to future health outcome in adult life through their health trajectory.

In introducing the topic of health psychology, I listed the goals of the British Psychological Society's Division of Health Psychology. These included promoting and maintaining health, preventing and managing illness, identifying psychological factors which contribute to physical illness, improving the health-care system and helping to formulate health policy (see www.health-psychology.org.uk). As applied to children and adolescents, health psychology has enormous potential for shaping the trajectory of health from childhood through to old age.

KEY CONCEPTS AND ISSUES

This whole chapter has been about the key concepts and issues in child health psychology which have occurred throughout this book, and are listed at the end of each chapter. For that reason I have refrained from repeating a long list here but central to the forward-looking perspective of this chapter, below are some key, overarching, food-for-thought concepts and issues:

- Adaptability
- Futurology
- Health trajectory
- Life-course perspective

FURTHER READING

A highly recommended children's book, which predicts what life might be like in the future, reported to be so popular it has a cult following and has been recently reprinted, updated to 2011 (see news article under 'Useful websites' below):

Hoyle, G. and Anderson, A. (2010) *2011: Living in the Future*. Seattle, WA: Blue Lantern.

USEFUL WEBSITES

For a review of the children's book referenced above, see the BBC news magazine article, 'Futurology: the tricky art of knowing what will happen next' (by Finlo Rohrer): www.bbc.co.uk/news/magazine-12058575

To find out more about the British Psychological Society (BPS) Division of Health Psychology (DHP), including current society aims and goals: www.health-psychology.org.uk

For more on the American Psychological Association (APA): www.apa.org

REFERENCES

Absolom, K., Eiser, C., Greco, V. and Davies, H. (2004) Health promotion for survivors of childhood cancer: a minimal intervention. *Patient Education and Counseling*, 55(3): 379–84.

Ajzen, I. (1985) From intentions to actions: a theory of planned behavior. In J. Kuhl and J. Beckmann (eds), *Action Control: From Cognition to Behavior*. Heidelberg: Springer-Verlag. pp. 11–39.

Ajzen, I. (1991) The theory of planned behavior. *Organizational Behavior and Human Decision Processes*, 50: 179–211.

Akinbami, L.J., Moorman, J.E., Garbe, P.L. and Sondik, E.J. (2009) Status of childhood asthma in the United States, 1980–2007. *Pediatrics*, 123 Suppl. 3: S131–45.

Al-Ansari, A.A., Perry, L.A., Smith, D.S. and Landon, J. (1982) Salivary cortisol determination: adaptation of a commercial serum cortisol kit. *Annals of Clinical Biochemistry*, 19: 163–6.

Alaszewski, A. (2006) *Using Diaries for Social Research*. London: Sage.

Alchin, L.K. (2009) Nursery rhymes lyrics and origins (www.rhymes.org.uk; retrieved 12 February 2011).

Alderson, A. and Morrow, V. (2004) *Ethics, Social Research and Consulting with Children and Young People*. Ilford, Essex: Barnardo's.

Anderson, N.B., Bennett Johnson, S., Belar, C.D., Breckler, S.J., Nordal, K.C., Ballard, D. and Kelley, K. (2010) Stress in America™: our health at risk. American Psychological Association (www.stressinamerica.org; retrieved 27 March, 2012).

Andre, M., Hedin, K., Hakansson, A., Molstad, S., Rodhe, N. and Petersson, C. (2007) More physician consultations and antibiotic prescriptions in families with high concern about infectious illness: adequate response to infection-prone child or self-fulfilling prophecy? *Family Practice*, 24(4): 302–7.

Andrews, K.R., Silk, K.S. and Eneli, I.U. (2010) Parents as health promoters: a theory of planned behavior perspective on the prevention of childhood obesity. *Journal of Health Communication*, 15(1): 95–107.

Antonucci, T.C. (1985) Social support: theoretical advances, recent findings and pressing issues. In I.G. Sarason and B.R. Sarason (eds), *Social Support:*

Theory, Research and Applications. Lancaster: Martinus Nijhoff. pp. 21–37.

Appleton, A.A., Buka, S.L., McCormick, M.C., Koenen, K.C., Loucks, E.B., Gilman, S.E. and Kubzansky, L.D. (2011) Emotional functioning at age 7 years is associated with C-reactive protein in middle adulthood. *Psychosomatic Medicine*, 73(4): 295–303.

Armitage, C.J. and Sprigg, C.A. (2010) The roles of behavioral and implementation intentions in changing physical activity in young children with low socioeconomic status. *Journal of Sport and Exercise Psychology*, 32(3): 359–76.

Ashman, S.B., Dawson, G., Panagiotides, H., Yamada, E. and Wilkinson, C.W. (2002) Stress hormone levels of children of depressed mothers. *Development and Psychopathology*, 14(2): 333–49.

Askelson, N.M., Campo, S., Lowe, J.B., Dennis, L.K., Smith, S. and Andsager, J. (2010) Factors related to physicians' willingness to vaccinate girls against HPV: the importance of subjective norms and perceived behavioral control. *Women and Health*, 50(2): 144–58.

Aujoulat, I., Simonelli, F. and Deccache, A. (2006) Health promotion needs of children and adolescents in hospitals: a review. *Patient Education and Counseling*, 61(1): 23–32.

Ayers, S., Joseph, S., McKenzie-McHarg, K., Slade, P. and Wijma, K. (2008) Post-traumatic stress disorder following childbirth: current issues and recommendations for future research. *Journal of Psychosomatic Obstetrics and Gynecology*, 29(4): 240–50.

Ball, T.M., Holberg, C.J., Aldous, M.B., Martinez, F.D. and Wright, A.L. (2002) Influence of attendance at day care on the common cold from birth through 13 years of age. *Archives of Pediatrics and Adolescent Medicine*, 156(2): 121–6.

Banks, P., Cogan, N., Riddell, S., Deeley, S., Hill, M. and Tisdall, K. (2002) Does the covert nature of caring prohibit the development of effective services for young carers? *British Journal of Guidance and Counselling*, 30(3): 229–46.

Barakat, L.P., Schwartz, L.A., Simon, K. and Radcliffe, J. (2007) Negative thinking as a coping strategy mediator of pain and internalizing symptoms in adolescents with sickle cell disease. *Journal of Behavioral Medicine*, 30(3): 199–208.

Barrera, M., Chassin, L. and Rogosch, F. (1993) Effects of social support and conflict on adolescent children of alcoholic and nonalcoholic fathers. *Journal of Personality and Social Psychology*, 64(4): 602–12.

Becker, M.H. (1974) The health belief model and personal health behaviour. *Health Education Monographs*, 2: 324–508.

Becker, M.H. and Maiman, L.A. (1975) Socio-behavioral determinants of compliance with health and medical care recommendations. *Medical Care*, 13: 10–14.

Becker, S. (2000) Young carers. In M. Davies (ed.), *The Blackwell Encyclopedia of Social Work*. Oxford: Blackwell. p. 378.

Becker, S. (2007) Global perspectives on children's unpaid caregiving in the family: research and policy on 'young carers' in the UK, Australia, the USA and sub-Saharan Africa. *Global Social Policy*, 7(1): 23–50.

Becker, S., Aldridge, J. and Dearden, C. (1998) *Young Carers and their Families*. Oxford: Blackwell Sciences.

Belanger, L.J., Plotnikoff, R.C., Clark, A. and Courneya, K.S. (2011) Physical activity and health-related quality of life in young adult cancer survivors: a Canadian provincial survey. *Journal of Cancer Survivorship*, 5(1): 44–53.

Bella, G.P., Garcia, M.C. and Spadari-Bratfisch, R.C. (2011) Salivary cortisol, stress, and health in primary caregivers (mothers) of children with cerebral palsy. *Psychoneuroendocrinology*, 36(6): 834–42.

Biank, N.M. and Werner-Lin, A. (2011) Growing up with grief: revisiting the death of a parent over the life course. *Omega: Journal of Death and Dying*, 63(3): 271–90.

Bibace, R. and Walsh, M.E. (1980) Development of children's concepts of illness. *Pediatrics*, 66(6): 912–17.

Bibace, R., Schmidt, L.R. and Walsh, M.E. (1994) Children's perceptions of illness. In G.N. Penny, P. Bennett and M. Herbert (eds), *Health Psychology: A Lifespan Perspective*. London: Harwood. pp. 13–30.

Black, D. (1976) What happens to bereaved children? *Proceedings of the Royal Society of Medicine*, 69(11): 842–4.

Bogosian, A., Moss-Morris, R. and Hadwin, J. (2010) Psychosocial adjustment in children and adolescents with a parent with multiple sclerosis: a systematic review. *Clinical Rehabilitation*, 24(9): 789–801.

Bolten, M.I., Wurmser, H., Buske-Kirschbaum, A., Papousek, M., Pirke, K.M. and Hellhammer, D. (2011) Cortisol levels in pregnancy as a psychobiological predictor for birth weight. *Archives of Women's Mental Health*, 14(1): 33–41.

Bosquet Enlow, M., Kullowatz, A., Staudenmayer, J., Spasojevic, J., Ritz, T. and Wright, R.J. (2009) Associations of maternal lifetime trauma and perinatal traumatic stress symptoms with infant cardiorespiratory reactivity to psychological challenge. *Psychosomatic Medicine*, 71(6): 607–14.

Boszormenyi-Nagy, I. and Spark, G.M. (1973) *Invisible Loyalties: Reciprocity in Intergenerational Family Therapy*. New York: Harper & Row.

Bovbjerg, D.H. (2003) Conditioning, cancer, and immune regulation. *Brain, Behavior, and Immunity*, 17 Suppl. 1: S58–61.

Bovbjerg, D.H. (2006) The continuing problem of post chemotherapy nausea and vomiting: contributions of classical conditioning. *Autonomic Neuroscience*, 129(1–2): 92–8.

Bowlby, J. (1969) *Attachment and Loss*, vol. 1: *Attachment*. London: The Hogarth Press and the Intstitute of Psychoanalysis.

Boyce, W.T., Adams, S., Tschann, J.M., Cohen, F., Wara, D. and Gunnar, M.R. (1995) Adrenocortical and behavioral predictors of immune responses to starting school. *Pediatric Research*, 38(6): 1009–17.

Boyce, W.T., Chesney, M., Alkon, A., Tschann, J.M., Adams, S., Chesterman, B. and Wara, D. (1995) Psychobiologic reactivity to stress and childhood respiratory illnesses: results of two prospective studies. *Psychosomatic Medicine*, 57(5): 411–22.

Boyle, C.A., Boulet, S., Schieve, L.A., Cohen, R.A., Blumberg, S.J., Yeargin-Allsopp, M. and Kogan, M.D. (2011) Trends in the prevalence of developmental disabilities in US children, 1997–2008. *Pediatrics*, 127(6): 1034–42.

Bracchitta, K.M. (2006) Factors influencing parental use of booster seats for their children. *Journal of Clinical Psychology in Medical Settings*, 13(3): 273–84.

Brand, S.R., Engel, S.M., Canfield, R.L. and Yehuda, R. (2006) The effect of maternal PTSD following *in utero* trauma exposure on behavior and temperament in the 9-month-old infant. *Annals of the New York Academy of Sciences*, 1071: 454–8.

Braveman, P. and Barclay, C. (2009) Health disparities beginning in childhood: a life-course perspective. *Pediatrics*, 124 (Suppl. 3): S163–75.

Bray, J.H. (2010) The future of psychology practice and science. *American Psychologist*, 65(5): 355–69.

Brewer, J.D. and Sparkes, A.C. (2011) Young people living with parental bereavement: insights from an ethnographic study of a UK childhood bereavement service. *Social Science and Medicine*, 72(2): 283–90.

Brook, C. and Marshall, N. (2001) *Essential Endocrinology*, 4th edn. Oxford: Blackwell Science.

Brown, D.F. and Moerenhout, R.G. (1991) The pain experience and psychological adjustment to orthodontic treatment of preadolescents, adolescents, and adults. *American Journal of Orthodontics and Dentofacial Orthopedics*, 100(4): 349–56.

Brown, J.A.C. (1972) *Freud and the Post-Freudians*. Harmondsworth, Middlesex: Penguin.

Brown, R.T., Wiener, L., Kupst, M.J., Brennan, T., Behrman, R., Compas, B.E. and Zeltzer, L. (2008) Single parents of children with chronic illness: an understudied phenomenon. *Journal of Pediatric Psychology*, 33(4): 408–21.

Bruce, J., Davis, E.P. and Gunnar, M.R. (2002) Individual differences in children's cortisol response to the beginning of a new school year. *Psychoneuroendocrinology*, 27(6): 635–50.

Buchbinder, D., Casillas, J., Krull, K.R., Goodman, P., Leisenring, W., Recklitis, C. and Zeltzer, L.K. (2011) Psychological outcomes of siblings of cancer survivors: a report from the Childhood Cancer Survivor Study. *Psychooncology*, 20(12): 1259–68.

Buenaver, L.F., Edwards, R.R. and Haythornthwaite, J.A. (2007) Pain-related catastrophizing and perceived social responses: inter-relationships in the context of chronic pain. *Pain*, 127(3): 234–42.

Bugental, D.B., Martorell, G.A. and Barraza, V. (2003) The hormonal costs of subtle forms of infant maltreatment. *Hormones and Behavior*, 43(1): 237–44.

Buitelaar, J.K., Huizink, A.C., Mulder, E.J., Robles de Medina, P.G. and Visser, G.H.A. (2003) Prenatal stress and cognitive development and temperament in infants. *Neurobiology of Aging*, 24 (Suppl. 1): S53–60.

Buske-Kirschbaum, A. (2009) Cortisol responses to stress in allergic children: interaction with the immune response. *Neuroimmunomodulation*, 16(5): 325–32.

Buske-Kirschbaum, A., Jobst, S., Wustmans, A., Kirschbaum, C., Rauh, W. and Hellhammer, D. (1997) Attenuated free cortisol response to psychosocial stress in children with atopic dermatitis. *Psychosomatic Medicine*, 59(4): 419–26.

Buske-Kirschbaum, A., von Auer, K., Krieger, S., Weis, S., Rauh, W. and Hellhammer, D. (2003) Blunted cortisol responses to psychosocial stress in asthmatic children: a general feature of atopic disease? *Psychosomatic Medicine*, 65(5): 806–10.

Buss, C., Davis, E.P., Muftuler, L.T., Head, K. and Sandman, C.A. (2010) High pregnancy anxiety during mid-gestation is associated with decreased gray matter density in 6–9-year-old children. *Psychoneuroendocrinology*, 35(1): 141–53.

Butler, A.H. and Astbury, G. (2005) The caring child: an evaluative case study of the Cornwall Young Carers project. *Children and Society*, 19: 292–303.

Caes, L., Vervoort, T., Eccleston, C., Vandenhende, M. and Goubert, L. (2011) Parental catastrophizing about child's pain and its relationship with activity restriction: the mediating role of parental distress. *Pain*, 152(1): 212–22.

Campbell, L.K., Scaduto, M., Van Slyke, D., Niarhos, F., Whitlock, J.A. and Compas, B.E. (2009) Executive function, coping, and behavior in survivors of childhood acute lymphocytic leukemia. *Journal of Pediatric Psychology*, 34(3): 317–27.

Cannon, W.B. (1929) *Bodily Changes in Pain, Hunger, Fear and Rage: An Account of Recent Researches into the Function of Emotional Excitement*, 2nd edn. New York: D. Appleton.

Carpenter, L.L., Shattuck, T.T., Tyrka, A.R., Geracioti, T.D. and Price, L.H. (2011) Effect of childhood physical abuse on cortisol stress response. *Psychopharmacology (Berl)*, 214(1): 367–75.

Carrion, V.G., Weems, C.F., Ray, R.D., Glaser, B., Hessl, D. and Reiss, A.L. (2002) Diurnal salivary cortisol in pediatric posttraumatic stress disorder. *Biological Psychiatry*, 51(7): 575–82.

CDC (Center for Disease Control and Prevention) (2010) Report: Child Health. (www.cdc.gov/nchs/fastats/children.htm; retrieved 8 June 2012).

Chase, N.D. (1999) *Burdened Children: Theory, Research and Treatment of Parentification*. Thousand Oaks, CA: Sage.

Chryssanthopoulou, C.C., Turner-Cobb, J.M., Lucas, A. and Jessop, D. (2005) Childcare as a stabilizing influence on HPA axis functioning: a reevaluation of maternal occupational patterns and familial relations. *Developmental Psychobiology*, 47(4): 354–68.

Cicchetti, D. (2010) Resilience under conditions of extreme stress: a multilevel perspective. *World Psychiatry*, 9(3): 145–54.

Cicchetti, D. and Rogosch, F.A. (2001) The impact of child maltreatment and psychopathology on neuroendocrine functioning. *Development and Psychopathology*, 13(4): 783–804.

Claar, R.L., Baber, K.F., Simons, L.E., Logan, D.E. and Walker, L.S. (2008) Pain coping profiles in adolescents with chronic pain. *Pain*, 140(2): 368–75.

Clanton, N.R., Klosky, J.L., Li, C., Jain, N., Srivastava, D.K., Mulrooney, D. and Krull, K.R. (2011) Fatigue, vitality, sleep, and neurocognitive functioning in adult survivors of childhood cancer: a report from the childhood cancer survivor study. *Cancer* (EPub: 13 April 2011).

Clarke, S.A. and Eiser, C. (2007) Health behaviours in childhood cancer survivors: a systematic review. *European Journal of Cancer*, 43(9): 1373–84.

Clarke, S.A., Davies, H., Jenney, M., Glaser, A. and Eiser, C. (2005) Parental communication and children's behaviour following diagnosis of childhood leukaemia. *Psychooncology*, 14(4): 274–81.

Clarke, S.A., Eiser, C. and Skinner, R. (2008) Health-related quality of life in survivors of BMT for paediatric malignancy: a systematic review of the literature. *Bone Marrow Transplant*, 42(2): 73–82.

Clarke, S.A., Sheppard, L. and Eiser, C. (2008) Mothers' explanations of communicating past health and future risks to survivors of childhood cancer. *Clinical Child Psychology and Psychiatry*, 13(1): 157–70.

Class, Q.A., Lichtenstein, P., Langstrom, N. and D'Onofrio, B.M. (2011) Timing of prenatal maternal exposure to severe life events and adverse pregnancy outcomes: a population study of 2.6 million pregnancies. *Psychosomatic Medicine*, 73(3): 234–41.

Clay, R.A. (2011) Stressed in America. *Monitor on Psychology*, 42: 60–3.

Clinch, J. and Eccleston, C. (2009) Chronic musculoskeletal pain in children: assessment and management. *Rheumatology (Oxford)*, 48(5): 466–74.

Clow, A., Thorn, L., Evans, P. and Hucklebridge, F. (2004) The awakening cortisol response: methodological issues and significance. *Stress: The International Journal on the Biology of Stress*, 7: 29–37.

Cobb, J.M. and Steptoe, A. (1996) Psychosocial stress and susceptibility to upper respiratory tract illness in an adult population sample. *Psychosomatic Medicine*, 58: 404–12.

Coddington, R.D. (1972) The significance of life events as etiologic factors in the diseases of children. *Journal of Psychosomatic Research*, 16: 205–13.

Coe, C.L. and Lubach, G.R. (2003) Critical periods of special health relevance for psychoneuroimmunology. *Brain, Behavior, and Immunity*, 17(1): 3–12.

Cohen, L.L., Vowles, K.E. and Eccleston, C. (2010) The impact of adolescent chronic pain on functioning: disentangling the complex role of anxiety. *Journal of Pain*, 11(11): 1039–46.

Cohen, S. and Herbert, T.B. (1996) Health psychology: psychological factors and physical disease from the perspective of human psychoneuroimmunology. *Annual Review of Psychology*, 47: 113–42.

Cohen, S. and Williamson, G. (1991) Stress and infectious disease in humans. *Psychological Bulletin*, 109: 5–24.

Cohen, S., Kamarck, T. and Mermelstein, R. (1983) A global measure of perceived stress. *Journal of Health and Social Behavior*, 24(4): 385–96.

Cohen, S., Tyrrell, D. and Smith, A.P. (1991) Psychological stress and susceptibility to the common cold. *New England Journal of Medicine*, 325(9): 606–12.

Colville, G. (2012) Paediatric intensive care. *The Psychologist*, 25(3): 206–9.

Comeaux, S.J. and Jaser, S.S. (2010) Autonomy and insulin in adolescents with type 1 diabetes. *Pediatric Diabetes*, 11(7): 498–504.

Compas, B.E. (2006) Psychobiological processes of stress and coping: implications for resilience in children and adolescents – comments on the papers of Romeo and McEwen and Fisher et al. *Annals of the New York Academy of Sciences*, 1094: 226–34.

Compas, B.E., Connor, J., Osowiecki, D. and Welch, A. (1997) Effortful and involuntary responses to stress: implications for coping with chronic stress. In B.H. Gottlieb (ed.), *Coping with Chronic Stress*. New York: Plenum Press. pp. 105–30.

Compas, B.E., Connor-Smith, J.K., Saltzman, H., Thomsen, A.H. and Wadsworth, M.E. (2001) Coping with stress during childhood and adolescence: problems, progress, and potential in theory and research. *Psychological Bulletin*, 127(1): 87–127.

Compas, B.E., Jaser, S.S., Dunn, M.J. and Rodriguez, E.M. (2012) Coping with chronic illness in childhood and adolescence. *Annual Review of Clinical Psychology*, 8: 455–80.

Connor-Smith, J.K., Compas, B.E., Wadsworth, M.E., Thomsen, A.H. and Saltzman, H. (2000) Responses to stress in adolescence: measurement of coping and involuntary stress responses. *Journal of Consulting and Clinical Psychology*, 68(6): 976–92.

Coyne, I. (2006) Children's experiences of hospitalization. *Journal of Child Health Care*, 10(4): 326–36.

Coyne, I. (2007) Disruption of parent participation: nurses' strategies to manage parents on children's wards. *Journal of Clinical Nursing*, 17: 3150–8.

Crandall, M., Kools, S., Miaskowski, C. and Savedra, M. (2007) Adolescents' pain experiences following acute blunt traumatic injury: struggle for internal control. *Journal for Specialists in Pediatric Nursing*, 12(4): 224–37.

Crandall, M., Lammers, C., Senders, C. and Braun, J.V. (2009) Children's tonsillectomy experiences: influencing factors. *Journal of Child Health Care*, 13(4): 308–21.

Creswell, J.W. (2009) *Research Design: Qualitative, Quantitative, and Mixed Methods Approaches*. London: Sage.

Crom, D.B. (2009) 'I think you are pretty; I don't know why everyone can't see that': reflections from a young adult brain tumor survivor camp. *Journal of Clinical Oncology*, 27(19): 3259–61.

Crom, D.B., Lensing, S.Y., Rai, S.N., Snider, M.A., Cash, D.K. and Hudson, M.M. (2007) Marriage, employment, and health insurance in adult survivors of childhood cancer. *Journal of Cancer Survivorship*, 1(3): 237–45.

Dahl, R.E. (2004) Adolescent brain development: a period of vulnerabilities and opportunities. Keynote address. *Annals of the New York Academy of Sciences*, 1021: 1–22.

Dahl, R.E. and Gunnar, M.R. (2009) Heightened stress responsiveness and emotional reactivity during pubertal maturation: implications for psychopathology. *Development and Psychopathology*, 21(1): 1–6.

D'Anna-Hernandez, K.L., Ross, R.G., Natvig, C.L. and Laudenslager, M.L. (2011) Hair cortisol levels as a retrospective marker of hypothalamic-pituitary axis activity throughout pregnancy: comparison to salivary cortisol. *Physiology and Behavior*, 104(2): 348–53.

Davies, R., Davis, B. and Sibert, J. (2003) Parents' stories of sensitive and insensitive care by paediatricians in the time leading up to and including diagnostic disclosure of a life-limiting condition in their child. *Child: Care, Health and Development*, 29(1): 77–82.

Davis, E.P., Donzella, B., Krueger, W.K. and Gunnar, M.R. (1999) The start of a new school year: individual differences in salivary cortisol response in relation to child temperament. *Developmental Psychobiology*, 35(3): 188–96.

Davis, E.P., Glynn, L.M., Schetter, C.D., Hobel, C., Chicz-Demet, A. and Sandman, C.A. (2007) Prenatal exposure to maternal depression and cortisol influences infant temperament. *Journal of the American Academy of Child and Adolescent Psychiatry*, 46(6): 737–46.

Davis, E.P. and Granger, D.A. (2009) Developmental differences in infant salivary alpha-amylase and cortisol responses to stress. *Psychoneuroendocrinology*, 34(6): 795–804.

Davis, E.P. and Sandman, C.A. (2010) The timing of prenatal exposure to maternal cortisol and psychosocial stress is associated with human infant cognitive development. *Child Development*, 81(1): 131–48.

Davis, E.P., Glynn, L.M., Waffarn, F. and Sandman, C.A. (2011) Prenatal maternal stress programs infant stress regulation. *Journal of Child Psychology and Psychiatry*, 52(2): 119–29.

Dawkins, R. (2006) *The God Delusion*. London: Bantam Press.

De Vriendt, T., Moreno, L.A. and De Henauw, S. (2009) Chronic stress and obesity in adolescents: scientific evidence and methodological issues for epidemiological research. *Nutrition, Metabolism and Cardiovascular Diseases*, 19(7): 511–19.

de Weerth, C. and Buitelaar, J.K. (2005) Physiological stress reactivity in human pregnancy: a review. *Neuroscience and Biobehavioral Reviews*, 29(2): 295–312.

de Weerth, C., van Hees, Y. and Buitelaar, J.K. (2003) Prenatal maternal cortisol levels and infant behavior during the first 5 months. *Early Human Development*, 74(2): 139–51.

Dearden, C. and Becker, S. (2004) *Young Carers in the UK: The 2004 Report*. London: Carers UK.

Deinzer, R., Kleineidam, C., Stiller Winkler, R., Idel, H. and Bachg, D. (2000) Prolonged reduction of salivary immunoglobulin A (sIgA) after major academic exam. *International Journal of Psychophysiology*, 37(3): 219–32.

Descartes, R. (1984) *A Discourse on Method*. London: J.M. Dent & Sons Ltd.

Detillion, C.E., Craft, T.K.S., Glasper, E.R., Prendergast, B.J. and DeVries, A.C. (2004) Social facilitation of wound healing. *Psychoneuroendocrinology*, 29(8): 1004–11.

Dettling, A.C., Parker, S.W., Lane, S., Sebanc, A. and Gunnar, M.R. (2000) Quality of care and temperament determine changes in cortisol concentrations over the day for young children in childcare. *Psychoneuroendocrinology*, 25(8): 819–36.

Devine, K.A., Reed-Knight, B., Loiselle, K.A., Fenton, N. and Blount, R.L. (2010) Posttraumatic growth in young adults who experienced serious childhood illness: a mixed-methods approach. *Journal of Clinical Psychology in Medical Settings*, 17(4): 340–8.

Dhabhar, F.S. and McEwen, B.S. (1997) Acute stress enhances while chronic stress suppresses cell-mediated immunity *in vivo*: a potential role for leukocyte trafficking. *Brain, Behavior, and Immunity*, 11(4): 286–306.

Dhabhar, F.S., Saul, A.N., Daugherty, C., Holmes, T.H., Bouley, D.M. and Oberyszyn, T.M. (2010) Short-term stress enhances cellular immunity and increases early resistance to squamous cell carcinoma. *Brain, Behavior, and Immunity*, 24(1): 127–37.

Di Gioia, C., Bracceschi, R., Copioli, C., Piccolo, B., Ziliani, P., Pisani, F. and Bevilacqua, G. (2011) Care to relieve pain-stress in preterm newborns. *Acta Bio Medica*, 82(1): 20–5.

Diamond, A., Barnett, W.S., Thomas, J. and Munro, S. (2007) Preschool program improves cognitive control. *Science*, 318(5855): 1387–8.

Dickerson, S.S. and Kemeny, M.E. (2004) Acute stressors and cortisol responses: a theoretical integration and synthesis of laboratory research. *Psychological Bulletin*, 130(3): 355–91.

Dickerson, S.S., Gruenewald, T.L. and Kemeny, M.E. (2009) Psychobiological responses to social self threat: functional or detrimental? *Self and Identity*, 8(2–3): 270–85.

DiClemente, C.C. and Prochaska, J.O. (1982) Self-change and therapy change of smoking behavior: a comparison of processes of change in cessation and maintenance. *Addictive Behaviors*, 7(2): 133–42.

Dobbs, D. (2005) Fact or phrenology? *Scientific American Mind*, 16(1): 24–31.

Doug, M., Adi, Y., Williams, J., Paul, M., Kelly, D., Petchey, R. and Carter, Y.H. (2011) Transition to adult services for children and young people with palliative care needs: a systematic review. *Archives of Disease in Childhood*, 96(1): 78–84.

Dowling, A.S. (2005) George Engel, M.D. (1913–1999). *American Journal of Psychiatry*, 162(11): 2039.

Dowling, E., Yabroff, K.R., Mariotto, A., McNeel, T., Zeruto, C. and Buckman, D. (2010) Burden of illness in adult survivors of childhood cancers: findings from a population-based national sample. *Cancer*, 116(15): 3712–21.

Dreger, L.C., Kozyrskyj, A.L., HayGlass, K.T., Becker, A.B. and MacNeil, B.J. (2010) Lower cortisol levels in children with asthma exposed to recurrent maternal distress from birth. *Journal of Allergy and Clinical Immunology*, 125(1): 116–22.

Dubé, E., Bettinger, J.A., Halperin, B., Bradet, R., Lavoie, F., Sauvageau, C., Gilca, V. and Boulianne, N. (2012) Determinants of parents' decision to vaccinate their children against rotavirus: results of a longitudinal study. *Health Education Research*, 27(6): 1069–80.

Dube, S.R., Fairweather, D., Pearson, W.S., Felitti, V.J., Anda, R.F. and Croft, J.B. (2009) Cumulative childhood stress and autoimmune diseases in adults. *Psychosomatic Medicine*, 71(2): 243–50.

Dubow, E.F. and Ullman, D.G. (1989) Assessing social support in elementary school children: the survey of children's social support. *Journal of Clinical Child Psychology*, 18: 52–64.

Duff, A.J., Gaskell, S.L., Jacobs, K. and Houghton, J.M. (2012) Management of distressing procedures in children and young people: time to adhere to the guidelines. *Archives of Disease in Childhood*, 97(1): 1–4.

Dufton, L.M., Dunn, M.J., Slosky, L.S. and Compas, B.E. (2011) Self-reported and laboratory-based responses to stress in children with recurrent pain and anxiety. *Journal of Pediatric Psychology*, 36(1): 95–105.

Dunn, M.J., Rodriguez, E.M., Barnwell, A.S., Grossenbacher, J.C., Vannatta, K., Gerhardt, C.A. and Compas, B.E. (2012) Posttraumatic stress symptoms in parents of children with cancer within six months of diagnosis. *Health Psychology*, 31(2): 176–85.

Earle, E.A., Clarke, S.A., Eiser, C. and Sheppard, L. (2006) 'Building a new normality': mothers' experiences of caring for a child with acute lymphoblastic leukaemia. *Child: Care, Health and Development*, 33(2): 155–60.

Eccleston, C., Jordan, A., McCracken, L.M., Sleed, M., Connell, H. and Clinch, J. (2005) The Bath Adolescent Pain Questionnaire (BAPQ): development and preliminary psychometric evaluation of an instrument to assess the impact of chronic pain on adolescents. *Pain*, 118(1–2): 263–70.

Eccleston, C., Jordan, A.L. and Crombez, G. (2006) The impact of chronic pain on adolescents: a review of previously used measures. *Journal of Pediatric Psychology*, 31(7): 684–97.

Eccleston, C., Palermo, T.M., Williams, A.C., Lewandowski, A. and Morley, S. (2009) Psychological therapies for the management of chronic and recurrent pain in children and adolescents. *Cochrane Database Syst Rev*(2): CD003968.

Ehrenreich, B. (2009) *Smile or Die: How Positive Thinking Fooled America and the World*. London: Granta.

Eiser, C. (1989) Coping with chronic childhood diseases: implications for counselling children and adolescents. *Counselling Psychology Quarterly*, 2(3): 323–36.

Eiser, C. (1990) *Chronic Childhood Disease: An Introduction to Psychological Theory and Research*. Cambridge: Cambridge University Press.

Eiser, C. (2004) *Children with Cancer: The Quality of Life*. New Jersey: Lawrence Erlbaum.

Eiser, C. (2007) Beyond survival: quality of life and follow-up after childhood cancer. *Journal of Pediatric Psychology*, 32(9): 1140–50.

Eiser, C. and Patterson, D. (1983) Slugs and snails and puppy-dog tails: children's ideas about the inside of their bodies. *Child: Care, Health and Development*, 9(4): 233–40.

Eiser, C., Patterson, D. and Eiser, J.R. (1983) Children's knowledge of health and illness: implications for health-education. *Child: Care, Health and Development*, 9(5): 285–92.

Eiser, C., Hill, J.J. and Blacklay, A. (2000) Surviving cancer: what does it mean for you? An evaluation of a clinic based intervention for survivors of childhood cancer. *Psychooncology*, 9(3): 214–20.

Eiser, C., Eiser, J.R. and Greco, V. (2004) Surviving childhood cancer: quality of life and parental regulatory focus. *Personality and Social Psychology Bulletin*, 30(2): 123–33.

Eiser, C., Absolom, K., Greenfield, D., Glaser, A., Horne, B., Waite, H. and Davies, H. (2006) Follow-up after childhood cancer: evaluation of a three-level model. *European Journal of Cancer*, 42(18): 3186–90.

Elborn, J.S., Shale, D.J. and Britton, J.R. (1991) Cystic fibrosis: current survival and population estimates to the year 2000. *Thorax*, 46(12): 881–5.

Elliott, G.R. and Eisdorfer, C. (eds) (1982) *Stress and Human Health*. New York: Springer-Verlag.

Ellman, L.M., Schetter, C.D., Hobel, C.J., Chicz-Demet, A., Glynn, L.M. and Sandman, C.A. (2008) Timing of fetal exposure to stress hormones: effects on newborn physical and neuromuscular maturation. *Developmental Psychobiology*, 50(3): 232–41.

Engel, G.L. (1977) The need for a new medical model: a challenge for biomedicine. *Science*, 196(4286): 129–36.

Engel, G.L., Reichsman, F.K. and Viederman, M. (1979) Monica: a 25-year longitudinal study of the consequences of trauma in infancy. *Journal of the American Psychoanalytic Association*, 27(1): 107–26.

Entringer, S., Buss, C., Andersen, J., Chicz-Demet, A. and Wadhwa, P.D. (2011) Ecological momentary assessment of maternal cortisol profiles over a multiple-day period predicts the length of human gestation. *Psychosomatic Medicine*, 73(6): 469–74.

Evans, P., Hucklebridge, F. and Clow, A. (2000) *Mind, Immunity and Health*. London: Free Association Books.

Exton, M.S., King, M.G. and Husband, A.J. (1999) Behavioral conditioning of immunity. In M. Schedlowski and U. Tewes (eds), *Psychoneuroimmunology: An Interdisciplinary Introduction*. New York: Kluwer Academic/Plenum. pp. 443–52.

Exton, M.S., von Auer, A.K., Buske-Kirschbaum, A., Stockhorst, U., Gobel, U. and Schedlowski, M. (2000) Pavlovian conditioning of immune function: animal investigation and the challenge of human application. *Behavioural Brain Research*, 110(1–2): 129–41.

Federenko, I., Wust, S., Hellhammer, D.H., Dechoux, R., Kumsta, R. and Kirschbaum, C. (2004) Free cortisol awakening responses are influenced by awakening time. *Psychoneuroendocrinology*, 29(2): 174–84.

Fink, N.S., Urech, C., Isabel, F., Meyer, A., Hoesli, I., Bitzer, J. and Alder, J. (2011) Fetal response to abbreviated relaxation techniques: a randomized controlled study. *Early Human Development*, 87(2): 121–7.

Fishbein, M. (1967) Attitude and the prediction of behavior. In M. Fishbein (ed.), *Readings in Attitude Theory and Measurement*. New York: Wiley. pp. 477–92.

Fishbein, M. (1980) A theory of reasoned action: some applications and implications. *Nebraska Symposium on Motivation*, 27: 65–116.

Fishbein, M. (2008) A reasoned action approach to health promotion. *Medical Decision Making*, 28(6): 834–44.

Flinn, M.V. and England, B.G. (1997) Social economics of childhood glucocorticoid stress response and health. *American Journal of Physical Anthropology*, 102(1): 33–53.

Folkman, S. (1997) Positive psychological states and coping with severe stress. *Social Science and Medicine*, 45(8): 1207–21.

Forsner, M., Jansson, L. and Sørlie, V. (2005a) Being ill as narrated by children aged 11–18 years. *Journal of Child Health Care*, 9(4): 314–23.

Forsner, M., Jansson, L. and Sørlie, V. (2005b) The experience of being ill as narrated by hospitalized children aged 7–10 years with short-term illness. *Journal of Child Health Care*, 9(2): 153–65.

Fowler, A., Stodberg, T., Eriksson, M. and Wickstrom, R. (2010) Long-term outcomes of acute encephalitis in childhood. *Pediatrics*, 126(4): e828–35.

Francis, R.D. (2009) *Ethics for Psychologists*, 2nd edn. Chichester: BPS Blackwell.

Francis, S.J., Walker, R.F., Riad-Fahmy, D., Hughes, D., Murphy, J.F. and Gray, O.P. (1987) Assessment of adrenocortical activity in term newborn infants using salivary cortisol determinations. *Journal of Pediatrics*, 111(1): 129–33.

Frank, J. (1995) *Couldn't Care More: A Study of Young Carers and their Needs*. London: The Children's Society.

Frank, J. and McLarnon, J. (2008) *Young Carers, Parents and their Families: Key Principles of Practice*. London: The Children's Society.

Frank, J., Tatum, C. and Tucker, S. (1999) *On Small Shoulders: Learning from the Experiences of Former Young Carers*. London: The Children's Society.

Friedrichsdorf, S.J. and Kang, T.I. (2007) The management of pain in children with life-limiting illnesses. *Pediatric Clinics of North America*, 54(5): 645–72.

Frobisher, C., Winter, D.L., Lancashire, E.R., Reulen, R.C., Taylor, A.J., Eiser, C. and Hawkins, M.M.

(2008) Extent of smoking and age at initiation of smoking among adult survivors of childhood cancer in Britain. *Journal of the National Cancer Institute*, 100(15): 1068–81.

Gaffney, A., McGrath, P.J. and Dick, B. (2003) Measuring pain in children: developmental and instrument issues. In N.L. Schechter, C.B. Berde and M. Yaster (eds), *Pain in Infants, Children and Adolescents*. Philadelphia: Lippincott Williams & Wilkins. pp. 130–41.

Gallagher, S., Phillips, A.C., Drayson, M.T. and Carroll, D. (2009) Parental caregivers of children with developmental disabilities mount a poor antibody response to pneumococcal vaccination. *Brain, Behavior, and Immunity*, 23(3): 338–46.

Gallagher, S., Phillips, A.C., Ferraro, A.J., Drayson, M.T. and Carroll, D. (2008) Social support is positively associated with the immunoglobulin M response to vaccination with pneumococcal polysaccharides. *Biological Psychology*, 78(2): 211–15.

Gaskell, S. (2010) Evidence-based guidelines for the management of invasive and/or distressing procedures with children. Position paper. Leicester: British Psychological Society.

Gatchel, R.J., Peng, Y.B., Peters, M.L., Fuchs, P.N. and Turk, D.C. (2007) The biopsychosocial approach to chronic pain: scientific advances and future directions. *Psychological Bulletin*, 133(4): 581–624.

Gauntlett-Gilbert, J. and Eccleston, C. (2007) Disability in adolescents with chronic pain: patterns and predictors across different domains of functioning. *Pain*, 131(1–2): 132–41.

Gehring, T.M. and Wyler, I.L. (1986) Family-system-test (fast): a 3-dimensional approach to investigate family relationships. *Child Psychiatry and Human Development*, 16(4): 235–48.

Gil, K.M., Thompson, R.J., Keith, B.R., Totafaucette, M., Noll, S. and Kinney, T.R. (1993) Sickle-cell disease pain in children and adolescents: change in pain frequency and coping strategies over time. *Journal of Pediatric Psychology*, 18(5): 621–37.

Gil, K.M., Phillips, G., Edens, J., Martin, N.J. and Abrams, M. (1994) Observation of pain behaviors during episodes of sickle cell disease pain. *Clinical Journal of Pain*, 10(2): 128–32.

Gil, K.M., Carson, J.W., Porter, L.S., Ready, J., Valrie, C., Redding-Lallinger, R. and Daeschner, C. (2003) Daily stress and mood and their association with pain, health-care use, and school activity in adolescents with sickle cell disease. *Journal of Pediatric Psychology*, 28(5): 363–73.

Gill, T. (2007) *No Fear: Growing Up in a Risk Averse Society*. London: Calouste Gulbenkian Foundation.

Gillies, M.L., Smith, L.N. and Parry-Jones, W.L. (2001) Postoperative pain: a comparison of adolescent inpatient and day patient experiences. *International Journal of Nursing Studies*, 38(3): 329–337.

Glaser, R., Pearson, G.R., Bonneau, R.H., Esterling, B.A., Atkinson, C. and Kiecolt-Glaser, J.K. (1993) Stress and the memory T-cell response to the Epstein-Barr virus in healthy medical students. *Health Psychology*, 12(6): 435–42.

Glover, J. (2009) *Bouncing Back: How Can Resilience be Promoted in Vulnerable Children and Young People?* Ilford, Essex: Barnardo's.

Glover, V., Bergman, K., Sarkar, P. and O'Connor, T.G. (2009) Association between maternal and amniotic fluid cortisol is moderated by maternal anxiety. *Psychoneuroendocrinology*, 34(3): 430–5.

Goedhart, G., Vrijkotte, T.G., Roseboom, T.J., van der Wal, M.F., Cuijpers, P. and Bonsel, G.J. (2010) Maternal cortisol and offspring birthweight: results from a large prospective cohort study. *Psychoneuroendocrinology*, 35(5): 644–52.

Goldacre, B. (2008) *Bad Science*. London: Fourth Estate.

Gollwitzer, P.M. and Oettingen, G. (1998) The emergence and implementation of health goals. *Psychology and Health*, 13: 687–715.

Gore-Felton, C. and Koopman, C. (2008) Behavioral mediation of the relationship between psychosocial factors and HIV disease progression. *Psychosomatic Medicine*, 70(5): 569–74.

Grandgeorge, M. and Hausberger, M. (2011) Human–animal relationships: from daily life to animal-assisted therapies. *Annali dell'Istituto Superiore di Sanità*, 47(4): 397–408.

Granger, D.A., Kivlighan, K.T., el-Sheikh, M., Gordis, E.B. and Stroud, L.R. (2007) Salivary alpha-amylase in biobehavioral research: recent developments and applications. *Annals of the New York Academy of Sciences*, 1098: 122–44.

Green, D.M., Cox, C.L., Zhu, L., Krull, K.R., Srivastava, D.K., Stovall, M. and Robison, L.L. (2012) Risk factors for obesity in adult survivors of childhood cancer: a report from the Childhood Cancer Survivor Study. *Journal of Clinical Oncology*, 30(3): 246–55.

Grodin, M.A. and Glantz, L.H. (1994) *Children as Research Subjects: Science, Ethics and Law*. Oxford: Oxford University Press.

Groschl, M., Rauh, M. and Dorr, H.G. (2003) Circadian rhythm of salivary cortisol, 17alpha-hydroxyprogesterone, and progesterone in healthy children. *Clinical Chemistry*, 49(10): 1688–91.

Guite, J.W., Logan, D.E., Sherry, D.D. and Rose, J.B. (2007) Adolescent self-perception: associations with chronic musculoskeletal pain and functional disability. *Journal of Pain*, 8(5): 379–86.

Gultekin, G. and Baran, G. (2007) A study of the self-concepts of 9–14-year-old children with acute and chronic diseases. *Social Behavior and Personality*, 35(3): 329–38.

Gunnar, M.R. (1992) Reactivity of the hypothalamic-pituitary-adrenocortical system to stressors in normal infants and children. *Pediatrics*, 90(3 pt 2): 491–7.

Gunnar, M.R. and Donzella, B. (2002) Social regulation of the cortisol levels in early human development. *Psychoneuroendocrinology*, 27(1): 199–220.

Gunnar, M.R. and Fisher, P.A. (2006) Bringing basic research on early experience and stress neurobiology to bear on preventive interventions for neglected and maltreated children. *Development and Psychopathology*, 18(3): 651–77.

Gunnar, M.R. and Quevedo, K. (2007) The neurobiology of stress and development. *Annual Review of Psychology*, 58: 145–73.

Gunnar, M.R. and Vazquez, D.M. (2001) Low cortisol and a flattening of expected daytime rhythm: potential indices of risk in human development. *Development and Psychopathology*, 13(3): 515–38.

Gunnar, M.R., Morison, S.J., Chisholm, K. and Schuder, M. (2001) Salivary cortisol levels in children adopted from Romanian orphanages. *Development and Psychopathology*, 13(3): 611–28.

Gunnar, M.R., Sebanc, A.M., Tout, K., Donzella, B., van Dulmen, M.M. (2003) Peer rejection, temperament, and cortisol activity in preschoolers. *Developmental Psychobiology*, 43: 346–58.

Gunnar, M.R., Frenn, K., Wewerka, S.S. and Van Ryzin, M.J. (2009) Moderate versus severe early life stress: associations with stress reactivity and regulation in 10–12-year-old children. *Psychoneuroendocrinology*, 34(1): 62–75.

Gunnar, M.R., Talge, N.M. and Herrera, A. (2009) Stressor paradigms in developmental studies: what does and does not work to produce mean increases in salivary cortisol. *Psychoneuroendocrinology*, 34(7): 953–67.

Gunnar, M.R., Wewerka, S., Frenn, K., Long, J.D. and Griggs, C. (2009) Developmental changes in hypothalamus-pituitary-adrenal activity over the transition to adolescence: normative changes and associations with puberty. *Development and Psychopathology*, 21(1): 69–85.

Gurney, J.G., Krull, K.R., Kadan-Lottick, N., Nicholson, H.S., Nathan, P.C., Zebrack, B. and Ness, K.K. (2009) Social outcomes in the Childhood Cancer Survivor Study cohort. *Journal of Clinical Oncology*, 27(14): 2390–5.

Gutteling, B.M., de Weerth, C. and Buitelaar, J.K. (2005) Prenatal stress and children's cortisol reaction to the first day of school. *Psychoneuroendocrinology*, 30(6): 541–9.

Gutteling, B.M., de Weerth, C., Willemsen-Swinkels, S.H., Huizink, A.C., Mulder, E.J., Visser, G.H. and Buitelaar, J.K. (2005) The effects of prenatal stress on temperament and problem behavior of 27-month-old toddlers. *European Child and Adolescent Psychiatry*, 14(1): 41–51.

Gutteling, B.M., de Weerth, C., Zandbelt, N., Mulder, E.J., Visser, G.H. and Buitelaar, J.K. (2006) Does maternal prenatal stress adversely affect the child's learning and memory at age six? *Journal of Abnormal Child Psychology*, 34(6): 789–98.

Hagan, M.J., Roubinov, D.S., Gress-Smith, J., Luecken, L.J., Sandler, I.N. and Wolchik, S. (2011) Positive parenting during childhood moderates the impact of recent negative events on cortisol activity in parentally bereaved youth. *Psychopharmacology (Berl)*, 214(1): 231–8.

Halligan, S.L., Herbert, J., Goodyer, I.M. and Murray, L. (2004) Exposure to postnatal depression predicts elevated cortisol in adolescent offspring. *Biological Psychiatry*, 55(4): 376–81.

Hamilton, K., Thomson, C.E. and White, K.M. (2013) Promoting active lifestyles in young children: investigating mothers' decisions about their child's physical activity and screen time behaviours. *Maternal and Child Health Journal*, 17(5): 968–76.

Hankin, B.L., Badanes, L.S., Abela, J.R. and Watamura, S.E. (2010) Hypothalamic-pituitary-adrenal axis dysregulation in dysphoric children and adolescents: cortisol reactivity to psychosocial stress from preschool through middle adolescence. *Biological Psychiatry*, 68(5): 484–90.

Harakeh, Z., Scholte, R.H.J., Vermulst, A.A., de Vries, H. and Engels, R.C.M.E. (2004) Parental factors and adolescents' smoking behavior: an extension of the theory of planned behavior. *Preventive Medicine*, 39(5): 951–61.

Harville, E., Xiong, X. and Buekens, P. (2010) Disasters and perinatal health: a systematic review. *Obstetrical and Gynecological Survey*, 65(11): 713–28.

Hatchette, J.E., McGrath, P.J., Murray, M. and Finley, G.A. (2008) The role of peer communication in the socialization of adolescents' pain experiences: a qualitative investigation. *BMC Pediatrics*, 8: 2.

Haupt, R., Spinetta, J.J., Ban, I., Barr, R.D., Beck, J.D., Byrne, J. and Jankovic, M. (2007) Long term survivors of childhood cancer: cure and care. The Erice statement. *European Journal of Cancer*, 43(12): 1778–80.

Hechler, T., Chalkiadis, G.A., Hasan, C., Kosfelder, J., Meyerhoff, U., Vocks, S. and Zernikow, B. (2009) Sex differences in pain intensity in adolescents suffering from cancer: differences in pain memories? *Journal of Pain*, 10(6): 586–93.

Hechler, T., Vervoort, T., Hamann, M., Tietze, A.L., Vocks, S., Goubert, L. and Zernikow, B. (2011) Parental catastrophizing about their child's chronic pain: are mothers and fathers different? *European Journal of Pain*, 15(5): 515.e1–515.e9.

Heim, C., Ehlert, U. and Hellhammer, D.H. (2000) The potential role of hypocortisolism in the pathophysiology of stress-related bodily disorders. *Psychoneuroendocrinology*, 25(1): 1–35.

Hepper, P.G. (1996) Fetal memory: does it exist? What does it do? *Acta Paediatrica Supplement*, 416: 16–20.

Hepper, P.G. (1997) Memory *in utero? Developmental Medicine and Child Neurology*, 39(5): 343–6.

Hermann, C., Hohmeister, J., Demirakca, S., Zohsel, K. and Flor, H. (2006) Long-term alteration of pain sensitivity in school-aged children with early pain experiences. *Pain*, 125(3): 278–85.

Hermann, C., Hohmeister, J., Zohsel, K., Ebinger, F. and Flor, H. (2007) The assessment of pain coping and pain-related cognitions in children and adolescents: current methods and further development. *Journal of Pain*, 8(10): 802–13.

Hermann, C., Hohmeister, J., Zohsel, K., Tuttas, M.L. and Flor, H. (2008) The impact of chronic pain in children and adolescents: development and initial validation of a child and parent version of the Pain Experience Questionnaire. *Pain*, 135(3): 251–61.

Hess, S.L., Johannsdottir, I.M., Hamre, H., Kiserud, C.E., Loge, J.H. and Fossa, S.D. (2011) Adult survivors of childhood malignant lymphoma are not aware of their risk of late effects. *Acta Oncologica*, 50(5): 653–9.

Hewitt, A.M. and Stephens, C. (2007) Healthy eating among 10–13-year-old New Zealand children: understanding choice using the theory of planned behaviour and the role of parental influence. *Psychology, Health and Medicine*, 12(5): 526–35.

Hiemstra, M., Otten, R., van Schayck, O.C. and Engels, R.C. (2012) Smoking-specific communication and children's smoking onset: an extension of the theory of planned behaviour. *Psychology and Health*, 27(9): 1100–17.

Hilgard, J.R. and LeBaron, S. (1982) Relief of anxiety and pain in children and adolescents with cancer: quantitative measures and clinical observations. *International Journal of Clinical and Experimental Hypnosis*, 30(4): 417–42.

Hill, K., Higgins, A., Dempster, M. and McCarthy, A. (2009) Fathers' views and understanding of their roles in families with a child with acute lymphoblastic leukaemia: an interpretative phenomenological analysis. *Journal of Health Psychology*, 14(8): 1268–80.

Himelstein, B.P. (2006) Palliative care for infants, children, adolescents, and their families. *Journal of Palliative Medicine*, 9(1): 163–81.

Himelstein, B.P., Hilden, J.M., Boldt, A.M. and Weissman, D. (2004) Pediatric palliative care. *New England Journal of Medicine*, 350(17): 1752–62.

Hobel, C.J., Dunkel-Schetter, C., Roesch, S.C., Castro, L.C. and Arora, C.P. (1999) Maternal plasma corticotropin-releasing hormone associated with stress at 20 weeks' gestation in pregnancies ending in preterm delivery. *American Journal of Obstetrics and Gynecology*, 180(1 pt 3): S257–63.

Hohmeister, J., Demirakca, S., Zohsel, K., Flor, H. and Hermann, C. (2009) Responses to pain in school-aged children with experience in a neonatal intensive care unit: cognitive aspects and maternal influences. *European Journal of Pain*, 13(1): 94–101.

Holdcroft, A. (2007) Gender bias in research: how does it affect evidence based medicine? *Journal of the Royal Society of Medicine*, 100(1): 2–3.

Holdcroft, A. and Jaggar, S. (eds) (2005) *Core Topics in Pain*. Cambridge: Cambridge University Press.

Holen, S., Lervag, A., Waaktaar, T. and Ystgaard, M. (2012) Exploring the associations between coping patterns for everyday stressors and mental health in young schoolchildren. *Journal of School Psychology*, 50(2): 167–93.

Holland, J.E. (1998) *Psycho-oncology*. New York: Oxford University Press.

Hollins, M., Stonerock, G.L., Kisaalita, N.R., Jones, S., Orringer, E. and Gil, K.M. (2012) Detecting the emergence of chronic pain in sickle cell disease. *Journal of Pain and Symptom Management*, 43(6): 1082–93.

Holmes, T.H. and Rahe, R.H. (1967) The social readjustment rating scale. *Journal of Psychosomatic Research*, 11: 213–18.

House, J.S., Landis, K.R. and Umberson, D. (1988) Social relationships and health. *Science*, 241(4865): 540–5.

Houtzager, B.A., Grootenhuis, M.A., Caron, H.N. and Last, B.F. (2004) Quality of life and psychological adaptation in siblings of paediatric cancer patients, 2 years after diagnosis. *Psychooncology*, 13(8): 499–511.

Hoyle, G. and Anderson, A. (1974) *2010: Living in the Future*. New York: Parents' Magazine Press.

Hudson, M.M., Tyc, V.L., Srivastava, D.K., Gattuso, J., Quargnenti, A., Crom, D.B. and Hinds, P. (2002)

Multi-component behavioral intervention to promote health protective behaviors in childhood cancer survivors: the protect study. *Medical and Pediatric Oncology*, 39(1): 2–1; discussion 2.

Hughes, J.M. and Callery, P. (2004) Parents' experiences of caring for their child following day case surgery: a diary study. *Journal of Child Health Care*, 8(1): 47–58.

Huguet, A., Stinson, J.N. and McGrath, P.J. (2010) Measurement of self-reported pain intensity in children and adolescents. *Journal of Psychosomatic Research*, 68(4): 329–36.

Huizink, A.C., Robles de Medina, P.G., Mulder, E.J., Visser, G.H. and Buitelaar, J.K. (2003) Stress during pregnancy is associated with developmental outcome in infancy. *Journal of Child Psychology and Psychiatry*, 44(6): 810–18.

Hunger, S.P., Lu, X., Devidas, M., Camitta, B.M., Gaynon, P.S., Winick, N.J., Reaman, G.H. and Carroll, W.L. (2012) Improved survival for children and adolescents with acute lymphoblastic leukemia between 1990 and 2005: a report from the children's oncology group. *Journal of Clinical Oncology*, 30(14): 1663–9.

Hunter, A.L., Minnis, H. and Wilson, P. (2011) Altered stress responses in children exposed to early adversity: a systematic review of salivary cortisol studies. *Stress: The International Journal on the Biology of Stress*, 14(6): 614–26.

Hurley, J.C. and Underwood, M.K. (2002) Children's understanding of their research rights before and after debriefing: informed assent, confidentiality, and stopping participation. *Child Development*, 73(1): 132–43.

Ireland, M.J. and Pakenham, K.I. (2010a) The nature of youth care tasks in families experiencing chronic illness/disability: development of the Youth Activities of Caregiving Scale (YACS). *Psychology and Health*, 25(6): 713–31.

Ireland, M.J. and Pakenham, K.I. (2010b) Youth adjustment to parental illness or disability: the role of illness characteristics, caregiving, and attachment. *Psychology, Health and Medicine*, 15(6): 632–45.

Jackson, C., Cheater, F.M. and Reid, I. (2008) A systematic review of decision support needs of parents making child health decisions. *Health Expectations*, 11(3): 232–51.

Jacobs, R.K., Anderson, V.A., Neale, J.L., Shield, L.K. and Kornberg, A.J. (2004) Neuropsychological outcome after acute disseminated encephalomyelitis: impact of age at illness onset. *Pediatric Neurology*, 31(3): 191–7.

Jaggar, S.I. (2005) Overview of pain pathways. In A. Holdcroft and S. Jaggar (eds), *Core Topics in Pain*. Cambridge: Cambridge University Press. pp. 3–5.

Jain, N., Brouwers, P., Okcu, M.F., Cirino, P.T. and Krull, K.R. (2009) Sex-specific attention problems in long-term survivors of pediatric acute lymphoblastic leukemia. *Cancer*, 115(18): 4238–45.

James, A.S., Tripp, M.K., Parcel, G.S., Sweeney, A. and Gritz, E.R. (2002) Psychosocial correlates of sun-protective practices of preschool staff toward their students. *Health Education Research*, 17(3): 305–14.

James, W. (1884) What is emotion? *Mind*, 9: 188–205.

Jansen, J., Beijers, R., Riksen-Walraven, M. and de Weerth, C. (2010) Cortisol reactivity in young infants. *Psychoneuroendocrinology*, 35(3): 329–38.

Janson, C., Leisenring, W., Cox, C., Termuhlen, A.M., Mertens, A.C., Whitton, J.A. and Kadan-Lottick, N.S. (2009) Predictors of marriage and divorce in adult survivors of childhood cancers: a report from the Childhood Cancer Survivor Study. *Cancer Epidemiology, Biomarkers and Prevention*, 18(10): 2626–35.

Jemal, A., Siegel, R., Xu, J. and Ward, E. (2010) Cancer statistics, 2010. *CA: Cancer Journal for Clinicians*, 60(5): 277–300.

Jenkins, S. and Wingate, C. (1994) Who cares for young carers? *British Medical Journal*, 308(6931): 733–4.

Jerrett, M.D. (1985) Children and their pain experience. *Children's Health Care*, 14(2): 83–9.

Jessop, D.S. and Turner-Cobb, J.M. (2008) Measurement and meaning of salivary cortisol: a focus on health and disease in children. *Stress: The International Journal on the Biology of Stress*, 11(1): 1–14.

Johannsdottir, I.M., Hjermstad, M.J., Moum, T., Wesenberg, F., Hjorth, L., Schroder, H. and Loge, J.H. (2010) Social outcomes in young adult survivors of low incidence childhood cancers. *Journal of Cancer Survivorship*, 4(2): 110–18.

Johannsdottir, I.M., Hjermstad, M.J., Moum, T., Wesenberg, F., Hjorth, L., Schroder, H. and Loge, J.H. (2012) Increased prevalence of chronic fatigue among survivors of childhood cancers: a population-based study. *Pediatric Blood and Cancer*, 58(3): 415–20.

Johnson, R.M., Runyan, C.W., Coyne-Beasley, T., Lewis, M.A. and Bowling, J.M. (2008) Storage of household firearms: an examination of the attitudes and beliefs of married women with children. *Health Education Research*, 23(4): 592–602.

Johnston, C.C., Rennick, J.E., Filion, F., Campbell-Yeo, M., Goulet, C., Bell, L. and Ranger, M. (2012) Maternal touch and talk for invasive procedures in infants and toddlers in the pediatric intensive care unit. *Journal of Pediatric Nursing*, 27(2): 144–53.

Johnston-Brookes, C.H., Lewis, M.A., Evans, G.W. and Whalen, C.K. (1998) Chronic stress and illness in children: the role of allostatic load. *Psychosomatic Medicine*, 60: 597–603.

Joseph, S., Becker, F. and Becker, S. (2009) *Manual for Measures of Caring Activities and Outcomes for Children and Young People*. Nottingham: University of Nottingham.

Joseph, S., Becker, S., Becker, F. and Regel, S. (2009) Assessment of caring and its effects in young people: development of the Multidimensional Assessment of Caring Activities Checklist (MACA-YC18) and the Positive and Negative Outcomes of Caring Questionnaire (PANOC-YC20) for young carers. *Child: Care, Health and Development*, 35(4): 510–20.

Kadan-Lottick, N.S., Zeltzer, L.K., Liu, Q., Yasui, Y., Ellenberg, L., Gioia, G. and Krull, K.R. (2010) Neurocognitive functioning in adult survivors of childhood non-central nervous system cancers. *Journal of the National Cancer Institute*, 102(12): 881–93.

Kajantie, E., Dunkel, L., Turpeinen, U., Stenman, U.H., Wood, P.J., Nuutila, M. and Andersson, S. (2003) Placental 11 beta-hydroxysteroid dehydrogenase-2 and fetal cortisol/cortisone shuttle in small preterm infants. *Journal of Clinical Endocrinology & Metabolism*, 88(1): 493–500.

Kalat, J.W. (2001) *Biological Psychology*. Belmont, CA: Wadsworth, Thomson Learning.

Kalra, S., Klein, J., Karaskov, T., Woodland, C., Einarson, A. and Koren, G. (2005) Use of hair cortisol as a biomarker for chronic stress in pregnancy. *Clinical Pharmacology and Therapeutics*, 77(2): P69.

Kalra, S., Einarson, A., Karaskov, T., Van Uum, S. and Koren, G. (2007) The relationship between stress and hair cortisol in healthy pregnant women. *Clinical and Investigative Medicine*, 30(2): E103–E107.

Kaminski, M.A., Pellino, T. and Wish, J. (2002) Play and pets: the physical and emotional impact of child-life and pet therapy on hospitalized children. *Children's Health Care*, 31(4): 321–35.

Kanner, A.D., Coyne, J.C., Schaefer, C. and Lazarus, R.S. (1981) Comparison of two modes of stress measurement: daily hassles and uplifts versus major life events. *Journal of Behavioral Medicine*, 4: 1–39.

Kanner, A.D., Feldman, S.S., Weinberger, D.A. and Ford, M. (1987) Uplifts, hassles, and adaptational outcomes in early adolescents. *Journal of Early Adolescence*, 7: 371–94.

Khamis, H.J. and Roche, A.F. (1994) Predicting adult stature without using skeletal age: the Khamis–Roche method. *Pediatrics*, 94(4 pt 1): 504–7.

Khashan, A.S., McNamee, R., Abel, K.M., Pedersen, M.G., Webb, R.T., Kenny, L.C. and Baker, P.N. (2008) Reduced infant birthweight consequent upon maternal exposure to severe life events. *Psychosomatic Medicine*, 70(6): 688–94.

Kiecolt-Glaser, J.K., Glaser, R., Gravenstein, S., Malarkey, W.B. and Sheridan, J. (1996) Chronic stress alters the immune response to influenza virus vaccine in older adults. *Proceedings of the National Academy of Sciences of the United States of America*, 93(7): 3043–7.

Kiecolt-Glaser, J.K., Gouin, J.P., Weng, N.P., Malarkey, W.B., Beversdorf, D.Q. and Glaser, R. (2011) Childhood adversity heightens the impact of later-life caregiving stress on telomere length and inflammation. *Psychosomatic Medicine*, 73(1): 16–22.

Kiecolt-Glaser, J.K., Marucha, P.T., Atkinson, C. and Glaser, R. (2001) Hypnosis as a modulator of cellular immune dysregulation during acute stress. *Journal of Consulting and Clinical Psychology*, 69(4): 674–82.

Kinahan, K.E., Sharp, L.K., Seidel, K., Leisenring, W., Didwania, A., Lacouture, M.E., Stovall, M., Haryani, A., Robison, L.L. and Krull, K.R. (2012) Scarring, disfigurement, and quality of life in long-term survivors of childhood cancer: a report from the Childhood Cancer Survivor Study. *Journal of Clinical Oncology*, 30(20): 2466–74.

King, J.A., Mandansky, D., King, S., Fletcher, K.E. and Brewer, J. (2001) Early sexual abuse and low cortisol. *Psychiatry and Clinical Neurosciences*, 55(1): 71–4.

Kirchhoff, A.C., Krull, K.R., Ness, K.K., Armstrong, G.T., Park, E.R., Stovall, M. and Leisenring, W. (2011) Physical, mental, and neurocognitive status and employment outcomes in the Childhood Cancer Survivor Study cohort. *Cancer Epidemiology, Biomarkers and Prevention*, 20(9): 1838–49.

Kirschbaum, C. and Hellhammer, D.H. (1994) Salivary cortisol in psychoneuroendocrine research: recent developments and applications. *Psychoneuroendocrinology*, 19(4): 313–33.

Kirschbaum, C., Pirke, K.M. and Hellhammer, D.H. (1993) The 'Trier Social Stress Test': a tool for investigating psychobiological stress responses in a laboratory setting. *Neuropsychobiology*, 28(1–2): 76–81.

Kirschbaum, C., Tietze, A., Skoluda, N. and Dettenborn, L. (2009) Hair as a retrospective calendar of cortisol production: increased cortisol incorporation into hair in the third trimester of pregnancy. *Psychoneuroendocrinology*, 34(1): 32–7.

Kirwin, K.M. and Hamrin, V. (2005) Decreasing the risk of complicated bereavement and future psychiatric disorders in children. *Journal of Child and Adolescent Psychiatric Nursing*, 18(2): 62–78.

Klinnert, M.D., Nelson, H.S., Price, M.R., Adinoff, A.D., Leung, D.Y. and Mrazek, D.A. (2001) Onset and persistence of childhood asthma: predictors from infancy. *Pediatrics*, 108(4): E69.

Knack, J.M., Jensen-Campbell, L.A. and Baum, A. (2011) Worse than sticks and stones? Bullying is associated with altered HPA axis functioning and poorer health. *Brain and Cognition*, 77(2): 183–90.

Knoll, B., Lassmann, B. and Temesgen, Z. (2007) Current status of HIV infection: a review for non-HIV-treating physicians. *International Journal of Dermatology*, 46(12): 1219–28.

Kohler, L. and Rigby, M. (2003) Indicators of children's development: considerations when constructing a set of national Child Health Indicators for the European Union. *Child: Care, Health and Development*, 29(6): 551–8.

Koopman, H.M., Baars, R.M., Chaplin, J. and Zwinderman, K.H. (2004) Illness through the eyes of the child: the development of children's understanding of the causes of illness. *Patient Education and Counseling*, 55(3): 363–70.

Koren, G., Klein, J., Karaskov, T., Stevens, B. and Yamada, J. (2003) Hair cortisol: a potential biological marker of chronic stress in neonates. *Therapeutic Drug Monitoring*, 25(4): 516.

Kramer, M.S., Lydon, J., Seguin, L., Goulet, L., Kahn, S.R., McNamara, H., Platt, R.W. (2009) Stress pathways to spontaneous preterm birth: the role of stressors, psychological distress, and stress hormones. *American Journal of Epidemiology*, 169(11): 1319–26.

Krull, K.R., Annett, R.D., Pan, Z., Ness, K.K., Nathan, P.C., Srivastava, D.K. and Hudson, M.M. (2011) Neurocognitive functioning and health-related behaviours in adult survivors of childhood cancer: a report from the Childhood Cancer Survivor Study. *European Journal of Cancer*, 47(9): 1380–8.

Kryski, K.R., Smith, H.J., Sheikh, H.I., Singh, S.M. and Hayden, E.P. (2011) Assessing stress reactivity indexed via salivary cortisol in preschool-aged children. *Psychoneuroendocrinology*, 36(8): 1127–36.

Kudielka, B.M., Buske-Kirschbaum, A., Hellhammer, D.H. and Kirschbaum, C. (2004) HPA axis responses to laboratory psychosocial stress in healthy elderly adults, younger adults, and children: impact of age and gender. *Psychoneuroendocrinology*, 29(1): 83–98.

Kurt, B.A., Nolan, V.G., Ness, K.K., Neglia, J.P., Tersak, J.M., Hudson, M.M., ... Arora, M. (2012) Hospitalization rates among survivors of childhood cancer in the childhood cancer survivor study cohort. *Pediatric Blood & Cancer*, 59(1): 126–32.

Lackey, N.R. and Gates, M.F. (2001) Adults' recollections of their experiences as young caregivers of family members with chronic physical illnesses. *Journal of Advanced Nursing*, 34(3): 320–8.

Langer, D.A., Chen, E. and Luhmann, J.D. (2005) Attributions and coping in children's pain experiences. *Journal of Pediatric Psychology*, 30(7): 615–22.

Layard, R. and Dunn, J. (2009) *A Good Childhood: Searching for Values in a Competitive Age*. London: Penguin.

Lazarus, R.S. and Folkman, S. (1984) *Stress, Appraisal and Coping*. New York: Springer-Verlag.

Leahey, T.H. (2004) *A History of Psychology: Main Currents in Psychological Thought*, 6th edn. Upper Saddle River, NJ: Pearson Prentice Hall.

Lederer, S.E. and Grodin, M.A. (1994) Historical overview: pediatric experimentation. In M.A. Grodin and L.H. Glantz (eds), *Children as Research Subjects: Science, Ethics and Law*. Oxford: Oxford University Press. pp. 3–25.

Levinson, B.M. (1962) The dog as a 'co-therapist'. *Mental Hygiene*, 46: 59–65.

Lindsay, B. (2003) *A Two-year-old Goes to Hospital*: A 50th anniversary reappraisal of the impact of James Robertson's film. *Journal of Child Health Care*, 7(1): 17–26.

Logan, D.E. and Rose, J.B. (2005) Is postoperative pain a self-fulfilling prophecy? Expectancy effects on postoperative pain and patient-controlled analgesia use among adolescent surgical patients. *Journal of Pediatric Psychology*, 30(2): 187–96.

Lorenz, K.Z. (1937) The companion in the bird's world. *Auk*, 54: 245–73.

Louv, R. (2010) *Last Child in the Woods*. New York: Workman.

Lu, Q., Krull, K.R., Leisenring, W., Owen, J.E., Kawashima, T., Tsao, J.C. and Zeltzer, L.K. (2011) Pain in long-term adult survivors of childhood cancers and their siblings: a report from the Childhood Cancer Survivor Study. *Pain*, 152(11): 2616–24.

Lu, Q., Tsao, J.C., Myers, C.D., Kim, S.C. and Zeltzer, L.K. (2007) Coping predictors of children's laboratory-induced pain tolerance, intensity, and unpleasantness. *Journal of Pain*, 8(9): 708–17.

Luecken, L.J., Kraft, A., Appelhans, B.M. and Enders, C. (2009) Emotional and cardiovascular sensitization to daily stress following childhood parental loss. *Developmental Psychology*, 45(1): 296–302.

Luecken, L.J., Hagan, M.J., Sandler, I.N., Tein, J.Y., Ayers, T.S. and Wolchik, S.A. (2010) Cortisol levels six-years after participation in the Family Bereavement Program. *Psychoneuroendocrinology*, 35(5): 785–9.

Lundberg, U., Westermark, O. and Rasch, B. (1993) Cardiovascular and neuroendocrine activity in pre-school children: comparison between day-care and home levels. *Scandinavian Journal of Psychology*, 34(4): 371–8.

Lupien, S., King, S., Meaney, M.J. and McEwen, B.S. (2000) Child's stress hormone levels correlate with mother's socioeconomic status and depressive state. *Biological Psychiatry*, 48: 976–80.

Lupien, S., King, S., Meaney, M.J. and McEwen, B.S. (2001) Can poverty get under your skin? Basal cortisol levels and cognitive function in children from low and high socioeconomic status. *Development and Psychopathology*, 13: 653–76.

Lupien, S.J., McEwen, B.S., Gunnar, M.R. and Heim, C. (2009) Effects of stress throughout the lifespan on the brain, behaviour and cognition. *Nature Reviews Neuroscience*, 10(6): 434–45.

Lutgendorf, S.K. and Costanzo, E.S. (2003) Psycho-neuroimmunology and health psychology: an integrative model. *Brain, Behavior, and Immunity*, 17(4): 225–32.

Lutgendorf, S.K., DeGeest, K., Sung, C.Y., Arevalo, J.M., Penedo, F., Lucci, J., III, Goodheart, M., Lubaroff, D., Farley, D.M., Sood, A.K. and Cole, S.W. (2009) Depression, social support, and beta-adrenergic transcription control in human ovarian cancer. *Brain, Behavior, and Immunity*, 23(2): 176–83.

Luthar, S.S., Cicchetti, D. and Becker, B. (2000) The construct of resilience: a critical evaluation and guidelines for future work. *Child Development*, 71(3): 543–62.

Lynch, A.M., Kashikar-Zuck, S., Goldschneider, K.R. and Jones, B.A. (2007) Sex and age differences in coping styles among children with chronic pain. *Journal of Pain and Symptom Management*, 33(2): 208–16.

McAndrew, S., Warne, T., Fallon, D. and Moran, P. (2012) Young, gifted, and caring: a project narrative of young carers, their mental health, and getting them involved in education, research and practice. *International Journal of Mental Health Nursing*, 21(1): 12–19.

McCracken, L.M., Gauntlett-Gilbert, J. and Eccleston, C. (2010) Acceptance of pain in adolescents with chronic pain: validation of an adapted assessment instrument and preliminary correlation analyses. *European Journal of Pain*, 14(3): 316–20.

McCubbin, H.I., Laresen, A. and Olson, D.H. (1985) F-COPES: Family Crises Oriented Personal Evaluation Scales. In D.H. Olson, H.I. McCubbin, H. Barnes, A. Larsen, M. Muxen and M. Wilson (eds),

Family Inventories: Inventories Used in a National Survey of Families across the Family Life Cycle. St Paul, MN: Family Social Science, University of Minnesota. pp. 143–9.

McDade, T.W., Chyu, L., Duncan, G.J., Hoyt, L.T., Doane, L.D. and Adam, E.K. (2011) Adolescents' expectations for the future predict health behaviors in early adulthood. *Social Science and Medicine*, 73(3): 391–8.

McEwen, B.S. (1998a) Protective and damaging effects of stress mediators. *New England Journal of Medicine*, 338(3): 171–9.

McEwen, B.S. (1998b) Stress, adaptation, and disease: allostasis and allostatic load. *Annals of the New York Academy of Sciences*, 840: 33–44.

McEwen, B.S. and Wingfield, J.C. (2003) The concept of allostasis in biology and biomedicine. *Hormones and Behavior*, 43: 2–15.

McGrath, A. and Collicut McGrath, J. (2007) *The Dawkins Delusion?: Atheist Fundamentalism and the Denial of the Divine*. London: SPCK.

McGrath, P. and Chesler, M. (2004) Fathers' perspectives on the treatment for pediatric hematology: extending the findings. *Issues in Comprehensive Pediatric Nursing*, 27(1): 39–61.

McGrath, P.A. and Hillier, L.M. (2003) Factors that modify children's pain. In N.L. Schechter, C.B. Berde and M. Yaster (eds), *Pain in Infants, Children, and Adolescents*. Philadelphia: Lippincott Williams & Wilkins. pp. 84–98.

McGrath, P. and Huff, N. (2001) 'What is it?': findings on preschoolers' responses to play with medical equipment. *Child: Care, Health and Development*, 27(5): 451–62.

McGrath, P. and Rawson-Huff, N. (2010) Corticosteroids during continuation therapy for acute lymphoblastic leukemia: the psycho-social impact. *Issues in Comprehensive Pediatric Nursing*, 33(1): 5–19.

McGrath, P.A., Speechley, K.N., Seifert, C.E., Biehn, J.T., Cairney, A.E.L., Gorodzinsky, F.P. and Morrissy, J.R. (2000) A survey of children's acute, recurrent, and chronic pain: validation of the Pain Experience Interview. *Pain*, 87(1): 59–73.

McGrath, P., Paton, M.A. and Huff, N. (2004) Beginning treatment for paediatric acute myeloid leukaemia: diagnosis and the early hospital experience. *Scandinavian Journal of Caring Science*, 18(4): 358–67.

McGrath, P., Paton, M.A. and Huff, N. (2005) Beginning treatment for pediatric acute myeloid leukemia: the family connection. *Issues in Comprehensive Pediatric Nursing*, 28(2): 97–114.

Macpherson, G. (ed.) (1999) *Black's Medical Dictionary*. London: A. & C. Black.

Marin, T.J., Chen, E., Munch, J.A. and Miller, G.E. (2009) Double-exposure to acute stress and chronic family stress is associated with immune changes in children with asthma. *Psychosomatic Medicine*, 71: 378–84.

Markell, A. and Markell, M.A. (2008) *The Children who Lived: Using Harry Potter and Other Fictional Characters to Help Grieving Children and Adolescents*. New York: Routledge.

Marsland, A.L., Cohen, S., Rabin, B.S. and Manuck, S.B. (2001) Associations between stress, trait negative affect, acute immune reactivity, and antibody response to hepatitis B injection in healthy young adults. *Health Psychology*, 20(1): 4–11.

Martin, A.L., McGrath, P.A., Brown, S.C. and Katz, J. (2007) Anxiety sensitivity, fear of pain and pain-related disability in children and adolescents with chronic pain. *Pain Research and Management*, 12(4): 267–72.

Mastorakos, G. and Ilias, I. (2000) Maternal hypothalamic-pituitary-adrenal axis in pregnancy and the postpartum period: postpartum-related disorders. *Annals of the New York Academy of Sciences*, 900: 95–106.

Mays, D., Black, J.D., Mosher, R.B., Shad, A.T. and Tercyak, K.P. (2011) Improving short-term sun safety practices among adolescent survivors of childhood cancer: a randomized controlled efficacy trial. *Journal of Cancer Survivorship*, 5(3): 247–54.

Meewisse, M.L., Reitsma, J.B., de Vries, G.J., Gersons, B.P. and Olff, M. (2007) Cortisol and post-traumatic stress disorder in adults: systematic review and meta-analysis. *British Journal of Psychiatry* 191: 387–92.

Melzack, R. (1999a) From the gate to the neuromatrix. *Pain*, Suppl. 6: S121–6.

Melzack, R. (1999b) Pain: an overview. *Acta Anaesthesiologica Scandinavica*, 43(9): 880–4.

Melzack, R. (2001) Pain and the neuromatrix in the brain. *Journal of Dental Education*, 65(12): 1378–82.

Melzack, R. (2005) Evolution of the neuromatrix theory of pain. The Prithvi Raj Lecture: presented at the Third World Congress of the World Institute of Pain, Barcelona 2004. *Pain Practice*, 5(2): 85–94.

Melzack, R. and Wall, P.D. (1965) Pain mechanisms: a new theory. *Science*, 150(3699): 971–9.

Melzack, R. and Wall, P.D. (2008) *The Challenge of Pain*, 2nd edn. London: Penguin.

Merlot, E., Couret, D. and Otten, W. (2008) Prenatal stress, fetal imprinting and immunity. *Brain, Behavior, and Immunity*, 22(1): 42–51.

Michaud, K., Matheson, K., Kelly, O. and Anisman, H. (2008) Impact of stressors in a natural context on release of cortisol in healthy adult humans: a meta-analysis. *Stress*, 11(3): 177–97. doi: 10.1080/10253890701727874.

Michel, G., Greenfield, D.M., Absolom, K., Ross, R.J., Davies, H. and Eiser, C. (2009) Follow-up care after childhood cancer: survivors' expectations and preferences for care. *European Journal of Cancer*, 45(9): 1616–23.

Michel, G., Kuehni, C.E., Rebholz, C.E., Zimmermann, K., Eiser, C., Rueegg, C.S. and von der Weid, N.X. (2011) Can health beliefs help in explaining attendance to follow-up care? The Swiss childhood cancer survivor study. *Psychooncology*, 20(10): 1034–43.

Miller, G.E., Chen, E. and Zhou, E.S. (2007) If it goes up, must it come down? Chronic stress and the hypothalamic-pituitary-adrenocortical axis in humans. *Psychological Bulletin*, 133(1): 25–45.

Miller, K.S., Vannatta, K., Compas, B.E., Vasey, M., McGoron, K.D., Salley, C.G. and Gerhardt, C.A. (2009) The role of coping and temperament in the adjustment of children with cancer. *Journal of Pediatric Psychology*, 34(10): 1135–43.

Millstein, S.G. and Irwin, C.E. (1987) Concepts of health and illness: different constructs or variations on a theme. *Health Psychology*, 6(6): 515–24.

Mitchell, M.J., Lemanek, K., Palermo, T.M., Crosby, L.E., Nichols, A. and Powers, S.W. (2007) Parent perspectives on pain management, coping, and family functioning in pediatric sickle cell disease. *Clinical Pediatrics (Philadelphia)*, 46(4): 311–19.

Mokkink, L.B., van der Lee, J.H., Grootenhuis, M.A., Offringa, M. and Heymans, H.S. (2008) Defining chronic diseases and health conditions in childhood (0–18 years of age): national consensus in the Netherlands. *European Journal of Pediatrics* 167(12): 1441–7.

Moore, T. and McArthur, M. (2007) We're all in it together: supporting young carers and their families in Australia. *Health and Social Care in the Community*, 15(6): 561–8.

Moore Ki, I.M., Hockenberry, M.J., Anhalt, C., McCarthy, K. and Kruss, K.R. (2012) Mathematics intervention for prevention of neurocognitive deficits in childhood leukemia. *Pediatric Blood and Cancer*, 59(2): 278–84.

Morgan, I.G., Ohno-Matsui, K. and Saw, S.M. (2012) Myopia. *Lancet*, 379(9827): 1739–48.

Morris, T., Greer, H.S. and White, P. (1977) Psychological and social adjustment to mastectomy: a 2-year follow-up study. *Cancer*, 40: 2381–7.

Morrison, D.M., Mar, C.M., Wells, E.A., Rogers Gillmore, M., Hoppe, M.J., Wilsdon, A., Murowchick, E.

and Archibald, M.E. (2002) The theory of reasoned action as a model of children's health behavior. *Journal of Applied Social Psychology*, 32(11): 2 266–95.

Morrison, V. and Bennett, P. (2012) *An Introduction to Health Psychology*, 3rd edn. Harlow, Essex: Pearson Education.

Moskowitz, D.S. and Young, S.N. (2006) Ecological momentary assessment: what it is and why it is a method of the future in clinical psychopharmacology. *Journal of Psychiatry & Neuroscience*, 31(1): 13–20.

Moss, H., Bose, S., Wolters, P. and Brouwers, P. (1998) A preliminary study of factors associated with psychological adjustment and disease course in school-age children infected with the human immunodeficiency virus. *Journal of Developmental and Behavioral Pediatrics*, 19(1): 18–25.

Moss, S. (2012) *Natural Childhood: A National Trust Report*. London: Park Lane Press.

Mulherin Engel, S., Berkowitz, G.S., Wolff, M.S. and Yehuda, R. (2005) Psychological trauma associated with the World Trade Center attacks and its effect on pregnancy outcome. *Paediatric and Perinatal Epidemiology*, 19(5): 334–41.

Myant, K.A. and Williams, J.M. (2005) Children's concepts of health and illness: understanding of contagious illnesses, non-contagious illnesses and injuries. *Journal of Health Psychology*, 10(6): 805–19.

National Scientific Council on the Developing Child (2005) *Excessive Stress Disrupts the Architecture of the Developing Brain*, Working Paper no. 3 (www.developingchild.net).

Ness, K.K., Hudson, M.M., Pui, C.H., Green, D.M., Krull, K.R., Huang, T.T. and Morris, E.B. (2012) Neuromuscular impairments in adult survivors of childhood acute lymphoblastic leukemia: associations with physical performance and chemotherapy doses. *Cancer*, 118(3): 828–38.

Newcomb, M.D. and Bentler, P.M. (1986) Loneliness and social support: a confirmatory hierarchical analysis. *Personality and Social Psychology Bulletin*, 12: 520–35.

Newport, D.J., Heim, C., Bonsall, R., Miller, A.H. and Nemeroff, C.B. (2004) Pituitary-adrenal responses to standard and low-dose dexamethasone suppression tests in adult survivors of child abuse. *Biological Psychiatry*, 55(1): 10–20.

NHS (National Health Service) (2012) Choices on-line document (www.nhs.uk/Conditions/Sickle-cell-anaemia/Pages/Introduction.aspx; retrieved 5 July 2012).

NHS Estates (2004) *Hospital Accommodation for Children and Young People*. London: The Stationery Office, Department of Health, UK.

Nickerson, R.S. (1992) *Looking Ahead: Human Factors Challenges in a Changing World*. Hillsdale, NJ: Lawrence Erlbaum Associates.

Nicolson, N.A. (2004) Childhood parental loss and cortisol levels in adult men. *Psychoneuroendocrinology*, 29(8): 1012–18.

Nicolson, N.A., Davis, M.C., Kruszewski, D. and Zautra, A.J. (2010) Childhood maltreatment and diurnal cortisol patterns in women with chronic pain. *Psychosomatic Medicine*, 72(5): 471–80.

Nicolson, R.H. (ed.) (1986) *Medical Research with Children: Ethics, Law and Practice*. Oxford: Oxford University Press.

Normandeau, S., Kalnins, I., Jutras, S. and Hanigan, D. (1998) A description of 5- to 12-year-old children's conception of health within the context of their daily life. *Psychology and Health*, 13(5): 883–96.

Novotney, A. (2010) The recession's toll on children. *Monitor on Psychology*, 41: 43–6.

O'Connor, T.G., Ben-Shlomo, Y., Heron, J., Golding, J., Adams, D. and Glover, V. (2005) Prenatal anxiety predicts individual differences in cortisol in pre-adolescent children. *Biological Psychiatry*, 58(3): 211–17.

O'Donnell, K., O'Connor, T.G. and Glover, V. (2009) Prenatal stress and neurodevelopment of the child: focus on the HPA axis and role of the placenta. *Developmental Neuroscience*, 31(4): 285–92.

O'Farrell, J. (2005) *May Contain Nuts*. New York: Doubleday.

ONS (Office for National Statistics) (2012) *Report: Childhood, Infant and Perinatal Mortality in England and Wales 2010* (www.ons.gov.uk/ons; retrieved 8 June 2012).

Painter, J.E., Sales, J.M., Pazol, K., Wingood, G.M., Windle, M., Orenstein, W.A. and DiClemente, R.J. (2010) Psychosocial correlates of intention to receive an influenza vaccination among rural adolescents. *Health Education Research*, 25(5): 853–64.

Pakenham, K.I. and Cox, S. (2012) The nature of caregiving in children of a parent with multiple sclerosis from multiple sources and the associations between caregiving activities and youth adjustment overtime. *Psychology and Health*, 27(3): 324–46.

Pakenham, K.I., Chiu, J., Bursnall, S. and Cannon, T. (2007) Relations between social support, appraisal and coping and both positive and negative outcomes in young carers. *Journal of Health Psychology*, 12(1): 89–102.

Palermo, T.M. and Eccleston, C. (2009) Parents of children and adolescents with chronic pain. *Pain*, 146(1–2): 15–17.

Palermo, T.M., Eccleston, C., Lewandowski, A.S., Williams, A.C. and Morley, S. (2010) Randomized controlled trials of psychological therapies for management of chronic pain in children and adolescents: an updated meta-analytic review. *Pain*, 148(3): 387–97.

Palermo, T.M., Wilson, A.C., Peters, M., Lewandowski, A. and Somhegyi, H. (2009) Randomized controlled trial of an Internet-delivered family cognitive-behavioral therapy intervention for children and adolescents with chronic pain. *Pain*, 146: 205–13.

Parke, R.D. and Gauvain, M. (2009) *Child Psychology: A Contemporary Viewpoint*, 7th edn. New York: McGraw-Hill.

Paul, F., Jones, M.C., Hendry, C. and Adair, P.M. (2007) The quality of written information for parents regarding the management of a febrile convulsion: a randomized controlled trial. *Journal of Clinical Nursing*, 16(12): 2308–22.

Peltzer, K. and Promtussananon, S. (2003) Black South African children's understanding of health and illness: colds, chicken pox, broken arms and AIDS. *Child: Care, Health and Development*, 29(5): 385–93.

Pence, L., Valrie, C.R., Gil, K.M., Redding-Lallinger, R. and Daeschner, C. (2007) Optimism predicting daily pain medication use in adolescents with sickle cell disease. *Journal of Pain and Symptom Management*, 33(3): 302–9.

Perquin, C.W., Hazebroek-Kampschreur, A.A., Hunfeld, J.A., Bohnen, A.M., van Suijlekom-Smit, L.W., Passchier, J. and van der Wouden, J.C. (2000) Pain in children and adolescents: a common experience. *Pain*, 87(1): 51–8.

Phillips, A.C., Burns, V.E., Carroll, D., Ring, C. and Drayson, M. (2005) The association between life events, social support, and antibody status following thymus-dependent and thymus-independent vaccinations in healthy young adults. *Brain, Behavior, and Immunity*, 19(4): 325–33.

Phillips, A.C., Carroll, D., Burns, V.E., Ring, C., Macleod, J. and Drayson, M. (2006) Bereavement and marriage are associated with antibody response to influenza vaccination in the elderly. *Brain, Behavior and Immunity*, 20(3): 279–89.

Piaget, J. and Inhelder, B. (1947) Diagnosis of mental operations and theory of the intelligence. *American Journal of Mental Deficiency*, 51(3): 401–6.

Piira, T., Hayes, B., Goodenough, B. and von Baeyer, C.L. (2006) Effects of attentional direction, age, and coping style on cold-pressor pain in children. *Behaviour Research and Therapy*, 44(6): 835–48.

Poresky, R.H. and Hendrix, C. (1990) Differential effects of pet presence and pet-bonding on young children. *Psychological Reports*, 67(1): 51–4.

Porter, R. (ed.) (2001) *Cambridge Illustrated History of Medicine*. Cambridge: Cambridge University Press.

Pruessner, J.C., Wolf, O.T., Hellhammer, D.H., Buske-Kirschbaum, A., von Auer, K., Jobst, S., Kaspers, F. and Kirschbaum, C. (1997) Free cortisol levels after awakening: a reliable biological marker for the assessment of adrenocortical activity. *Life Sciences*, 61(26): 2539–49.

Pui, C.H. and Evans, W.E. (2006) Treatment of acute lymphoblastic leukemia. *New England Journal of Medicine*, 354(2): 166–78.

Quas, J.A., Yim, I.S., Edelstein, R.S., Cahill, L. and Rush, E.B. (2011) The role of cortisol reactivity in children's and adults' memory of a prior stressful experience. *Developmental Psychobiology*, 53(2): 166–74.

Quesada, A.A., Wiemers, U.S., Schoofs, D. and Wolf, O.T. (2012) Psychosocial stress exposure impairs memory retrieval in children. *Psychoneuroendocrinology*, 37(1): 125–36.

Quinn, G.P., Huang, I.C., Murphy, D., Zidonik-Eddelton, K. and Krull, K.R. (2012) Missing content from health-related quality of life instruments: interviews with young adult survivors of childhood cancer. *Quality of Life Research* (EPub date: 31 January).

Ranmal, R., Prictor, M. and Scott, J. (2012) *Interventions for Improving Communication with Children and Adolescents about their Cancer (Review)*. The Cochrane Collaboration, Wiley Online Library.

Rask, C.U., Olsen, E.M., Elberling, H., Christensen, M.F., Ornbol, E., Fink, P. and Skovgaard, A.M. (2009) Functional somatic symptoms and associated impairment in 5–7-year-old children: the Copenhagen Child Cohort 2000. *European Journal of Epidemiology*, 24(10): 625–34.

Reed-Knight, B., McCormick, M., Lewis, J.D. and Blount, R.L. (2012) Participation and attrition in a coping skills intervention for adolescent girls with inflammatory bowel disease. *Journal of Clinical Psychology in Medical Settings*, 19(2): 188–96.

Reichsman, F., Engel, G.L., Harway, V. and Escalona, S. (1957) Monica, an infant with gastric fistula and depression: an interim report on her development to the age four years. *Psychiatric Research Reports of the American Psychiatric Association*, 8: 12–27.

Reid, M., Landesman, S., Treder, R. and Jaccard, J. (1989) 'My family and friends': six- to twelve-year-old children's perceptions of social support. *Child Development*, 60(4): 896–910.

Reiter, P.L., Brewer, N.T., Gottlieb, S.L., McRee, A.L. and Smith, J.S. (2009) Parents' health beliefs and HPV vaccination of their adolescent daughters. *Social Science and Medicine*, 69(3): 475–80.

Rempel, G.R., Ravindran, V., Rogers, L.G. and Magill-Evans, J. (2013) Parenting under pressure: a grounded theory of parenting young children with life-threatening congenital heart disease. *Journal of Advanced Nursing*, 69(3): 619–30.

Riad-Fahmy, D., Read, G.F. and Griffiths, K. (1982) Steroids in saliva for assessing endocrine function. *Endocrine Reviews*, 3: 367–95.

Ribera, J.M. and Oriol, A. (2009) Acute lymphoblastic leukemia in adolescents and young adults. *Hematology/Oncology Clinics of North America*, 23(5): 1033–42.

Robertson, J. (1958) *Young Children in Hospital*. London: Tavistock.

Robinson, K.E., Livesay, K.L., Campbell, L.K., Scaduto, M., Cannistraci, C.J., Anderson, A.W. and Compas, B.E. (2010) Working memory in survivors of childhood acute lymphocytic leukemia: functional neuroimaging analyses. *Pediatric Blood and Cancer*, 54(4): 585–90.

Robison, L.L., Mertens, A.C., Boice, J.D., Breslow, N.E., Donaldson, S.S., Green, D.M. and Zeltzer, L.K. (2002) Study design and cohort characteristics of the Childhood Cancer Survivor Study: a multi-institutional collaborative project. *Medical and Pediatric Oncology*, 38(4): 229–39.

Rodriguez, E.M., Dunn, M.J., Zuckerman, T., Vannatta, K., Gerhardt, C.A. and Compas, B.E. (2012) Cancer-related sources of stress for children with cancer and their parents. *Journal of Pediatric Psychology*, 37(2): 185–97.

Rokach, A. and Matalon, R. (2007) 'Tails' – A fairy tale on furry tails: a 15-year theatre experience for hospitalized children created by health professionals. *Paediatrics and Child Health*, 12(4): 301–4.

Rokach, A. and Parvini, M. (2011) Experience of adults and children in hospitals. *Early Child Development and Care*, 181(5): 707–15.

Rolls, L. and Payne, S. (2003) Childhood bereavement services: a survey of UK provision. *Palliative Medicine*, 17(5): 423–32.

Ronicle, J. and Kendall, S. (2011) Improving support for young carers: family focused approaches. Department for Education, Research Report DFE-RR084, York Consulting LLP.

Rosenstock, I.M. (1974) The health belief model and preventive health behaviour. *Health Education Monographs*, 2: 354–86.

Rosmalen, J.G.M., Oldehinkle, A.J., Ormel, J., de Winter, A.F., Buitelaar, J.K. and Verhulst, F.C. (2005) Determinants of salivary cortisol levels in 10–12 year old children: a population-based study of individual differences. *Psychoneuroendocrinology*, 30: 483–95.

Rothenberger, S.E., Resch, F., Doszpod, N. and Moehler, E. (2011) Prenatal stress and infant affective reactivity at five months of age. *Early Human Development*, 87(2): 129–136.

Roth-Isigkeit, A., Thyen, U., Raspe, H.H., Stoven, H. and Schmucker, P. (2004) Reports of pain among German children and adolescents: an epidemiological study. *Acta Paediatrica*, 93(2): 258–63.

Roth-Isigkeit, A., Thyen, U., Stoven, H., Schwarzenberger, J. and Schmucker, P. (2005) Pain among children and adolescents: restrictions in daily living and triggering factors. *Pediatrics*, 115(2): e152–62.

Roy, A., Janal, M.N. and Roy, M. (2010) Childhood trauma and prevalence of cardiovascular disease in patients with type 1 diabetes. *Psychosomatic Medicine*, 72(8): 833–8.

Rozenzweig, M.R., Breedlove, S.M. and Leiman, A.L. (2002) *Biological Psychology*, 3rd edn. Sunderland, MA: Sinauer Associates.

Rudolph, K.D., Dennig, M.D. and Weisz, J.R. (1995) Determinants and consequences of children's coping in the medical setting: conceptualization, review, and critique. *Psychological Bulletin*, 118(3): 328–57.

Rushforth, H. (1999) Practitioner review: communicating with hospitalised children: review and application of research pertaining to children's understanding of health and illness. *Journal of Child Psychology and Psychiatry*, 40(5): 683–91.

Ryder, C.S. (2007) *Take your Pediatrician with You: Keeping your Child Healthy at Home and on the Road*. Baltimore, MD: The Johns Hopkins University Press.

Sallfors, C., Fasth, A. and Hallberg, L.R. (2002) Oscillating between hope and despair: a qualitative study. *Child: Care, Health and Development*, 28(6): 495–505.

Sallfors, C., Hallberg, L.R. and Fasth, A. (2003) Gender and age differences in pain, coping and health status among children with chronic arthritis. *Clinical and Experimental Rheumatology*, 21(6): 785–93.

Samuelsson, M., Thernlund, G. and Ringstrom, J. (1996) Using the five field map to describe the social network of children: a methodological study. *International Journal of Behavioral Development*, 19(2): 327–45.

Sandler, I.N., Ayers, T.S., Wolchik, S.A., Tein, J.Y., Kwok, O.M., Haine, R.A. and Griffin, W.A. (2003) The family bereavement program: efficacy evaluation of a theory-based prevention program for parentally bereaved children and adolescents. *Journal of Consulting and Clinical Psychology*, 71(3): 587–600.

Sandman, C.A., Wadhwa, P.D., Chicz-DeMet, A., Dunkel-Schetter, C. and Porto, M. (1997) Maternal stress, HPA activity, and fetal/infant outcome. *Annals of the New York Academy of Sciences*, 814: 266–75.

Sandman, C.A., Davis, E.P., Buss, C. and Glynn, L.M. (2011) Exposure to prenatal psychobiological stress exerts programming influences on the mother and her fetus. *Neuroendocrinology*, 95(1): 8–21.

Santiago, L.B., Jorge, S.M. and Moreira, A.C. (1996) Longitudinal evaluation of the development of salivary cortisol circadian rhythm in infancy. *Clinical Endocrinology*, 44(2): 157–61.

Sapolsky, R. (1994) *Why Zebras Don't Get Ulcers: A Guide to Stress, Stress-related Diseases, and Coping.* New York: W.H. Freeman.

Sarafino, E.P. (1998) *Health Psychology: Biopsychosocial Interactions*, 3rd edn. New York: John Wiley & Sons.

Sarafino, E.P. and Smith, T.W. (2012) *Health Psychology: Biopsychosocial Interactions*, 7th edn. New York: John Wiley & Sons.

Sarkar, P., Bergman, K., Fisk, N.M., O'Connor, T.G. and Glover, V. (2007) Amniotic fluid testosterone: relationship with cortisol and gestational age. *Clinical Endocrinology*, 67(5): 743–7.

Sauve, B., Koren, G., Walsh, G., Tokmakejian, S. and Van Uum, S.H.M. (2007) Measurement of cortisol in human hair as a biomarker of systemic exposure. *Clinical and Investigative Medicine*, 30(5): E183–E181.

Schanberg, L.E., Lefebvre, J.C., Keefe, F.J., Kredich, D.W. and Gil, K.M. (1997) Pain coping and the pain experience in children with juvenile chronic arthritis. *Pain*, 73(2): 181–9.

Schechter, N.L., Berde, C.B. and Yaster, M. (2003) Pain in infants, children and adolescents: an overview. In N.L. Schechter, C.B. Berde and M. Yaster (eds), *Pain in Infants, Children and Adolescents*. Philadelphia: Lippincott Williams & Wilkins. pp. 2–16.

Schedlowski, M. and Pacheco-Lopez, G. (2010) The learned immune response: Pavlov and beyond. *Brain, Behavior, and Immunity*, 24(2): 176–85.

Schedlowski, M. and Tewes, U. (eds) (1999) *Psychoneuroimmunology: An Interdisciplinary Introduction*. New York: Kluwer Academic/Plenum.

Schreier, A. and Evans, G.W. (2003) Adrenal cortical response of young children to modern and ancient stressors. *Current Anthropology*, 44(2): 306–9.

Schulte, I.E. and Petermann, F. (2011) Somatoform disorders: 30 years of debate about criteria! What about children and adolescents? *Journal of Psychosomatic Research*, 70(3): 218–28.

Schulz, M.S. and Masek, B.J. (1996) Medical crisis intervention with children and adolescents with chronic pain. *Professional Psychology: Research and Practice*, 27(2): 121–9.

Sclare, I. (1997) *Child Psychology Portfolio*. Windsor: NFER-Nelson.

Seiffge-Krenke, I. (1995) *Stress, Coping, and Relationships in Adolescence*. Mahway, NJ: Lawrence Erlbaum.

Selye, H. (1956) *The Stress of Life*. New York: McGraw-Hill.

Selye, H. (1974) *Stress without Distress*. Philadelphia: Lipincott.

Selye, H. (1976a) *Stress in Health and Disease*. Boston: Butterworths.

Selye, H. (1976b) *The Stress of Life*, rev. edn. New York: McGraw-Hill.

Sephton, S.E., Sapolsky, R.M., Kraemer, H. and Spiegel, D. (2000) Diurnal cortisol rhythm as a predictor of breast cancer survival. *Journal of the National Cancer Institute.*, 92(12): 994–1000.

Shepherd, E., Woodgate, R.L. and Sawatzky, J.A. (2010) Pain in children with central nervous system cancer: a review of the literature. *Oncology Nursing Forum*, 37(4): E318–30.

Sheppard, L., Eiser, C. and Kingston, J. (2005) Mothers' perceptions of children's quality of life following early diagnosis and treatment for retinoblastoma (Rb). *Child: Care, Health and Development*, 31(2): 137–42.

Sherman, B.F., Bonanno, G.A., Wiener, L.S. and Battles, H.B. (2000) When children tell their friends they have AIDS: possible consequences for psychological well-being and disease progression. *Psychosomatic Medicine*, 62(2): 238–47.

Shirakawa, T., Enomoto, T., Shimazu, S. and Hopkin, J.M. (1997) The inverse association between tuberculin responses and atopic disorder. *Science*, 275(5296): 77–9.

Shirtcliff, E.A., Coe, C.L. and Pollak, S.D. (2009) Early childhood stress is associated with elevated antibody levels to herpes simplex virus type 1. *Proceedings of the National Academy of Sciences of the United States of America*, 106(8): 2963–7.

Shonkoff, J.P., Boyce, W.T. and McEwen, B.S. (2009) Neuroscience, molecular biology, and the childhood roots of health disparities: building a new framework for health promotion and disease prevention. *Journal of the American Medical Association*, 301(21): 2252–9.

Sieberg, C.B., Huguet, A., von Baeyer, C.L. and Seshia, S. (2012) Psychological interventions for headache in children and adolescents. *Canadian Journal of Neurological Sciences*, 39(1): 26–34.

Sigelman, C.K. and Rider, E.A. (2009) *Life-Span Human Development*, 6th edn. Belmont, CA: Thomson/Wadsworth.

Signorello, L.B., Mulvihill, J.J., Green, D.M., Munro, H.M., Stovall, M., Weathers, R.E., ... Boice, J.D., Jr. (2012) Congenital anomalies in the children of cancer survivors: a report from the childhood cancer survivor study. *Journal of Clinical Oncology*, 30(3): 239–45.

Simons, L.E., Sieberg, C.B., Carpino, E., Logan, D. and Berde, C. (2011) The Fear of Pain Questionnaire (FOPQ): assessment of pain-related fear among children and adolescents with chronic pain. *Journal of Pain*, 12(6): 677–86.

Slopen, N., Lewis, T.T., Gruenewald, T.L., Mujahid, M.S., Ryff, C.D., Albert, M.A. and Williams, D.R. (2010) Early life adversity and inflammation in African Americans and whites in the midlife in the United States survey. *Psychosomatic Medicine*, 72(7): 694–701.

Small, F., Alderdice, F., McCusker, C., Stevenson, M. and Stewart, M. (2005) A prospective cohort study comparing hospital admission for gastro-enteritis with home management. *Child: Care, Health and Development*, 31(5): 555–62.

Sourkes, B.M. (1995) *Armfuls of Time: The Psychological Experience of the Child with a Life-threatening Illness*. London: Routledge.

Spiegel, D. (1999) Healing words: emotional expression and disease outcome. *Journal of the American Medical Association*, 281(14): 1328–9.

Spirito, A., Stark, L.J. and Williams, C. (1988) Development of a brief coping checklist for use with pediatric patients. *Journal of Pediatric Psychology*, 13: 555–74.

Spitzer, C., Bouchain, M., Winkler, L.Y., Wingenfeld, K., Gold, S.M., Grabe, H.J. and Heesen, C. (2012) Childhood trauma in multiple sclerosis: a case-control study. *Psychosomatic Medicine*, 74(3): 312–18.

Stanulla, M. and Schrauder, A. (2009) Bridging the gap between the north and the south of the world: the case of treatment response in childhood acute lymphoblastic leukemia. *Hematologica*, 94(6): 748–52.

Steadman, L. and Quine, L. (2004) Encouraging young males to perform testicular self-examination: a simple, but effective, implementation intentions intervention. *British Journal of Health Psychology*, 9(4): 479–87.

Steele, R.G., Anderson, B., Rindel, B., Dreyer, M.L., Perrin, K., Christensen, R., Tyc, V. and Flynn, P.M. (2001) Adherence to antiretroviral therapy among HIV-positive children: examination of the role of caregiver health beliefs. *AIDS Care*, 13(5): 617–29.

Sterling, P. and Eyer, J. (1988) Allostasis: a new paradigm to explain arousal pathology. In S. Fisher and J. Reason (eds), *Handbook of Life Stress, Cognition and Health*. New York: Wiley. pp. 629–49.

Stockhorst, U., Spennes-Saleh, S., Körholz, D., Göbel, U., Schneider, M.E., Steingrüber, H.-J. and Klosterhalfen, S. (2000) Anticipatory symptoms and anticipatory immune responses in pediatric cancer patients receiving chemotherapy: features of a classically conditioned response? *Brain, Behavior, and Immunity*, 14(3): 198–218.

Stokes, J.A. (2004) *Then, Now and Always. Supporting Children through Grief: A Guide for Practitioners*. Cheltenham: Portfolio/Winston's Wish.

Streisand, R., Braniecki, S., Tercyak, K.P. and Kazak, A.E. (2001) Childhood illness-related parenting stress: the pediatric inventory for parents. *Journal of Pediatric Psychology*, 26(3): 155–62.

Stroebe, M.S. (2008) *Handbook of Bereavement Research and Practice: Advances in Theory and Intervention*. Washington, DC: American Psychological Association.

Stroud, L.R., Foster, E., Papandonatos, G.D., Handwerger, K., Granger, D.A., Kivlighan, K.T. and Niaura, R. (2009) Stress response and the adolescent transition: performance versus peer rejection stressors. *Developmental Psychopathology*, 21(1): 47–68.

Stuber, M.L., Meeske, K.A., Krull, K.R., Leisenring, W., Stratton, K., Kazak, A.E. and Zeltzer, L.K. (2010) Prevalence and predictors of posttraumatic stress disorder in adult survivors of childhood cancer. *Pediatrics*, 125(5): e1124–34.

Sturgess, W. (2001) Young children's perception of their relationships with family members: links with family care setting, friendships, and adjustment. *International Journal of Behavioral Development*, 25(6): 521–9.

Sullivan, M.J., Thorn, B., Haythornthwaite, J.A., Keefe, F., Martin, M., Bradley, L.A. and Lefebvre, J.C. (2001) Theoretical perspectives on the relation between catastrophizing and pain. *Clinical Journal of Pain*, 17(1): 52–64.

Sumpter, R., Brunklaus, A., McWilliam, R. and Dorris, L. (2011) Health-related quality-of-life and behavioural outcome in survivors of childhood meningitis. *Brain Injury*, 25(13–14): 1288–95.

Sumter, S.R., Bokhorst, C.L., Miers, A.C., Van Pelt, J. and Westenberg, P.M. (2010) Age and puberty differences in stress responses during a public speaking task: do adolescents grow more sensitive to social evaluation? *Psychoneuroendocrinology*, 35(10): 1510–16.

Susman, E.J., Dockray, S., Granger, D.A., Blades, K.T., Randazzo, W., Heaton, J.A. and Dorn, L.D. (2010)

Cortisol and alpha amylase reactivity and timing of puberty: vulnerabilities for antisocial behaviour in young adolescents. *Psychoneuroendocrinology*, 35(4): 557–69.

Sutton, S. (2008) How does the health action process approach (HAPA) bridge the intention-behavior gap? An examination of the model's causal structure. *Applied Psychology: An International Review*, 57(1): 66–74.

Swanson, V., Power, K.G., Crombie, I.K., Irvine, L., Kiezebrink, K., Wrieden, W. and Slane, P.W. (2011) Maternal feeding behaviour and young children's dietary quality: a cross-sectional study of socially disadvantaged mothers of two-year old children using the theory of planned behaviour. *International Journal of Behavioral Nutrition and Physical Activity* 8: 65.

Sweet, E. (2010) 'If your shoes are raggedy you get talked about': symbolic and material dimensions of adolescent social status and health. *Social Science and Medicine*, 70: 2029–35.

Syse, A., Aas, G.B. and Loge, J.H. (2012) Children and young adults with parents with cancer: a population-based study. *Clinical Epidemiology*, 4: 41–52.

Tallis, R. (2011) *Aping Mankind: Neuromania, Darwinitis and the Misrepresentation of Humanity*. Durham: Acumen.

Tan, C.E., Li, H.J., Zhang, X.G., Zhang, H., Han, P.Y., An, Q. and Wang, M.Q. (2009) The impact of the Wenchuan earthquake on birth outcomes. *PLoS One*, 4(12): e8200.

Tarullo, A.R. and Gunnar, M.R. (2006) Child maltreatment and the developing HPA axis. *Hormones and Behavior*, 50(4): 632–9.

Taylor, N., Absolom, K., Snowden, J. and Eiser, C. (2012) Need for psychological follow-up among young adult survivors of childhood cancer. *European Journal of Cancer Care*, 21(1): 52–8.

Taylor, S.E., Cousino Klein, L., Lewis, B.P., Gruenwald, T.L., Gurung, R.A.R. and Updegraff, J.A. (2000) Biobehavioral responses to stress in females: tend-and-befriend, not flight-or-fight. *Psychological Review*, 107(3): 411–29.

Tegethoff, M., Greene, N., Olsen, J., Meyer, A.H. and Meinlschmidt, G. (2010) Maternal psychosocial adversity during pregnancy is associated with length of gestation and offspring size at birth: evidence from a population-based cohort study. *Psychosomatic Medicine*, 72(4): 419–26.

Tetlock, P.E. (1994) The psychology of futurology and the future of psychology. *Psychological Science*, 5(1): 1–7.

Thastum, M. and Herlin, T. (2011) Pain-specific beliefs and pain experience in children with juvenile idiopathic arthritis: a longitudinal study. *Journal of Rheumatology*, 38(1): 155–60.

Thastum, M., Herlin, T. and Zachariae, R. (2005) Relationship of pain-coping strategies and pain-specific beliefs to pain experience in children with juvenile idiopathic arthritis. *Arthritis and Rheumatism*, 53(2): 178–84.

Thompson, R.J., Jr., Gil, K.M., Gustafson, K.E., George, L.K., Keith, B.R., Spock, A. and Kinney, T.R. (1994) Stability and change in the psychological adjustment of mothers of children and adolescents with cystic fibrosis and sickle cell disease. *Journal of Pediatric Psychology*, 19(2): 171–88.

Thomsen, A.H., Compas, B.E., Colletti, R.B., Stanger, C., Boyer, M.C. and Konik, B.S. (2002) Parent reports of coping and stress responses in children with recurrent abdominal pain. *Journal of Pediatric Psychology*, 27(3): 215–26.

Tinson, J. (2009) *Conducting Research with Children and Adolescents: Design, Methods and Empirical Cases*. Oxford: Goodfellow.

Tonkin, L. (1996) Growing around grief: another way of looking at grief and recovery. *Bereavement Care*, 15(1): 10 (published online 2009; www.tandfonline.com).

Torpy, J.M., Campbell, A. and Glass, R.M. (2010) JAMA patient page: chronic diseases of children. *Journal of the American Medical Association*, 303(7): 682.

Tovey, H. (2007) *Playing Outdoors: Places and Spaces, Risks and Challenge*. Milton Keynes: Open University Press.

Tracy, E.M. and Abell, N. (1994) Social network map: some further refinements on administration. *Social Work Research*, 18(1): 56–60.

Tracy, E.M. and Whittaker, J.K. (1990) The social network map: assessing social support in clinical practice. *Families in Society: The Journal of Contemporary Human Services*, 71: 461–70.

Trajanovska, M., Manias, E., Cranswick, N. and Johnston, L. (2010) Parental management of childhood complaints: over-the-counter medicine use and advice-seeking behaviours. *Journal of Clinical Nursing*, 19(13–14): 2065–75.

Tucci, F. and Arico, M. (2008) Treatment of pediatric acute lymphoblastic leukemia. *Hematologica*, 93(8): 1124–8.

Turner-Cobb, J.M. and Steptoe, A. (1998) Psychosocial influences on upper respiratory infectious illness in children. *Journal of Psychosomatic Research*, 45(4): 319–30.

Turner-Cobb, J.M., Steptoe, A., Perry, L. and Axford, J. (1998) Adjustment in patients with rheumatoid arthritis and their children. *Journal of Rheumatology*, 25(3): 565–71.

Turner-Cobb, J.M., Rixon, L. and Jessop, D.S. (2008) A prospective study of diurnal cortisol responses to the social experience of school transition in four-year-old children: anticipation, exposure, and adaptation. *Developmental Psychobiology*, 50(4): 377–89.

Turner-Cobb, J.M., Osborn, M., da Silva, L., Keogh, E. and Jessop, D.S. (2010) Sex differences in hypothalamic-pituitary-adrenal axis function in patients with chronic pain syndrome. *Stress: The International Journal on the Biology of Stress*, 13(4): 293–301.

Turner-Cobb, J.M., Rixon, L. and Jessop, D.S. (2011) Hypothalamic-pituitary-adrenal axis activity and upper respiratory tract infection in young children transitioning to primary school. *Psychopharmacology*, 214(1): 309–17.

Turner-Cobb, J.M., Smith, P.C., Ramchandani, P., Begen, F., Osborn, M., Jessop, D.S. and Padkin, A. (2013) Psychobiological impact of the ICU experience in relatives of patients: a mixed methods assessment of stress, emotional response, coping and support. Manuscript submitted for publication.

Tyrrell, D. (1970) Hunting common cold viruses by some new methods. *Journal of Infectious Diseases*, 121(5): 561–71.

Tyrrell, D. and Fielder, M. (2002) *Cold Wars: The Fight against the Common Cold*. Oxford: Oxford University Press.

Upton, P. and Eiser, C. (2006) School experiences after treatment for a brain tumour. *Child: Care, Health and Development*, 32(1): 9–17.

Urizar, G.G., Jr, and Muñoz, R.F. (2011) Impact of a prenatal cognitive-behavioral stress management intervention on salivary cortisol levels in low-income mothers and their infants. *Psychoneuroendocrinology*, 36(10): 1480–94.

Urizar, G.G., Jr, Milazzo, M., Le, H.N., Delucchi, K., Sotelo, R. and Munoz, R.F. (2004) Impact of stress reduction instructions on stress and cortisol levels during pregnancy. *Biological Psychology*, 67(3): 275–82.

Valentine, A., Buchanan, H. and Knibb, R. (2010) A preliminary investigation of 4 to 11-year-old children's knowledge and understanding of stress. *Patient Education and Counseling*, 79(2): 255–7.

Van Cleave, J., Gortmaker, S.L. and Perrin, J.M. (2010) Dynamics of obesity and chronic health conditions among children and youth. *Journal of the American Medical Association*, 303(7): 623–30.

Van Cleve, L., Bossert, E.A., Beecroft, P., Adlard, K., Alvarez, O. and Savedra, M.C. (2004) The pain experience of children with leukaemia during the first years after diagnosis. *Nursing Research*, 53(1): 1–10.

Van den Bergh, B.R. (2005) Antenatal maternal anxiety and stress and the neurobehavioural development of the fetus and child: links and possible mechanisms. A review. *Neuroscience and Biobehavioral Reviews*, 29: 237–58.

Van den Bergh, B.R., Van Calster, B., Smits, T., Van Huffel, S. and Lagae, L. (2008) Antenatal maternal anxiety is related to HPA-axis dysregulation and self-reported depressive symptoms in adolescence: a prospective study on the fetal origins of depressed mood. *Neuropsychopharmacology*, 33(3): 536–45.

van der Lee, J.H., Mokkink, L.B., Grootenhuis, M.A., Heymans, H.S. and Offringa, M. (2007) Definitions and measurement of chronic health conditions in childhood: a systematic review. *Journal of the American Medical Association*, 297(24): 2741–51.

van Dijk, A., McGrath, P.A., Pickett, W. and VanDen-Kerkhof, E.G. (2006) Pain prevalence in nine- to 13-year-old schoolchildren. *Pain Research and Management*, 11(4): 234–40.

Van Meurs, P., Howard, K.E., Versloot, J., Veerkamp, J.S. and Freeman, R. (2005) Child coping strategies, dental anxiety and dental treatment: the influence of age, gender and childhood caries prevalence. *European Journal of Paediatric Dentistry*, 6(4): 173–8.

Varni, J.W., Rapoff, M.A., Waldron, S.A., Gragg, R.A., Bernstein, B.H. and Lindsley, C.B. (1996) Effects of perceived stress on pediatric chronic pain. *Journal of Behavioral Medicine*, 19(6): 515–28.

Varni, J.W., Walco, G.A. and Katz, E.R. (1989) Assessment and management of chronic and recurrent pain in children with chronic diseases. *Pediatrician*, 16(1–2): 56–63.

Vedhara, K. and Irwin, M. (eds) (2005) *Human Psychoneuroimmunology*. New York: Oxford University Press.

Vedhara, K., Cox, N.K., Wilcock, G.K., Perks, P., Hunt, M., Anderson, S., Lightman, S.L. and Shanks, S.M. (1999) Chronic stress in elderly carers of dementia patients and antibody response to influenza vaccination. *Lancet*, 353(9153): 627–31.

Vedhara, K., Miles, J., Crown, A., McCarthy, A., Shanks, N., Davies, D. and Ben-Shlomo, Y. (2007) Relationship of early childhood illness with adult cortisol in the Barry Caerphilly Growth (BCG) cohort. *Psychoneuroendocrinology*, 32(8–10): 865–73.

Vegni, E., Fiori, L., Riva, E., Giovannini, M. and Moja, E.A. (2010) How individuals with phenylketonuria experience their illness: an age-related qualitative study. *Child: Care, Health and Development*, 36(4): 539–48.

Velleman, S., Stallard, P. and Richardson, T. (2010) A review and meta-analysis of computerized cognitive behaviour therapy for the treatment of pain in children and adolescents. *Child: Care, Health and Development*, 36(4): 465–72.

Ventura, T., Gomes, M.C. and Carreira, T. (2012) Cortisol and anxiety response to a relaxing intervention on pregnant women awaiting amniocentesis. *Psychoneuroendocrinology*, 37(1): 148–56.

Vermeer, H.J., van Ijzendoorn, M.H., Groeneveld, M.G. and Granger, D.A. (2012) Downregulation of the immune system in low-quality child care: the case of secretory immunoglobulin A (SIgA) in toddlers. *Physiology and Behavior*, 105(2): 161–7.

Versloot, J., Veerkamp, J.S.J., Hoogstraten, J. and Martens, L.C. (2004) Children's coping with pain during dental care. *Community Dentistry and Oral Epidemiology*, 32(6): 456–61.

Vervoort, T., Craig, K.D., Goubert, L., Dehoorne, J., Joos, R., Matthys, D. and Crombez, G. (2008) Expressive dimensions of pain catastrophizing: a comparative analysis of school children and children with clinical pain. *Pain*, 134(1–2): 59–68.

Vervoort, T., Goubert, L., Eccleston, C., Vandenhende, M., Claeys, O., Clarke, J. and Crombez, G. (2009) Expressive dimensions of pain catastrophizing: an observational study in adolescents with chronic pain. *Pain* 146(1): 170–6.

Vetter, T.R. (2012) Pediatric chronic pain. In R.J. Moore (ed.), *Handbook of Pain and Palliative Care*. New York: Springer-Verlag. pp. 139–68.

Viau, R., Arsenault-Lapierre, G., Fecteau, S., Champagne, N., Walker, C.D. and Lupien, S. (2010) Effect of service dogs on salivary cortisol secretion in autistic children. *Psychoneuroendocrinology*, 35(8): 1187–93.

Vowles, K.E., Cohen, L.L., McCracken, L.M. and Eccleston, C. (2010) Disentangling the complex relations among caregiver and adolescent responses to adolescent chronic pain. *Pain*, 151(3): 680–6.

Wadhwa, P.D., Dunkel-Schetter, C., Chicz-DeMet, A., Porto, M. and Sandman, C.A. (1996) Prenatal psychosocial factors and the neuroendocrine axis in human pregnancy. *Psychosomatic Medicine*, 58(5): 432–46.

Wakefield, A.J., Murch, S.H., Anthony, A., Linnell, J., Casson, D.M., Malik, M., Berelowitz, M., Dhillon, A.P., Thomson, M.A., Harvey, P., Valentine, A., Davies, S.E. and Walker-Smith, J.A. (1998) Ileal-lymphoid-nodular hyperplasia, non-specific colitis, and pervasive developmental disorder in children. *Lancet*, 351(9103): 637–41.

Wallace, D.P., Sim, L.A., Harrison, T.E., Bruce, B.K. and Harbeck-Weber, C. (2012) Covert video monitoring in the assessment of medically unexplained symptoms in children. *Journal of Pediatric Psychology*, 37(3): 329–37.

Wallace, W.H., Blacklay, A., Eiser, C., Davies, H., Hawkins, M., Levitt, G.A. and Jenney, M.E. (2001) Developing strategies for long term follow up of survivors of childhood cancer. *British Medical Journal*, 323(7307): 271–4.

Walsh, M.E. and Bibace, R. (1991) Children's conceptions of AIDS: a developmental analysis. *Journal of Pediatric Psychology*, 16(3): 273–85.

Watamura, S.E., Donzella, B., Alwin, J. and Gunnar, M.R. (2003) Morning-to-afternoon increases in cortisol concentrations for infants and toddlers at child care: age differences and behavioral correlates. *Child Development*, 74(4): 1006–20.

Watamura, S.E., Donzella, B., Kertes, D.A. and Gunnar, M.R. (2004) Developmental changes in baseline cortisol activity in early childhood: relations with napping and effortful control. *Developmental Psychobiology*, 45(3): 125–33.

Wegman, H.L. and Stetler, C. (2009) A meta-analytic review of the effects of childhood abuse on medical outcomes in adulthood. *Psychosomatic Medicine*, 71(8): 805–12.

Weisz, J.R., McCabe, M.A. and Dennig, M.D. (1994) Primary and secondary control among children undergoing medical procedures: adjustment as a function of coping style. *Journal of Consulting and Clinical Psychology*, 62(2): 324–32.

Weithorn, L.A. and Scherer, D.G. (1994) Children's involvement in research participation decisions: psychological considerations. In M.A. Grodinand and L.H. Glantz (eds), *Children as Research Subjects: Science, Ethics and Law*. Oxford: Oxford University Press. pp. 133–79.

Wells, D. (2011) The value of pets for human health. *The Psychologist*, 24(3): 172–6.

Werner, H. (1948) *Comparative Psychology of Mental Development*. New York: Harper and Row.

White, K.M., Hyde, M.K., O'Connor, E.L., Naumann, L. and Hawkes, A.L. (2010) Testing a belief-based intervention encouraging sun-safety among adolescents in a high risk area. *Preventive Medicine*, 51(3–4): 325–8.

WHO (1948) Constitution of the World Health Organization. Source: WHO *Basic Documents*, 45th edn, Supplement, October 2006, page 1. http://www.who.int/governance/eb/who_constitution_en.pdf. The Constitution was adopted by the International Health Conference held in New York from 19 June to 22 July 1946, signed on 22 July 1946 by the representatives of 61 States (*Off. Rec. Wld*

Hlth Org., 2, 100), and entered into force on 7 April 1948.

WHO/UNAIDS (2011) World AIDS Day report 2011 (www.who.int/hiv/data/en/; retrieved 2 September 2012).

Widmaier, E.P., Raff, H. and Strang, K.T. (2010) *Vander's Human Physiology: The Mechansims of Body Function*, 12th edn. New York: McGraw-Hill Higher Education.

Wiebe, D.J., Berg, C.A., Korbel, C., Palmer, D.L., Beveridge, R.M., Upchurch, R. and Donaldson, D.L. (2005) Children's appraisals of maternal involvement in coping with diabetes: enhancing our understanding of adherence, metabolic control, and quality of life across adolescence. *Journal of Pediatric Psychology*, 30(2): 167–78.

Wilder, R.L. (1998) Hormones, pregnancy and autoimmune diseases. *Annals of the New York Academy of Sciences*, 840: 45–50.

Wills, T.A., Vaccaro, D. and McNamara, G. (1992) The role of life events, family support, and competence in adolescent substance use: a test of vulnerability and protective factors. *American Journal of Community Psychology*, 20(3): 349–74.

Wolchik, S.A., Coxe, S., Tein, J.Y., Sandler, I.N. and Ayers, T.S. (2008) Six-year longitudinal predictors of posttraumatic growth in parentally bereaved adolescents and young adults. *Omega: Journal of Death and Dying*, 58(2): 107–28.

Wolchik, S.A., Ruehlman, L.S., Braver, S.L. and Sandler, I.N. (1989) Social support of children of divorce: direct and stress buffering effects. *American Journal of Community Psychology*, 17(4): 485–501.

Wolf, J.M., Miller, G.E. and Chen, E. (2008) Parent psychological states predict changes in inflammatory markers in children with asthma and healthy children. *Brain, Behavior, and Immunity*, 22(4): 433–41.

Wollgarten-Hadamek, I., Hohmeister, J., Demirakca, S., Zohsel, K., Flor, H. and Hermann, C. (2009) Do burn injuries during infancy affect pain and sensory sensitivity in later childhood? *Pain*, 141(1–2): 165–72.

Wong, W.Y., Donfield, S.M., Rains, E., FitzGerald, G., Pearson, S.K. and Gomperts, E.D. (2004) Frequency and causes of hospitalization in HIV-negative children and adolescents with haemophilia A or B and its effect on academic achievement. *Haemophilia*, 10(1): 27–33.

Woodgate, R. and Kristjanson, L.J. (1996) 'Getting better from my hurts': toward a model of the young child's pain experience. *Journal of Pediatric Nursing*, 11(4): 233–42.

Woolston, J.L., Gianfredi, S., Gertner, J.M., Paugus, J.A. and Mason, J.W. (1983) Salivary cortisol: a non-traumatic sampling technique for assaying cortisol dynamics. *Journal of the American Academy of Child and Adolescent Psychiatry*, 22(5): 474–6.

Wust, S., Entringer, S., Federenko, I.S., Schlotz, W. and Hellhammer, D.H. (2005) Birth weight is associated with salivary cortisol responses to psychosocial stress in adult life. *Psychoneuroendocrinology*, 30(6): 591–8.

Xiong, X., Harville, E.W., Mattison, D.R., Elkind-Hirsch, K., Pridjian, G. and Buekens, P. (2008) Exposure to Hurricane Katrina, post-traumatic stress disorder and birth outcomes. *American Journal of the Medical Sciences*, 336(2): 111–15.

Yamada, J., Stevens, B., de Silva, N., Klein, J. and Koren, G. (2003) Hair cortisol as a biologic marker of chronic stress in neonates: a pilot study. *Pediatric Research*, 53(4): 454a.

Yamada, J., Stevens, B., de Silva, N., Gibbins, S., Beyene, J., Taddio, A., Newman, C. and Koren, G. (2007) Hair cortisol as a potential biologic marker of chronic stress in hospitalized neonates. *Neonatology*, 92(1): 42–9.

Yehuda, R., Kahana, B., Binder-Brynes, K. and Southwick, S.M. (1995) Low urinary cortisol excretion in Holocaust survivors with posttraumatic stress disorder. *American Journal of Psychiatry*, 152(7): 982–6.

Yehuda, R., Bierer, L.M., Schmeidler, J., Aferiat, D.H., Breslau, I. and Dolan, S. (2000) Low cortisol and risk for PTSD in adult offspring of Holocaust survivors. *American Journal of Psychiatry*, 157(8): 1252–9.

Yehuda, R., Halligan, S.L. and Grossman, R. (2001) Childhood trauma and risk for PTSD: relationship to intergenerational effects of trauma, parental PTSD, and cortisol excretion. *Development and Psychopathology*, 13(3): 733–53.

Yehuda, R., Engel, S.M., Brand, S.R., Seckl, J., Marcus, S.M. and Berkowitz, G.S. (2005) Transgenerational effects of posttraumatic stress disorder in babies of mothers exposed to the World Trade Center attacks during pregnancy. *Journal of Clinical Endocrinology and Metabolism*, 90(7): 4115–18.

Yehuda, R., Bell, A., Bierer, L.M. and Schmeidler, J. (2008) Maternal, not paternal, PTSD is related to increased risk for PTSD in offspring of Holocaust survivors. *Journal of Psychiatric Research*, 42(13): 1104–11.

Yim, I.S., Quas, J.A., Cahill, L. and Hayakawa, C.M. (2010) Children's and adults' salivary cortisol responses to an identical psychosocial laboratory stressor. *Psychoneuroendocrinology*, 35(2): 241–8.

Zebrack, B.J., Stuber, M.L., Meeske, K.A., Phipps, S., Krull, K.R., Liu, Q. and Zeltzer, L.K. (2012) Perceived positive impact of cancer among long-term survivors of childhood cancer: a report from the Childhood Cancer Survivor Study. *Psychooncology*, 21(6): 630–9.

Zernikow, B., Wager, J., Hechler, T., Hasan, C., Rohr, U., Dobe, M., ... Blankenburg, M. (2012) Characteristics of highly impaired children with severe chronic pain: a 5-year retrospective study on 2249 pediatric pain patients. *BMC Pediatrics*, 12(1): 54.

Ziadni, M.S., Patterson, C.A., Pulgaron, E.R., Robinson, M.R. and Barakat, L.P. (2011) Health-related quality of life and adaptive behaviors of adolescents with sickle cell disease: stress processing moderators. *Journal of Clinical Psychology in Medical Settings*, 18(4): 335–44.

Zimet, G.D., Dahlen, N.W., Zimet, S.G. and Farley, G.K. (1988) Multidimensional scale of perceived social support. *Journal of Personality Assessment*, 52(1): 30–41.

Zimmermann, L.K. and Stansbury, K. (2004) The influence of emotion regulation, level of shyness, and habituation on the neuroendocrine response of three-year-old children. *Psychoneuroendocrinology*, 29(8): 973–82.

INDEX

References in **bold** are to tables and in *italic* are to figures.